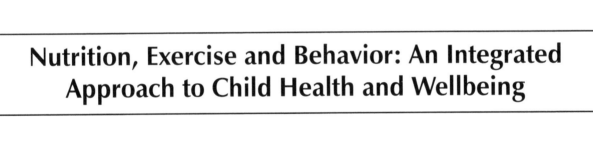

Nutrition, Exercise and Behavior: An Integrated Approach to Child Health and Wellbeing

Nutrition, Exercise and Behavior: An Integrated Approach to Child Health and Wellbeing

Editor: Duncan Bayer

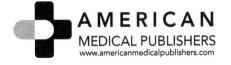

AMERICAN
MEDICAL PUBLISHERS
www.americanmedicalpublishers.com

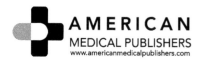

Cataloging-in-Publication Data

Nutrition, exercise and behavior : an integrated approach to child health and wellbeing / edited by Duncan Bayer.
    p. cm.
Includes bibliographical references and index.
ISBN 978-1-63927-764-3
1. Children--Health and hygiene. 2. Children--Nutrition. 3. Exercise for children.
4. Child psychology. 5. Child health services. I. Bayer, Duncan.
RJ101 .N88 2023
362.198 92--dc23

American Medical Publishers,
41 Flatbush Avenue,
1st Floor, New York,
NY 11217, USA

ISBN 978-1-63927-764-3 (Hardback)

Contents

Preface

Nutrition is critical to the physical, mental, behavioral and social development of children. In addition to nutrition, balanced diet and exercise form the foundation of children's healthy development, strong growth and long-term wellbeing. Infants require breastfeeding as well as a variety of nutritious foods to grow and stay healthy, including vegetables and fruits, fish, eggs, meat, grains, and pulses. Iodized salt is crucial for children to avoid delayed development and learning impairments. Physical activity is essential for brain development and supporting necessary mental functions. It maintains physical fitness and boosts mental health by reducing the signs of pain, depression, loneliness and anxiety. Furthermore, academic performance, energy levels, concentration and sleep quality can all be enhanced by physical activity and exercise. It also improves learning, thinking and problem-solving abilities, attention span and motor skills. This book aims to shed light on the role of nutrition and exercise in child health and wellbeing. It will also provide interesting topics for research which interested readers can take up. Those with an interest in this field would find this book helpful.

This book is a comprehensive compilation of works of different researchers from varied parts of the world. It includes valuable experiences of the researchers with the sole objective of providing the readers (learners) with a proper knowledge of the concerned field. This book will be beneficial in evoking inspiration and enhancing the knowledge of the interested readers.

In the end, I would like to extend my heartiest thanks to the authors who worked with great determination on their chapters. I also appreciate the publisher's support in the course of the book. I would also like to deeply acknowledge my family who stood by me as a source of inspiration during the project.

Editor

Dietary Patterns and their Association with Body Composition and Cardiometabolic Markers in Children and Adolescents: Genobox Cohort

Miriam Latorre-Millán [1,2,†] ⓘ, Azahara I. Rupérez [1,3,†] ⓘ, Esther M. González-Gil [1,4,5], Alba Santaliestra-Pasías [1,3,4], Rocío Vázquez-Cobela [6], Mercedes Gil-Campos [4,7] ⓘ, Concepción M. Aguilera [4,5,8] ⓘ, Ángel Gil [4,5,8] ⓘ, Luis A. Moreno [1,3,4] ⓘ, Rosaura Leis [4,6,9,*] ⓘ and Gloria Bueno [1,2,3,4]

[1] GENUD Research group, Instituto de Investigación Sanitaria de Aragón (IIS Aragón), Universidad de Zaragoza, 50013 Zaragoza, Spain; latorremiriam0@gmail.com (M.L.-M.); airuperez@unizar.es (A.I.R.); esthergg@ugr.es (E.M.G.-G.); albasant@unizar.es (A.S.-P.); lmoreno@unizar.es (L.A.M.); mgbuenol@unizar.es (G.B.)

[2] Unidad de Endocrinología Pediátrica, Hospital Clínico Universitario Lozano Blesa, 50009 Zaragoza, Spain

[3] Instituto Agroalimentario de Aragón (IA2), 50013 Zaragoza, Spain

[4] Centro de Investigación Biomédica en Red de Fisiopatología de la Obesidad y Nutrición (CIBEROBN), Instituto de Salud Carlos III, 28029 Madrid, Spain; mercedes_gil_campos@yahoo.es (M.G.-C.); caguiler@ugr.es (C.M.A.); agil@ugr.es (Á.G.)

[5] Departamento de Bioquímica y Biología Molecular II, Instituto de Nutrición y Tecnología de los Alimentos, Centro de Investigación Biomédica, Universidad de Granada, 18016 Granada, Spain

[6] Unidad de Gastroenterología, Hepatología y Nutrición Pediátrica, Grupo de Investigación Nutrición Pediátrica, Instituto de Investigación Sanitaria de Santiago de Compostela (IDIS), Complejo Hospitalario Universitario de Santiago, 15706 Santiago de Compostela, Spain; cobela.rocio@gmail.com

[7] Unidad de Metabolismo e Investigación Pediátrica, Hospital Universitario Reina Sofía, Instituto Maimónides de Investigación Biomédica de Córdoba (IMIBIC), 14071 Córdoba, Spain

[8] Instituto de Investigación Biosanitaria IBS.GRANADA, Complejo Hospitalario Universitario de Granada, 18014 Granada, Spain

[9] Unidad de Investigación en Nutrición, Crecimiento y Desarrollo Humano de Galicia (GALINUT), Universidad de Santiago de Compostela, 15706 Santiago de Compostela, Spain

* Correspondence: mariarosaura.leis@usc.es;
† These authors contributed equally to this work.

Abstract: Diet is a key factor for obesity development; however, limited data are available on dietary cluster analysis in children with obesity. We aimed to assess the associations between dietary patterns and obesity and several cardiometabolic markers. Anthropometry, bioelectrical impedance, blood pressure and plasma biomarkers of oxidative stress, inflammation and endothelial damage were determined in 674 Caucasian children, aged 5–16, with normal or excess weight. Using a food frequency questionnaire and cluster analysis, two consistent dietary patterns were shown, labeled as health conscious (HC) and sweet and processed (SP). The HC pattern included a greater proportion of participants with overweight/obesity than the SP cluster (80.1% vs. 63.8%). However, children with obesity within the HC cluster, showed less abdominal fat, through waist to hip (0.93 vs. 0.94) and waist to height (0.61 vs. 0.63) indexes ($p < 0.01$). Univariate general models showed several additional differences in cardiometabolic risk biomarkers in the global and stratified analyses, with a healthier profile being observed mainly in the HC cluster. However, multivariate models questioned these findings and pointed out the need for further studies in this field. Anyhow, our findings support the benefits of a healthy diet and highlight the importance of dietary patterns in the cardiometabolic risk assessment of children with overweight/obesity, beyond weight control.

Keywords: cluster analysis; obesity; diet; anthropometry; inflammation; oxidative stress; cardiovascular disease

1. Introduction

The World Health Organization (WHO) stated that the prevalence of overweight and obesity has risen dramatically worldwide from 1975 to 2016, as it has nearly triplicated among adults, and even more among children and adolescents (aged 5–19), increasing from 4% to 18% [1]. WHO also highlighted Spain among the European countries with the highest prevalence [1], and although national studies suggested that it has stabilized in the last few years, it continues to be high in this country, at over 40% (for children seven and eight years old) [2]. This is a concern as obesity is related to a wide range of negative health outcomes in adults and children [3]. In the pediatric age, priorities include considering diet in relation to excess weight and over-feeding complications [4]. High intake of energy-dense foods is a significant contributor to excess body mass index (BMI), being considered as a leading risk factor to the global burden of disease [5].

Dietary patterns analysis is considered one of the best dietary approaches [6,7], as it accounts for the overall diet, by including the interactive effect of individual food items, macro- and micro- nutrients, and bioactive compounds. It has been increasingly applied in recent years to evaluate diet and its relationship to health outcomes, linking specific dietary habits to chronic diseases, including obesity and related phenotypes such as body composition and cardiometabolic markers [6–10]. However, as some reviews have highlighted [11,12], the association between dietary patterns and BMI has shown inconsistent results in cross-sectional studies in children and adolescents. Additionally, there is still scarce literature on these populations regarding the associations between dietary patterns and other variables of body composition beyond BMI, and metabolic indicators, especially biochemical ones related to oxidative stress, inflammation or endothelial damage [11,12]. Indeed, in Spain the enKid [13], the ANIBES [14], the EsNuPi [15], and the SI! [16] studies had large sample sizes (n > 400), and all considered BMI exclusively as an obesity phenotype indicator in relation to dietary patterns (except SI! [16], which also included a few other parameters but in participants of a very small age range) and were not performed in a clinical care environment. Hence, there is little information available on dietary patterns related to obesity phenotype among children and adolescents.

Therefore, the main objective of this study was to assess the associations between dietary patterns identified by cluster analysis and obesity and several cardiometabolic markers of body composition, blood pressure, general metabolism, oxidative stress, inflammation and endothelial damage, in children and adolescents.

2. Materials and Methods

2.1. Study Sample

A total of 793 children from those recruited in the GENOBOX clinic cohort participated in this study after applying the inclusion and exclusion criteria. The GENOBOX study was carried out in three hospitals from cities located in different Spanish areas: Hospital Clínico Universitario de Santiago (Santiago de Compostela), Hospital Clínico Universitario Lozano Blesa (Zaragoza), and Hospital Universitario Reina Sofía (Córdoba). Participants were recruited after attending the hospital for diagnosis of minor disorders that were not confirmed after clinical and laboratory investigations or suspecting overweight or obesity. For the current study, children with any BMI classification were eligible, other inclusion criteria included: 5–16 years old, being Caucasian, absence of endogenous obesity, and having a minimal amount of useful dietary intake data. Exclusion criteria were disease and the use of medications that altered blood pressure, glucose or lipid metabolism, having exercised intensely in the 24 h previous to the examination, having participated in a research study in the last three months, having not signed the written informed consent, or not meeting the inclusion criteria.

All participants and their families were informed about the purpose of the study before giving their written consent. The study was developed following the Declaration of Helsinki recommendations (as well as the Edinburgh review) and was approved by the ethics committees of each participating center (Code IDs: Santiago 2011/198, Zaragoza 10/2010, Córdoba 01/2017).

2.2. Body Composition Indicators

Trained staff performed the body composition measurements, according to the International Society for the Advancement of the Kinanthropometry (ISAK) standardized procedures and criteria [17]. All measurements were made in the anatomical position and in underwear. Height, body circumferences and skinfolds were recorded at a 1 mm accuracy.

Height (floor to vertex distance) was measured with a standing stadiometer (SECA® 225 model, Seca gmbh & co, Hamburg, Germany). Waist and hip circumferences were measured with a Cescorf® inelastic tape (Cescorf Equipamentos para Esportes, Porto Alegre, Brazil). Waist to hip, and waist to height indexes were calculated. Skinfolds (biceps, triceps, subscapular and supraspinal) were determined with a caliper (Holtain®, Crosswell, UK). The sum of these four skinfolds was calculated to perform the subsequent analyses.

A scale adapted for children (BC420SMA, Tanita®, Tokio, Japan) was used to perform the bioelectrical impedance analysis (BIA) and to determine weight. Weight was recorded in kg with an accuracy of one decimal. BMI was calculated as the ratio between weight (kg) and the square of height (m^2) and its Z-scores related to national reference values [18]. Children were classified as having normal weight, overweight or obesity, according to BMI by using the Cole et al. sex and age cut-offs for children [19]. BIA was used to obtain body fat mass (FM) and fat free mass (FFM) values (grams and percentage). Fat mass index (FMI) and free fat mass index (FFMI) Z-scores were calculated according to Wells et al. [20].

2.3. Blood Pressure

Systolic (SBP) and diastolic (DBP) blood pressure were measured twice in the participants' right arm, using an electronic manometer (M6, HEM-7001-E, Omron®, Tokio, Japan), with a 5 min interval. If measures differed more than 20%, an additional measurement was taken. The mean value was calculated as the average of the two closest measurements.

2.4. Blood Samples and Biomarkers

Blood samples were collected from the antecubital vein after at least 8 h of overnight fasting. General biochemical analyses were done at the participating university hospitals using automatic analyzers. These analytes were: glucose (mg/dL), insulin (mU/L), triglycerides (TG, mg/dL), total cholesterol (mg/dL), high-density lipoprotein cholesterol (HDLc, mg/dL), low-density lipoprotein cholesterol (LDLc, mg/dL), creatinine (mg/dL), aspartate transaminase (AST, U/L), alanine transaminase (ALT, U/L), and gamma-glutamyl transferase (GGT, U/L).

Biomarkers of oxidative stress, inflammation and endothelial damage were determined in laboratories of the University of Granada. Tocopherols and carotenes levels (nmol/L) were analyzed by high-performance liquid chromatography [21], expressed as tocopherols/TG and carotenes/TG. Total plasma antioxidant capacity (TAC, mM Eq Trolox®) was studied using an antioxidant spectrophotometric assay kit (709001, Cayman Chemical®, Ann Arbor, MI, USA). Catalase activity (CAT, U/g hemoglobin) was determined in erythrocytes as described [22], by a colorimetric method (K033-H1, DetectX® Arbor Assays, Ann Arbor MI, USA). The remaining biomarkers were analyzed with X-Map technology and LINCO-plexTM kits for human monoclonal antibodies (Linco Research, St Charles, MO, USA), using a Luminex® 200TM device (Luminex Corporation, Austin, TX, USA), following the manufacturer's instructions. The kits used were as follows: panel A of human serum adipokines

(HADK1-61K-A-03): adiponectin (mg/L) and resistin (µg/L); panel B of human serum adipokines (HADK2-61K-B-07): leptin (µg/L), monocyte chemoattractant protein-1 (MCP-1, pg/L), and tumor necrosis factor alpha (TNFα, pg/L); panel 1 of human cardiovascular disease (CVD) (HCVD1-67AK-06): selectin (ng/L), soluble vascular cell adhesion molecule-1 (sVCAM-1, ng/L), myeloperoxidase (MPO, µg/L), and total plasminogen activator inhibitor-1 (tPAI-1, µg/L).

Additionally, two biochemical indexes were calculated: HDLc/LDLc, and the homeostasis model assessment for insulin resistant (HOMA-IR) [23].

2.5. Dietary Assessment

Dietary intake was assessed using a qualitative food frequency questionnaire (FFQ), which included common foods consumed in Spain. The children and their caregivers were interviewed by a trained dietician, and consumption frequency of each one of the 83 food items in the last four weeks was recorded as never or hardly ever; 1–3 times per month; once, 2–4 or 5–6 times per week; and once, 2–3, 4–6 or >6 times per day. These answers were converted into times per week (ranging 0 to 42) for their use in further analyses.

2.6. Covariates

Covariates were collected in a questionnaire that included questions regarding lifestyle behaviors, medical history, and socioeconomic status. Recruitment center, age and gender were recorded. Participants were classified as children or adolescents according to their age, since traditionally dietary guidelines establish a difference between school age and adolescence, and also energy requirements increase significantly from 12 years [24]. Maternal education reported by parents was classified according to the International Standard Classification of Education (ISCED) criteria, as low (primary school), medium (high school) or high (bachelor's degree or higher) [25]. The regular performance of moderate-to-vigorous physical activity was evaluated from two questions: (1) "Does your child practice any extracurricular sport?" and (2) "Is your child member of any sports club?" [26]. If either one of the answers was positive, the child was considered a regularly active child, with the opposite, if both were negative, the child was considered a non-active child. In addition, pubertal stage was determined according to Tanner's criteria [27] by a pediatrician. Children in stage I were considered as prepubertal, and children in stages II-V as pubertal.

2.7. Statistical Analyses

The sample size estimation was calculated for the GENOBOX study, based on the principal cardiometabolic risk factors associated with obesity, as previously described [28]. Figure S1 shows a flow diagram that reflects the evolution of the sample.

Dietary patterns were identified through cluster analysis (CA). First, a data cleaning process was performed. Initially, 793 children and adolescents with available FFQ data were included. The 83 food items were grouped into 44 study variables (as shown in Table S1). After removing individuals with more than 50% of missing values for those variables, 765 subjects remained for subsequent analyses. Multiple imputations were applied to estimate missing values using gender, age, BMI, and origin (recruitment center) as predictors for missing values, and the pooled data from the imputed databases were retrieved. Out of the 44 food items included in the FFQ, "meat substitute products and soy products" were excluded from the analysis as more than 95% of the subjects reported to consume them "never or almost never" or "1–3 times per month". Correlations between the single items were calculated to assess multi-collinearity, and no redundant variables were identified. Standardized Z-scores were obtained for the remaining 43 food items, as variance differences of the variables may otherwise affect the resulting clusters. Additionally, univariate ($n = 28$) and multivariate ($n = 63$) outliers were removed. Finally, 674 subjects remained for the following analyses.

A combination of hierarchical and non-hierarchical CA was used to identify individuals with similar dietary patterns. First, hierarchical CA was performed using Ward's method, based on squared Euclidian distances. Several possible cluster solutions were identified and compared to inform the next step, considering the coefficients and fusion level. A non-hierarchical k-means clustering procedure was used, specifying the number of clusters identified in the first step, using a random initial seed and ten iterations to further refine the preliminary solution by optimizing classification. The solution of the number of clusters was identified through the widely used dendrogram and elbow graphical methods. The dendrogram method illustrates the groupings derived from the application of the hierarchical clustering algorithm in an arboreal way, whereas the elbow method represents, in a linear way, the inertia (sum of the squared distances of each cluster object from its centroid) for the different solutions proposed, allowing a sudden change in the slope or flexion (elbow) coinciding with the appropriate number of solutions to be seen. The final cluster solution was selected based on interpretability, stability, and the proportion of the study population in each dietary pattern. Randomly splitting the database in two halves to repeat the same procedure in a subsample (50%) was used to examine the stability and reliability of the final solution, obtaining a Cohen's kappa value of 0.950. Radar plots showing the maximum and minimum Z-score values of each dietary pattern were compared to describe the clusters and study their interpretability.

Additionally, further analyses were performed in the total sample, as well as stratifying by dietary pattern and subgroups according to BMI status (normal weight, overweight, obesity), age (children 5–11 years, adolescents 12–16 years), and gender (male, female). Normal distribution of the variables was assessed using the Kolmogorov–Smirnov test, and non-normally distributed variables (SBP, DBP, HDLc, resistin, TNFα, selectin, and sVCAM1) were transformed into a logarithm scale for analyses.

Means and standard deviation were calculated for the studied continuous variables, then Levene's and Student's t test were used for simple comparisons between pair of groups. Likewise, Pearson's chi-square (χ^2) test was used to study categorical variables.

Finally, differences in the means of body composition and cardiometabolic indicators by dietary pattern were estimated by models adjusted for gender, recruitment center, sport practice and Tanner stage. Additionally, maternal education and BMI Z-score were used as confounders in body composition and cardiometabolic variables, respectively. As some dependent variables might be related, to avoid the chance of making a type error I, we carried out a multivariate analysis of covariance (MANCOVA) for combined variables of the same group, taking into account the covariates. Levene's test and Box's M test were used for checking assumptions of homogeneity of variances and variance–covariance matrices, respectively. Later, as the second step for MANCOVA, we performed follow-up univariate analysis of covariance (ANCOVA) on stepwise generalized linear models (GLM) on each dependent variable and discriminant analysis.

All statistical analyses were carried out with SPSS 19.0, (IBM, Chicago, IL, USA). Graphics were performed with Excel 2016 (Microsoft, Redmon, Washington, DC, USA).

3. Results

The general characteristics of the total study population and BMI ranged subgroups are shown in Table 1. Compared with the normal weight group, those with overweight/obesity were more likely to be female and to have mothers with a low or medium education level, and they showed significantly greater values for BMI and BMI Z-score. No differences by BMI status were found for pubertal stage and age.

Table 1. Descriptive characteristics of children and adolescents by body mass index (BMI) status (GENOBOX cohort).

	All n = 674 (100%)	Normal Weight n = 178 (26.4%)	Overweight and Obesity n = 496 (73.6%)	p
Gender				**0.018**
Male	307 (45.5%)	95 (53.4%)	212 (42.7%)	
Female	367 (54.5%)	83 (46.6%)	284 (57.3%)	
Pubertal stage (Tanner)				0.163
Prepubertal	333 (49.4%)	96 (53.9%)	237 (47.8%)	
Pubertal	341 (50.6%)	82 (46.1%)	259 (52.2%)	
Maternal education level				**<0.001**
Low	58 (8.9%)	9 (5.2%)	49 (10.3%)	
Medium	480 (73.8%)	116 (66.7%)	364 (76.5%)	
High	112 (17.2%)	49 (28.2%)	63 (13.2%)	
Age				0.273
Children (5–11 years)	439 (65.1%)	122 (68.5%)	317 (63.9%)	
Adolescents (12–16 years)	235 (304.9%)	56 (31.5%)	179 (36.1%)	
Age (years) Mean ± SD	10.7 (2.5)	10.5 (2.7)	10.7 (2.5)	0.297
BMI				**<0.001**
Normal weight	178 (26.4%)	178 (100%)	0 (0%)	
Overweight	165 (24.5%)	0 (0%)	165 (33.3%)	
Obesity	331 (49.1%)	0 (0%)	331 (66.7%)	
BMI (kg/m^2) Mean (SD)	24.0 (5.6)	17.3 (2.3)	26.4 (4.3)	**<0.001**
BMI Z-score (kg/m^2) Mean (SD)	1.8 (1.7)	−0.3 (0.6)	2.6 (1.3)	**<0.001**

p: significance of the χ^2 test for categorical variables and Student's t test for continuous variables, assessing differences between normal weight and overweight/obese groups. Bold letters in p values mean significant differences between BMI subgroups. Abbreviations: BMI, body mass index; SD, standard deviation.

3.1. Dietary Patterns

A two clusters solution for dietary patterns was considered the most interpretable and stable. These patterns were labeled as "Health Conscious" (HC) and "Sweet and Processed" (SP). Radar plots shown in Figure 1 and Table S2 show the differences in Z-scores of the food items for each pattern. The relative frequency of most food items differed significantly between the clusters. Compared with the SP pattern, the HC pattern showed significantly ($p < 0.001$) lower mean FFQ Z-scores for salty snacks, vegetable oils, savory pastries, chocolate or nut-based spreads, fried meat, nuts and seeds, fried potatoes, ketchup, cold cuts, pizza, chocolate, added sugar, sweetened starches, ice creams, candies and trinkets, fast food, fried fish, sweetened milk products, mayonnaise, white bread, butter and margarine. Whereas the foods showing the most significantly ($p < 0.001$) higher mean FFQ Z-scores in the HC pattern were raw vegetables, fruit with no added sugar, hot drinks, fish (not fried), unsweetened breakfast cereals, diet drinks and whole grain bread. There were no significant differences for sweetened breakfast cereals, water, rice and pasta, cheese, meat (not fried) and sweetened drinks.

As the bar plot in Figure 2 shows, compared to the SP cluster, the HC cluster included a greater proportion of participants with overweight or obesity (29.0% and 51.1% vs. 17.7% and 46.1%, $p < 0.001$). In addition, Table 2 shows higher age, BMI and BMI Z-score in children allocated to the HC cluster than in those in the SP cluster, as well as more pubertals and adolescents. However, no significant differences were found between clusters related to gender and maternal education level.

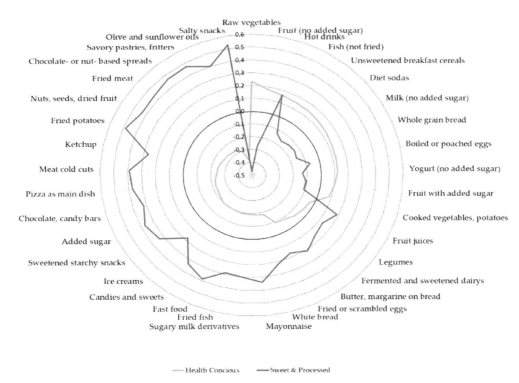

Figure 1. Radar plot of the significant differences ($p < 0.05$) in food frequency questionnaire (FFQ) items that characterize each dietary pattern in Spanish children and adolescents.

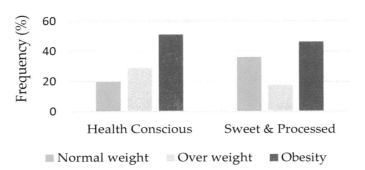

Figure 2. Frequency distribution of BMI subgroups in children and adolescents in each dietary cluster (GENOBOX cohort).

Table 2. Descriptive characteristics of Spanish children and adolescents by dietary cluster (GENOBOX cohort).

	Health Conscious $n = 403$ (59.8%)	Sweet and Processed $n = 271$ (40.2%)	p
Gender			0.102
Male	175 (43.4%)	132 (48.7%)	
Female	228 (56.6%)	139 (51.3%)	
Pubertal stage (Tanner)			**0.019**
Prepubertal	184 (45.7%)	149 (55.0%)	
Pubertal	219 (54.3%)	122 (45.0%)	
Maternal education level			0.288
Low	29 (7.5%)	29 (11.1%)	
Medium	291 (75.0%)	189 (72.1%)	
High	68 (17.5%)	44 (16.8%)	

Table 2. *Cont.*

	Health Conscious $n = 403$ (59.8%)	Sweet and Processed $n = 271$ (40.2%)	p
Age			**0.004**
Children (5–11 years)	245 (60.8%)	194 (71.6%)	
Adolescents (12–16 years)	158 (39.2%)	77 (28.4%)	
Age (years) Mean (SD)	10.9 (2.5)	10.3 (2.5)	0.002
BMI			**<0.001**
Normal weight	80 (19.9%)	98 (36.2%)	
Overweight	117 (29.0%)	48 (17.7%)	
Obesity	206 (51.1%)	125 (46.1%)	

p: significance of the χ^2 test for categorical variables and Student's t test for continuous variables, assessing differences between dietary clusters. Bold letters in p values mean significant differences between dietary clusters. Abbreviations: BMI, body mass index; SD, standard deviation.

3.2. Obesity Related Cardiometabolic Risk Indicators and Dietary Patterns

When applying the multivariate analysis, there was a statistically significant difference between the dietary clusters on combined body composition variables (BMI Z-score, skinfold sum and hip circumference) after controlling for covariates (recruitment center, sport practice, pubertal stage, gender, and maternal education) in the total sample, F(3, 491) = 4,290, $p = 0.005$, Wilks' $\lambda = 0.974$, partial $\eta^2 = 0.026$ (Box's M p-value = 0.062, Wilks' λ p-value for discriminant analysis < 0.001). However, no significant results were found for the rest of the biomarkers.

Table 3 shows mean and standard deviation values for body composition parameters, blood pressure and circulating biomarkers for each cluster in the total sample and in subgroups by BMI status when GLM were applied. Significant differences were found in the total sample, compared to the SP cluster, being allocated to the HC cluster was associated with higher mean values for age, hip circumference, skinfold sum, carotenes/TG, catalase activity, leptin, and MPO; and lower mean values for DBP, resistin, TNFα, MCP-1, tPAI-1, and sVCAM-1.

When stratifying by BMI, additional differences between clusters were observed. In the normal weight subgroup, children in the HC cluster showed lower mean values for DBP and HDLc/LDLc index than those in the SP cluster. In the overweight subgroup, those allocated to the HC cluster showed higher mean values for age, BMI, BMI Z-score, weight, and hip circumference; and lower mean values for AST, GGT, catalase, tPAI-1 and selectin, than children in the SP cluster. Lastly, in the obesity subgroup, those allocated to the HC cluster showed lower mean values for waist to hip and waist to height indexes, and MCP-1, than children in the SP cluster.

Table S3 shows mean and standard deviation values for body composition parameters, blood pressure and circulating biomarkers for each dietary cluster, stratified by age and gender. On one hand, compared to the SP cluster, those younger children allocated to the HC cluster showed higher mean values for BMI, BMI Z-score, weight, hip and waist circumference, skinfold sum, FMI Z-score, ALT, GGT, carotenes/TG, leptin and adiponectin/leptin index; and lower mean values for catalase, MCP-1, tPAI-1, sVCAM-1 than those allocated to the SP cluster. Whereas adolescents allocated to the HC cluster showed higher mean values for waist to height index; and lower mean values for HDLc/LDLc index, adiponectin, TNFα and MCP-1 than those in the SP cluster. On the other hand, males allocated to the HC cluster showed higher mean values for hip circumference, skinfold sum, ALT, and leptin; and lower mean values for DBP, MCP-1 and tPAI-1 than those in the SP cluster. However, females allocated to the HC cluster showed higher mean values for age, waist to hip index, total cholesterol, LDLc, and MPO; and lower mean values for HDLc/LDLc index than those in the SP cluster.

Table 3. Mean differences of cardiometabolic and health risk indicators between dietary clusters in the three BMI subgroups of children and adolescents (GENOBOX cohort).

	All (n = 674)		Normal Weight (n = 178)		Overweight (n = 165)		Obesity (n = 331)	
	Health Conscious (n = 403)	Sweet and Processed (n = 271)	Health Conscious (n = 80)	Sweet and Processed (n = 98)	Health Conscious (n = 117)	Sweet and Processed (n = 48)	Health Conscious (n = 206)	Sweet and Processed (n = 125)
Age (years)	10.9 (2.5)	**10.3 (2.5) ****	10.8 (2.9)	10.2 (2.5)	11.7 (2.1)	**10.2 (2.1) *****	10.5 (2.5)	10.4 (2.6)
Body composition indicators								
BMI (kg/m^2)	24.6 (5.1)	23.2 (6.3)	17.7 (2.6)	17.0 (2.0)	**23.7 (2.4)**	**21.8 (2.3) ****	27.7 (3.9)	28.5 (4.4)
BMI Z-score (kg/m^2)	2.0 (1.6)	1.6 (1.9)	-0.21 (0.56)	-0.33 (0.54)	**1.44 (0.49)**	**1.22 (0.42) ***	3.11 (1.06)	3.35 (1.18)
Body mass (kg)	54.6 (18.5)	49.5 (20.6)	38.7 (14.0)	34.3 (11.0)	**54.4 (12.2)**	**45.9 (11.9) ***	60.9 (19.2)	62.8 (20.3)
Hip circumference (cm)	**90.2 (13.6)**	**83.2 (15.2) ****	76.5 (11.4)	72.0 (9.5)	**91.2 (9.0)**	**83.5 (8.6) ***	95.5 (12.8)	95.3 (13.7)
Waist circumference (cm)	82.3 (15.0)	77.1 (17.6)	64.8 (11.8)	60.8 (5.9)	81.7 (9.7)	75.4 (9.4)	89.5 (12.6)	91.3 (14.4)
Waist to hip index	0.56 (0.08)	0.54 (0.10)	0.85 (0.08)	0.85 (0.07)	0.90 (0.08)	0.90 (0.07)	0.93 (0.07)	**0.94 (0.09) ****
Waist to height index	83.7 (30.1)	68.1 (35.7)	0.45 (0.05)	0.44 (0.04)	0.54 (0.05)	0.52 (0.04)	**0.61 (0.06)**	**0.63 (0.06) ****
Skinfold sum (mm)	**38.3 (10.0)**	**33.9 (9.5) ****	42.1 (18.7)	37.2 (17.3)	88.4 (17.7)	77.0 (22.1)	102.4 (18.8)	103.0 (22.6)
FMI Z-score (kg/m^2)	11.6 (5.1)	10.4 (5.6)	3.5 (2.7)	2.7 (1.8)	6.4 (2.3)	5.7 (2.4)	9.7 (4.06)	9.3 (4.0)
FFMI Z-score (kg/m^2)	10.9 (2.5)	10.3 (2.5)	8.1 (4.2)	7.2 (3.9)	11.6 (4.7)	10.3 (4.1)	13.6 (4.9)	14.7 (5.2)
Cardiometabolic indicators								
Blood pressure								
SBP (mm Hg)^	109 (13)	108 (14)	104 (12)	100 (12)	108 (12)	106 (13)	112 (14)	121
DBP (mm Hg)^	**65 (11)**	**66 (10) ***	**61 (9)**	**63 (10) ***	64 (11)	63 (8)	67 (11)	121
General metabolic biomarkers								
Glucose (mg/dL)	84 (8)	86 (8)	84 (8)	86 (7)	85 (8)	88 (8)	84 (8)	85 (8)
Insulin (mU/L)	12.20 (8.42)	11.52 (9.92)	8.00 (4.54)	7.27 (4.87)	11.11 (7.78)	10.55 (6.12)	14.47 (9.18)	15.4 (12.44)
HOMA-IR	2.57 (1.84)	2.48 (2.18)	1.68 (1.00)	1.56 (1.08)	2.35 (1.73)	2.36 (1.53)	3.05 (2.00)	3.27 (2.70)
TG (mg/dL)	69 (34)	69 (35)	57 (23)	54 (23)	66 (30)	77 (44)	76 (38)	77 (34)
Cholesterol (mg/dL)	165 (30)	161 (28)	169 (26)	164 (28)	166 (33)	163 (31)	162 (30)	159 (26)
LDLc (mg/dL)	97 (26)	92 (25)	95 (22)	87 (26)	99 (30)	93 (25)	97 (26)	94 (24)
HDLc (mg/dL)^	50 (13)	55 (15)	59 (13)	65 (15)	49 (11)	54 (14)	47 (12)	47 (11)
HDLc/LDLc index	0.61 (0.46)	0.81 (0.67)	0.66 (0.22)	**0.94 (0.6) ****	0.59 (0.43)	0.78 (0.65)	0.6 (0.54)	0.72 (0.73)
AST (U/L)	22 (9)	23 (7)	24 (8)	25 (6)	**20 (6)**	**24 (9) ***	22 (10)	22 (7)
ALT (U/L)	20 (12)	19 (11)	17 (9)	16 (6)	18 (9)	21 (21)	22 (14)	20 (8)
GGT (U/L)	12 (7)	13 (7)	10 (3)	10 (3)	**11 (5)**	**14 (13) ***	14 (9)	15 (5)
Oxidative stress biomarkers								
Carotenes/TG	**1.71 (1.65)**	**1.53 (1.25) ***	2.70 (2.32)	2.55 (1.56)	1.43 (1.12)	1.34 (0.81)	1.38 (1.36)	1.00 (0.76)
Tocopherols/TG	0.14 (0.07)	0.15 (0.07)	0.17 (0.07)	0.19 (0.07)	0.13 (0.06)	0.12 (0.06)	0.13 (0.08)	0.13 (0.05)
TAC (mM Eq Trolox®)	2.05 (0.87)	2.09 (0.91)	1.88 (0.66)	1.99 (0.75)	2.06 (0.85)	2.19 (1.13)	2.11 (0.97)	2.17 (0.96)
Catalase (U/g Hb)	**164.68 (103.66)**	**163.94 (153.67) ****	119.65 (71.23)	136.22 (119.74)	**165.71 (83.01)**	**232.91 (283.63) ***	180.90 (118.02)	162.27 (74.02)
Adipokines and biomarkers of inflammation and endothelial damage								
Adiponectin (mg/L)	14.58 (8.67)	15.18 (8.31)	17.27 (11.37)	17.08 (9.52)	14.91 (7.86)	14.51 (8.86)	13.13 (7.31)	13.51 (6.05)
Leptin (ug/L)	**15.56 (12.96)**	**14.09 (15.82) ****	4.59 (4.89)	3.95 (4.26)	12.44 (5.83)	12.47 (9.57)	22.47 (14.32)	25.13 (18.36)
Resistin (ug/L)^	**20.18 (14.89)**	**21.06 (14.47) ****	24.07 (21.24)	23.85 (17.18)	18.43 (10.37)	18.80 (14.73)	19.4 (13.27)	19.24 (10.32)
TNFα (ng/L)^	**2.82 (1.72)**	**2.89 (1.58) ***	2.27 (1.20)	2.4 (1.34)	2.67 (2.11)	3.26 (1.95)	3.15 (1.59)	3.23 (1.48)
MCP-1 (ng/L)	**88.47 (37.69)**	**92.81 (38.84) ****	83.54 (28.28)	85.21 (39.62)	88.01 (48.11)	89.70 (32.51)	**91.01 (34.32)**	**102.26 (39.22) ***
tPAI-1 (ug/L)	**22.9 (14.29)**	**25.48 (17.31) *****	16.31 (12.21)	17.8 (12.94)	**21.76 (12.64)**	**28.85 (17.23) ****	26.61 (14.93)	31.92 (18.34)
Selectin (ug/L)^	27.34 (14.7)	30.38 (16.59)	27.86 (15.66)	24.51 (11.69)	**22.45 (11.9)**	**34.89 (20.32) ***	31.06 (15.25)	33.6 (17.38)
sVCAM-1 (mg/L)^	**1.04 (0.32)**	**1.14 (0.25) ***	1.07 (0.33)	1.20 (0.27)	1.00 (0.27)	1.15 (0.28)	1.04 (0.34)	1.07 (0.22)
MPO (ug/L)	**39.99 (83.94)**	**32.95 (42.29) ***	42.25 (77.48)	36.98 (50.22)	27.96 (29.79)	29.97 (39.36)	46.15 (105.63)	30.18 (33.95)

^ Logarithm transformed variable used for analyses. Bold letters mean significant differences (*: $p \leq 0.05$; **: $p \leq 0.01$; ***: $p \leq 0.001$) between dietary patterns in the stepwise generalized linear models adjusted for recruitment center, sport practice, pubertal stage, gender and, additionally, maternal education level for body composition or BMI Z-score for metabolic variables. Student's t-test was used to analyze age differences. Abbreviations: BMI: body mass index; circ.: circumference; FMI: fat mass index; FFMI: free fat mass index; SBP: systolic blood pressure; DBP: diastolic blood pressure; HOMA-IR: homeostatic model assessment for insulin resistance; TG: triglycerides; HDL: high-density lipoprotein cholesterol; LDLc: low-density lipoprotein cholesterol; AST: aspartate transaminase; ALT: alanine transaminase; GGT: gamma-glutamyl transferase; TAC: total antioxidant capacity; TNFα: tumor necrosis factor alpha; MCP-1: monocyte chemoattractant protein-1; tPAI-1: total plasminogen activator inhibitor-1; sVCAM1: soluble vascular cell adhesion molecule-1; MPO: myeloperoxidase.

4. Discussion

In the present study, we have observed that those children allocated to the HC pattern showed higher BMI than those in the SP pattern. However, being allocated to the HC cluster was associated with a mainly healthier cardiometabolic profile, although we will also discuss some conflictive results. Overall, these results suggest that other factors could influence health status beyond BMI and current food consumption frequency but also highlight that having a healthy dietary pattern could help prevent future cardiometabolic risk.

Dietary patterns have been previously explored using two types of analytical approaches. On the one hand, a priori driven methods, which focus on constructing dietary scores using a predefined combination of diet quality based on dietary guidelines. On the other hand, a posteriori exploratory methods, which reduce large datasets into smaller ones to summarize total dietary exposure by the use of multivariate statistical techniques. In relation to the latter group, CA has been increasingly applied in recent years, mainly because it provides an intuitive picture of the whole diet. CA reduces behaviors into patterns and categorizes individuals according to continuous and mutually exclusive differences. In contrast, principal component analysis (PCA) or reduced rank regression (RRR) assign scores of the derived factors to each individual according to the intercorrelations of behaviors, which can also be influenced by a larger subjective component in decision making, especially in the way in which the researchers code and define the dietary pattern groups [7]. Hence, CA allows the completion of global assessments of the quality of the diet referring to identifiable groups of individuals, as well as their association with health outcomes and nutritional biomarkers, in a more understandable and applicable way in the field of dietary recommendations [6].

The conducted CA showed two dietary patterns, HC and SP, in the present sample of Spanish children and adolescents, with opposite characteristics regarding the consumption of the main food and beverage groups. The HC pattern was characterized by having higher consumption frequency (CF) of fruits and vegetables, whole grains, and dairy, being closer to compliance with the FFQ dietary guidelines [29]. In contrast, the SP pattern was characterized by having higher CF of snacks, sweets, fat, and processed foods. According to previous reviews regarding the use of CA or other approaches to study children and adolescents' dietary patterns [11,12], definitions and labels of unhealthy eating patterns are wide, although they have been mainly characterized by a high consumption of high energy dense foods and beverages or ready-to-eat food, similar to our SP pattern. Otherwise, healthy and HC dietary patterns have been quite frequently described too, with a consistent characterization similar to ours and are generally considered to be protective against weight gain [3]. Specifically, in Spain, there have been four previous studies including large samples of children or adolescents, which also found healthy dietary patterns in their study populations by using different approaches, labeling them as "healthy" (enKID [13,30] and SI! [16]), or "Mediterranean-like" (ANIBES [14,31,32] and EsNuPi [15]), including a high intake of vegetables, fruits and fish, similar to our HC.

Regarding obesity, these healthy patterns in Spanish children and adolescents generated conflicting results. ANIBES [14,31,32] and enKID [13,30] found a negative association, EsNuPi [13] found different associations according to age, and SI! [15] found a positive association, as did we. Indeed, we found that the HC cluster included a higher proportion of children with obesity (51.1% vs. 46.1%) and overweight (29.0% vs. 19.7%), and a lower proportion with normal weight (19.9% vs. 36.2%) than the SP cluster. However, there are also abroad studies that observed this counterintuitive cluster's association in children and adolescents, such as a healthy one associated with a higher percentage of overweight/obesity in a cross-sectional study in Europe [33]. Similar findings have been reported through both cross-sectional and longitudinal approaches, in which healthier patterns were found to be related to higher BMI and BMI gain in Norway [34] and to higher obesity odds ratios in the U.S. [35]. In addition, it is interesting to note that children with excess weight were included in a high proportion in both clusters. This can be explained by the higher proportion of children with excess weight in the total sample. However, a second potential conclusion can be drawn, in which there could be two types of children with obesity, those who are conscious of the importance of a healthy diet and those who consume a lot of processed foods and sweets. The association between healthy dietary patterns and obesity has already been discussed in previous reviews [11,12], where all kinds of directions have been described, as well as highlighting the difficulty in comparing studies. In fact, explaining this controversy would require accounting for all determinants of energy balance and their interactions, as well as for differences in methodology, including the specific studied sample and bias [6,11,12].

First, associations such as the one described in the present study have been previously explained by other authors as reverse causation. This has been attributed to an attempt by the individuals to control their excess weight or the disease burden, and patterns have been described and labeled related to restrictive eating behaviors [11,12]. Indeed, HC patterns are in agreement with several interventions for obesity treatment, which recommend a high intake of foods considered to be protective against weight gain, such as vegetables and fruits, and a low intake of foods considered obesogenic, with a high fat and carbohydrate content [4,12,36,37].

Interestingly, sampling differences with previous studies are not negligible, as most of these were not based on cohort studies conducted in a clinical setting, but population cross-sectional studies (frequently using random multistage census- and school-based sampling procedures). In contrast, the present study has been performed in a specialized hospital environment and included subjects with excess weight attending health care services. This could imply a higher interest of the participants in improving their health, since non-attendance to health care visits has been associated with long-term excess weight in school children [38].

However, it could be possible that subjects with excess weight allocated to the HC cluster had some negative dietary-related behaviors not considered in the current analysis, which could contribute to a high energy imbalance. Indeed, a review highlighted the co-occurrence of both healthy and unhealthy behaviors, or even compensatory ones, or the use of ineffective dieting methods [35]. These behaviors could include differences in portion size, preparation, serving style, skipping breakfast or other meals, and having a high total energy intake. In fact, children with excess weight tend to have higher energy intake requirements, due in part also to higher fat-free mass [35]. However, in our study, we found no difference in FFMI between children from both clusters.

Otherwise, our analysis accounted for the main non-dietary confounders, considering physical activity due to its influence on obesity, along with diet [1], and the high prevalence of insufficient physical activity in Spanish adolescents (around three quarters) [39]. We also included origin (recruitment center) and maternal education level as covariates, as the main socio-economic and demographic factors in obesity susceptibility [30,40]. We found maternal education level was associated with obesity, but not to the HC cluster, as observed in previous studies [13,41]. Finally we took into account gender, age and puberty stage, due to the existing differences in obesity prevalence (higher in 6–13-year-old boys) [1,30], physiology of eating [42,43], cognitive behaviors [44,45], and the effect of diet on development [46]. Indeed, we found a HC cluster with a higher proportion of females and younger children, in agreement with previous literature [11], and with a lower consumption frequency of food puberty accelerators, such as sweetened soft beverages and meat products [46]. Somehow, as could be expected, we observed small differences in the results when stratifying the analyses between clusters by age or puberty, suggesting a possible presence of this effect on our findings.

Moreover, some authors consider the report bias to explain this association between obesity and a healthy pattern. They could include socially acceptable responses tending to under- or over- report food intake, or omit some foods they perceived as unhealthy, which are more common among subjects with an unhealthy diet, excess weight and males [47,48]. Additionally, reports about meals out of parental control would be missed as information was provided mainly by parents, while both a more frequent use of the school meals canteen (associated with healthier dietary intakes [49]) and a low family presence during the main meals have been reported in Spanish children and adolescents [50,51], with food intakes outside of parental control increasing with age [52]. However, our study used trained dieticians/nutritionists and imputation to minimize missing data, and, more importantly, we also found associations between the identified dietary patterns and several fat distribution and cardiometabolic markers reflecting a better health profile in all the subgroups of the HC cluster (including BMI as a covariate in the biomarkers analysis), so a strong effect of these bias reports should not be considered in the present study.

When analyzing the wide range of cardiometabolic risk biomarkers, we must take into consideration that some of the observed differences between the clusters may be due to chance. With this in mind, we conducted a multivariate analysis. Its results allowed us to support the differences related to body composition, but not those associated with the rest of biomarkers. However, the use of several dichotomous or ordinal variables as covariates (recruitment center, sport practice, gender, and maternal education) could have subtracted strength from the model. Thus, further studies are encouraged to search for the potential association of diet with these cardiometabolic risk biomarkers using more suitable continuous covariates.

Despite the lack of overall association, the individual generalized linear models showed interesting findings. Compared to the SP cluster, the HC cluster showed higher several subcutaneous and general fat mass indicators beyond BMI especially in those with overweight, children and males when stratifying analyses by BMI, age, and gender, respectively. However, after stratifying by BMI, age and gender, the SP cluster was found to be associated with a worse cardiometabolic profile. Within those in the obesity subgroup, participants allocated to the SP cluster showed higher indicators of abdominal/visceral fat mass (waist to hip and waist to height indexes), and therefore, a worse phenotype related to higher metabolic risk [53–55] than those in the HC cluster. Although it is the first time that this scenario has been described in Spanish children and adolescents with excess weight, our findings are supported by the available literature. Previous studies have reported a stronger influence of diet on fat mass than on muscle mass in overweight children [9], which is in line with our findings, since we found no differences related to fat free mass between the identified dietary clusters. However, other authors have described the positive association between BMI and healthy dietary patterns as being mediated by a higher muscle mass [56]. In contrast, when stratifying the body composition analysis by age and gender, we found some confusing results, as abdominal fat indicators such as waist to hip and waist to height were higher in the HC clustered females and adolescents, respectively. As other authors had found healthy and restrictive patterns to be more likely in this population [11,12], and considering the lower levels of physical activity in Spanish female adolescents [39], this could be explained in terms of the same reverse causation. This way, it could be possible that higher abdominal fat makes this population subgroup more conscious to follow a healthy dietary pattern. In addition, we also find the HC cluster associated with a worse lipid profile specifically in these subgroups, allowing us to suggest that the dietary pattern may less strongly influence a worse cholesterol metabolic profile than type of fat distribution (and physical activity levels) [57]. The SP cluster showed a worse CVD profile, indicated through higher DBP figures, when analyzed in the total population and the normal weight group, in agreement with a previous analysis carried out by our team, which identified a higher DBP in children with a higher consumption frequency of energy dense salty foods [58]. Additionally, the SP cluster was associated with a mainly worse metabolic phenotype through several biochemical indicators, both in the total sample and the age- gender- and BMI-stratified analyses. Hence, although the HC cluster was associated with higher obesity subcutaneous indicators (especially when analyzing the total sample and the overweight subgroup), it was also associated with a better phenotype in terms of oxidative stress, inflammatory and endothelial damage biomarkers. For example, compared to those with a SP pattern in the total sample, children with a HC pattern showed higher serum levels of carotenes/TG, as well as lower resistin, TNFα, MCP-1, tPAI-1, sVCAM1, although higher leptin and MPO. Moreover, the difference in MCP-1 was also found in the subgroup of participants with obesity, as well as in children, adolescents, and males, in the stratified analyses.

Regarding these results, the HC pattern was characterized by high frequency of consumption of vegetables, fruit, fish, low-fat dairy products, with a high content in antioxidants, micronutrients, fiber, and essential fatty acids. These exert antioxidant, anti-inflammatory and antithrombotic effects [59] and are known to contribute to the delay of CVD initiation and progression [59]. In this way, our results are in agreement with the previous ones of our team [60], showing plasma levels of carotenes/TAG to be correlated with the consumption frequency of carotene-rich foods in normal weight children, and decreased by a cumulative effect of obesity and unhealthy metabolic status, as well as negatively associated with BMI status, endothelial and glucose metabolism biomarkers in children and adolescents. In contrast, the SP pattern was characterized by high frequency of consumption of food items with a higher content in saturated fatty acids, salt, high glycemic index and low content in fiber and micronutrients. This kind of food contributes to higher levels of circulating free fat acids and glucose, and consequently to the increased generation of free radicals, which deplete the antioxidant defense systems and further contribute to inflammation, causing disruption in several metabolic pathways. The SP pattern is similar to other ones often labeled as western patterns, which have been related to undesirable health outcomes, including central obesity and weight gain, with moderate evidence in children and adolescents, but strong evidence in adults [12]. Indeed, although with a shorter list of biomarkers, a previous review on dietary patterns studies worldwide [12], and other European prospective studies using CA [10–61] have described similar associations in children and adolescents.

Our phenotype related findings support an effect of diet on the molecular mechanisms related to the "obesity paradox", in which adipose tissue expansion is feasible without the accompanying adipocyte dysfunction [62], in children and adolescents. Indeed, mechanisms involving oxidative stress and inflammation have been described in childhood obesity [63], as well as the modulating role of diet over them [59,64–66]. Thus, our findings suggest that a HC dietary pattern can be associated with the metabolically healthy phenotype and a low cardiometabolic risk in children and adolescents with excess weight through both classic and novel indicators—most of them not commonly available in routine health control procedures. Otherwise, we found a SP pattern present in a high proportion of children and adolescents associated with a worse phenotype, both through fat distribution and cardiometabolic markers.

Limitations of this study must be acknowledged. The cross-sectional design does not allow the establishment of causal associations. Selection bias also cannot be ruled out given the voluntary nature of participation, which may involve under representation of certain population groups such as those who have no need for care from the social services [38] (possibly due to not being aware of having a health problem or, even if they were aware, this could make them want to avoid the negative results from an evaluation because they do not want the confirmation or to hear it from others, or to accept the consequences or initiate a change or intervention), or those with lower parental education levels or higher incomes. The inclusion of only Caucasian children could also be seen as a limitation, as dietary patterns may differ according to race and ethnicity, so this work does not reflect all Spanish children and adolescents. However, since the Caucasian ethnic group is the one that predominates our environment, it was considered as an inclusion criterion to homogenize the study population. The direction of these possible selection biases cannot be predicted as no information on non-participants is available. The possible effect of some reporting bias has already been discussed above. The used FFQ was not quantitative so it did not assess the total food intake, although when comparing dietary patterns obtained with and without energy adjustment it is unlikely that energy intake influences the membership results, as found by other authors [6,7]. In addition, it only covered the previous four weeks, and potential differences due to seasonality could have affected the results. However, reports and measurements were performed in the same period of time. Body composition measurement by BIA is not as accurate as other methods (such as DXA or BodPod®), but it is easier to apply when studying large clinical populations. Physical activity was assessed according to two questions characterizing sports activity, which could miss children that devote a substantial amount of time to recreational physical activity outside of planned sport lessons. Finally, the non-significant multivariate analysis regarding cardiometabolic risk biomarkers forces the individual significant findings to be considered as preliminary observations, which could be due to chance, and therefore that should be investigated further in future studies.

As for strengths, to our knowledge, this is the first Spanish study applying cluster analysis to identify dietary patterns in a cohort study on childhood obesity. Likewise, the use of a wide range of body composition and biochemical cardiometabolic risk indicators should also be considered a strength as there is a lack of studies assessing the effect of diet on these cardiometabolic risk indicators. In addition, the study was performed using standardized and harmonized information from clinical care centers of three different Spanish regions, providing comparable food consumption frequency estimates in a large sample size.

5. Conclusions

Our results suggest a mainly better cardiometabolic health for those children and adolescents who follow a healthy dietary pattern independently of BMI, and especially for those male children with overweight (who are the subpopulation with the highest prevalence of excess weight); however, multivariate analyses call these findings into question. Likewise, there is an HC dietary pattern that could be associated with a worse fat distribution and cholesterol metabolism in females and adolescents, which requires us to take into account further considerations and involved factors. Otherwise, there is also a SP dietary pattern linked to a mainly worse cardiometabolic profile that could lead to greater excess weight and worse health status in overweight children and adolescents. Consequently, our findings highlight the importance of the association between dietary patterns and cardiometabolic risk markers related to oxidative stress, inflammation, and endothelial damage, which may be already present in childhood, and determine the appearance of future cardiometabolic diseases. Longitudinal studies would be useful to corroborate and evaluate long-term implications of these findings. Diet along with other approaches should be considered in prevention studies aiming to reduce cardiometabolic risk, beyond weight control.

Author Contributions: Conceptualization, M.G.-C., R.L., C.M.A., Á.G., L.A.M. and G.B.; data collection, M.L.-M., R.V.-C., M.G.-C., R.L., G.B.; statistical analyses, M.L.-M., A.I.R., A.S.-P.; writing—original draft preparation, M.L.-M., A.I.R.; writing—review and editing, M.L.-M., A.I.R., E.M.G.-G., A.S.-P., M.G.-C., C.M.A., Á.G., L.A.M., R.L., G.B. All authors have read and agreed to the published version of the manuscript.

Acknowledgments: The authors would like to thank the children and their parents for their participation in the study. The authors also acknowledge the University of Granada "Plan Propio de Investigacion 2016-Excellence actions: Unit of Excellence on Exercise and Health (UCEES)".

References

1. WHO. Obesity and Overweight. Available online: https://www.who.int/news-room/fact-sheets/detail/ obesity-and-overweight (accessed on 29 October 2020).
2. Perez-Farinos, N.; Lopez-Sobaler, A.M.; Dal Re, M.A.; Villar, C.; Labrado, E.; Robledo, T.; Ortega, R.M. The ALADINO study: A national study of prevalence of overweight and obesity in Spanish children in 2011. *Biomed. Res. Int.* **2013**, *2013*, 163687. [CrossRef] [PubMed]
3. Han, J.C.; Lawlor, D.A.; Kimm, S.Y. Childhood obesity. *Lancet* **2010**, *375*, 1737–1748. [CrossRef]

4. Consultation, W.F.E. *Joint WHO/FAO Expert Consultation: Diet, Nutrition and the Prevention of Chronic Diseases*; WHO: Geneva, Switzerland, 2003.

5. GBD-Collaborators. Global, regional, and national comparative risk assessment of 84 behavioural, environmental and occupational, and metabolic risks or clusters of risks, 1990–2016: A systematic analysis for the Global Burden of Disease Study 2016. *Lancet* **2017**, *390*, 1345–1422. [CrossRef]

6. Devlin, U.M.; McNulty, B.A.; Nugent, A.P.; Gibney, M.J. The use of cluster analysis to derive dietary patterns: Methodological considerations, reproducibility, validity and the effect of energy mis-reporting. *Proc. Nutr. Soc.* **2012**, *71*, 599–609. [CrossRef] [PubMed]

7. Newby, P.K.; Tucker, K.L. Empirically derived eating patterns using factor or cluster analysis: A review. *Nutr. Rev.* **2004**, *62*, 177–203. [CrossRef]

8. Wirfalt, E.; Drake, I.; Wallstrom, P. What do review papers conclude about food and dietary patterns? *Food Nutr. Res.* **2013**, *57*. [CrossRef]

9. Smith, A.D.; Emmett, P.M.; Newby, P.K.; Northstone, K. Dietary patterns and changes in body composition in children between 9 and 11 years. *Food Nutr. Res.* **2014**, *58*. [CrossRef]

10. Fernandez-Alvira, J.M.; Bammann, K.; Eiben, G.; Hebestreit, A.; Kourides, Y.A.; Kovacs, E.; Michels, N.; Pala, V.; Reisch, L.; Russo, P.; et al. Prospective associations between dietary patterns and body composition changes in European children: The IDEFICS study. *Public Health Nutr.* **2017**, *20*, 3257–3265. [CrossRef]

11. Leech, R.M.; McNaughton, S.A.; Timperio, A. The clustering of diet, physical activity and sedentary behavior in children and adolescents: A review. *Int. J. Behav. Nutr. Phys. Act.* **2014**, *11*, 4. [CrossRef]

12. Cunha, C.M.; Costa, P.R.F.; de Oliveira, L.P.M.; Queiroz, V.A.O.; Pitangueira, J.C.D.; Oliveira, A.M. Dietary patterns and cardiometabolic risk factors among adolescents: Systematic review and meta-analysis. *Br. J. Nutr.* **2018**, *119*, 859–879. [CrossRef]

13. Aranceta, J.; Perez-Rodrigo, C.; Ribas, L.; Serra-Majem, L. Sociodemographic and lifestyle determinants of food patterns in Spanish children and adolescents: The enKid study. *Eur. J. Clin. Nutr.* **2003**, *57* (Suppl. 1), S40–S44. [CrossRef]

14. Perez-Rodrigo, C.; Gil, A.; Gonzalez-Gross, M.; Ortega, R.M.; Serra-Majem, L.; Varela-Moreiras, G.; Aranceta-Bartrina, J. Clustering of Dietary Patterns, Lifestyles, and Overweight among Spanish Children and Adolescents in the ANIBES Study. *Nutrients* **2015**, *8*, 11. [CrossRef] [PubMed]

15. Plaza-Díaz, J.; Molina-Montes, E.; Soto-Méndez, M.J.; Madrigal, C.; Hernández-Ruiz, Á.; Valero, T.; Lara Villoslada, F.; Leis, R.; Martínez de Victoria, E.; Moreno, J.M.; et al. Clustering of Dietary Patterns and Lifestyles Among Spanish Children in the EsNuPI Study. *Nutrients* **2020**, *12*, 2536. [CrossRef]

16. Bodega, P.; Fernández-Alvira, J.M.; Santos-Beneit, G.; de Cos-Gandoy, A.; Fernández-Jiménez, R.; Moreno, L.A.; de Miguel, M.; Carral, V.; Orrit, X.; Carvajal, I.; et al. Dietary Patterns and Cardiovascular Risk Factors in Spanish Adolescents: A Cross-Sectional Analysis of the SI! Program for Health Promotion in Secondary Schools. *Nutrients* **2019**, *11*, 2297. [CrossRef]

17. Stewart, A.; Marfell-Jones, M.; Olds, T.; de Ridder, H. *Protocolo Internacional Para la Valoración Antropométrica*; Sociedad internacional para el avance de la cineantropometría, Universidad Católica de Murcia, Campus de los Jerónimos: Guadalupe (Murcia), España, Spain, 2011.

18. Sobradillo, B.; Aguirre, A.; Aresti, U.; Bilbao, A.; Fernández-Ramos, C.; Lizárraga, A.; Lorenzo, H.; Madariaga, L.; Rica, I.; Ruiz, I. Curvas y tablas de crecimiento (estudios longitudinal y transversal). Fundación Faustino Orbegozo Eizaguirre. In *Curvas y Tablas de Crecimiento (Estudios Longitudinal y Transversal)*; Sobradillo, B., Aguirre, A., Aresti, U., Bilbao, A., Fernández-Ramos, C., Lizárraga, A., Lorenzo, H., Madariaga, L., Rica, I.I.R., Eds.; Fundación Faustino Orbegozo Eizaguirre: Madrid, Spain, 2004.

19. Cole, T.J.; Bellizzi, M.C.; Flegal, K.M.; Dietz, W.H. Establishing a standard definition for child overweight and obesity worldwide: International survey. *BMJ* **2000**, *320*, 1240–1243. [CrossRef]

20. Wells, J.C.; Williams, J.E.; Chomtho, S.; Darch, T.; Grijalva-Eternod, C.; Kennedy, K.; Haroun, D.; Wilson, C.; Cole, T.J.; Fewtrell, M.S. Body-composition reference data for simple and reference techniques and a 4-component model: A new UK reference child. *Am. J. Clin. Nutr.* **2012**, *96*, 1316–1326. [CrossRef]

21. Garcia-Rodriguez, C.E.; Mesa, M.D.; Olza, J.; Vlachava, M.; Kremmyda, L.S.; Diaper, N.D.; Noakes, P.S.; Miles, E.A.; Ramirez-Tortosa, M.C.; Liaset, B.; et al. Does consumption of two portions of salmon per week enhance the antioxidant defense system in pregnant women? *Antioxid. Redox Signal.* **2012**, *16*, 1401–1406. [CrossRef] [PubMed]

22. Aebi, H. Catalase in vitro. *Methods Enzymol.* **1984**, *105*, 121–126.

23. Matthews, D.R.; Hosker, J.P.; Rudenski, A.S.; Naylor, B.A.; Treacher, D.F.; Turner, R.C. Homeostasis model assessment: Insulin resistance and beta-cell function from fasting plasma glucose and insulin concentrations in man. *Diabetologia* **1985**, *28*, 412–419. [CrossRef]

24. Tojo, R.; Leis, R. Alimentación del niño escolar. In *Manual Práctico de Nutrición en Pediatría*; Pediatría, A., Ed.; Ergón: Jackson, MS, USA, 2007; pp. 91–106.

25. UNESCO. *International Standard Classification of Education (ISCED)*; UNESCO: Paris, France, 2011.

26. Verbestel, V.; De Henauw, S.; Bammann, K.; Barba, G.; Hadjigeorgiou, C.; Eiben, G.; Konstabel, K.; Kovács, E.; Pitsiladis, Y.; Reisch, L.; et al. Are context-specific measures of parental-reported physical activity and sedentary behaviour associated with accelerometer data in 2-9-year-old European children? *Public Health Nutr.* **2015**, *18*, 860–868. [CrossRef]

27. Tanner, J.M.; Whitehouse, R.H. Clinical longitudinal standards for height, weight, height velocity, weight velocity, and stages of puberty. *Arch. Dis. Child.* **1976**, *51*, 170–179. [CrossRef] [PubMed]

28. Leis, R.; Jurado-Castro, J.M.; Llorente-Cantarero, F.J.; Anguita-Ruiz, A.; Iris-Rupérez, A.; Bedoya-Carpente, J.J.; Vázquez-Cobela, R.; Aguilera, C.M.; Bueno, G.; Gil-Campos, M. Cluster Analysis of Physical Activity Patterns, and Relationship with Sedentary Behavior and Healthy Lifestyles in Prepubertal Children: Genobox Cohort. *Nutrients* **2020**, *12*, 1288. [CrossRef]

29. Aranceta-Bartrina, J.; Partearroyo, T.; López-Sobaler, A.M.; Ortega, R.M.; Varela-Moreiras, G.; Serra-Majem, L.; Pérez-Rodrigo, C. Updating the Food-Based Dietary Guidelines for the Spanish Population: The Spanish Society of Community Nutrition (SENC) Proposal. *Nutrients* **2019**, *11*, 2675. [CrossRef] [PubMed]

30. Serra-Majem, L.; Aranceta Bartrina, J.; Perez-Rodrigo, C.; Ribas-Barba, L.; Delgado-Rubio, A. Prevalence and deteminants of obesity in Spanish children and young people. *Br. J. Nutr.* **2006**, *96* (Suppl. 1), S67–S72. [CrossRef]

31. Aranceta-Bartrina, J.; Perez-Rodrigo, C. Determinants of childhood obesity: ANIBES study. *Nutr. Hosp.* **2016**, *33*, 339. [CrossRef]

32. Samaniego-Vaesken, M.L.; Partearroyo, T.; Ruiz, E.; Aranceta-Bartrina, J.; Gil, A.; Gonzalez-Gross, M.; Ortega, R.M.; Serra-Majem, L.; Varela-Moreiras, G. The Influence of Place of Residence, Gender and Age Influence on Food Group Choices in the Spanish Population: Findings from the ANIBES Study. *Nutrients* **2018**, *10*, 392. [CrossRef]

33. Fernández-Alvira, J.M.; Börnhorst, C.; Bammann, K.; Gwozdz, W.; Krogh, V.; Hebestreit, A.; Barba, G.; Reisch, L.; Eiben, G.; Iglesia, I.; et al. Prospective associations between socio-economic status and dietary patterns in European children: The Identification and Prevention of Dietary- and Lifestyle-induced Health Effects in Children and Infants (IDEFICS) Study. *Br. J. Nutr.* **2015**, *113*, 517–525. [CrossRef]

34. Van der Sluis, M.E.; Lien, N.; Twisk, J.W.; Steenhuis, I.H.; Bere, E.; Klepp, K.I.; Wind, M. Longitudinal associations of energy balance-related behaviours and cross-sectional associations of clusters and body mass index in Norwegian adolescents. *Public Health Nutr.* **2010**, *13*, 1716–1721. [CrossRef]

35. Boone-Heinonen, J.; Gordon-Larsen, P.; Adair, L.S. Obesogenic clusters: Multidimensional adolescent obesity-related behaviors in the U.S. *Ann. Behav. Med.* **2008**, *36*, 217–230. [CrossRef]

36. Patel, C.; Ghanim, H.; Ravishankar, S.; Sia, C.L.; Viswanathan, P.; Mohanty, P.; Dandona, P. Prolonged reactive oxygen species generation and nuclear factor-kappaB activation after a high-fat, high-carbohydrate meal in the obese. *J. Clin. Endocrinol. Metab.* **2007**, *92*, 4476–4479. [CrossRef]

37. Yip, C.S.C.; Chan, W.; Fielding, R. The Associations of Fruit and Vegetable Intakes with Burden of Diseases: A Systematic Review of Meta-Analyses. *J. Acad. Nutr. Diet.* **2019**, *119*, 464–481. [CrossRef] [PubMed]

38. Aguila, Q.; Ramon, M.A.; Matesanz, S.; Vilatimo, R.; Del Moral, I.; Brotons, C.; Ulied, A. Assessment study of the nutritional status, eating habits and physical activity of the schooled population of Centelles, Hostalets de Balenya and Sant Marti de Centelles (ALIN 2014 Study). *Endocrinol. Diabetes Nutr.* **2017**, *64*, 138–145. [CrossRef]

39. Guthold, R.; Stevens, G.A.; Riley, L.M.; Bull, F.C. Global trends in insufficient physical activity among adolescents: A pooled analysis of 298 population-based surveys with 1·6 million participants. *Lancet Child Adolesc. Health* **2020**, *4*, 23–35. [CrossRef]

40. Ortega Anta, R.M.; Lopez-Solaber, A.M.; Perez-Farinos, N. Associated factors of obesity in Spanish representative samples. *Nutr. Hosp.* **2013**, *28* (Suppl. 5), 56–62. [CrossRef]

41. Fernandez-Alvira, J.M.; De Bourdeaudhuij, I.; Singh, A.S.; Vik, F.N.; Manios, Y.; Kovacs, E.; Jan, N.; Brug, J.; Moreno, L.A. Clustering of energy balance-related behaviors and parental education in European children: The ENERGY-project. *Int. J. Behav. Nutr. Phys. Act.* **2013**, *10*, 5. [CrossRef]

42. Asarian, L.; Geary, N. Sex differences in the physiology of eating. *Am. J. Physiol. Regul. Integr. Comp. Physiol.* **2013**, *305*, R1215–R1267. [CrossRef] [PubMed]

43. De Cosmi, V.; Scaglioni, S.; Agostoni, C. Early Taste Experiences and Later Food Choices. *Nutrients* **2017**, *9*, 107. [CrossRef]

44. Huon, G.; Lim, J. The emergence of dieting among female adolescents: Age, body mass index, and seasonal effects. *Int. J. Eat. Disord.* **2000**, *28*, 221–225. [CrossRef]

45. Sichert-Hellert, W.; Beghin, L.; De Henauw, S.; Grammatikaki, E.; Hallstrom, L.; Manios, Y.; Mesana, M.I.; Molnar, D.; Dietrich, S.; Piccinelli, R.; et al. Nutritional knowledge in European adolescents: Results from the HELENA (Healthy Lifestyle in Europe by Nutrition in Adolescence) study. *Public Health Nutr.* **2011**, *14*, 2083–2091. [CrossRef]

46. Villamor, E.; Jansen, E.C. Nutritional Determinants of the Timing of Puberty. *Annu. Rev. Public Health* **2016**, *37*, 33–46. [CrossRef]

47. Bandini, L.G.; Schoeller, D.A.; Cyr, H.N.; Dietz, W.H. Validity of reported energy intake in obese and nonobese adolescents. *Am. J. Clin. Nutr.* **1990**, *52*, 421–425. [CrossRef]

48. Ventura, A.K.; Loken, E.; Mitchell, D.C.; Smiciklas-Wright, H.; Birch, L.L. Understanding reporting bias in the dietary recall data of 11-year-old girls. *Obesity* **2006**, *14*, 1073–1084. [CrossRef]

49. Coon, K.A.; Goldberg, J.; Rogers, B.L.; Tucker, K.L. Relationships between use of television during meals and children's food consumption patterns. *Pediatrics* **2001**, *107*, E7. [CrossRef] [PubMed]

50. Castells Cuixart, M.; Capdevila Prim, C.; Girbau Sola, T.; Rodriguez Caba, C. Study on feeding behavior in school children aged 11-13 years from Barcelona. *Nutr. Hosp.* **2006**, *21*, 517–532.

51. Varela-Moreiras, G.; Requejo, A.; Ortega, R.; Zamora, S.; Salas, J.; Cabrerizo, L.; Aranceta, J.; Ávila, J.; Murillo, J.; Belmonte, S.; et al. *Libro Blanco de la Nutrición en España*; Fundación Española de la Nutrición; Lesinguer: Madrid, Spain, 2013.

52. Taillie, L.S.; Afeiche, M.C.; Eldridge, A.L.; Popkin, B.M. The contribution of at-home and away-from-home food to dietary intake among 2-13-year-old Mexican children. *Public Health Nutr.* **2017**, *20*, 2559–2568. [CrossRef]

53. Marcano, M.; Solano, L.; Pontiles, M. Hyperlipidemia and hyperglycemia prevalence in obese children: Increased risk of cardiovascular disease? *Nutr. Hosp.* **2006**, *21*, 474–483.

54. Cruz, M.L.; Bergman, R.N.; Goran, M.I. Unique effect of visceral fat on insulin sensitivity in obese Hispanic children with a family history of type 2 diabetes. *Diabetes Care* **2002**, *25*, 1631–1636. [CrossRef]

55. Weiss, R.; Dufour, S.; Taksali, S.E.; Tamborlane, W.V.; Petersen, K.F.; Bonadonna, R.C.; Boselli, L.; Barbetta, G.; Allen, K.; Rife, F.; et al. Prediabetes in obese youth: A syndrome of impaired glucose tolerance, severe insulin resistance, and altered myocellular and abdominal fat partitioning. *Lancet* **2003**, *362*, 951–957. [CrossRef]

56. Stevens, J.; McClain, J.E.; Truesdale, K.P. Selection of measures in epidemiologic studies of the consequences of obesity. *Int. J. Obes.* **2008**, *32* (Suppl. 3), S60–S66. [CrossRef]

57. Revenga-Frauca, J.; González-Gil, E.M.; Bueno-Lozano, G.; de Miguel-Etayo, P.; Velasco-Martínez, P.; Rey-López, J.P.; Bueno-Lozano, O.; Moreno, L.A. Abdominal fat and metabolic risk in obese children and adolescents. *J. Physiol. Biochem.* **2009**, *65*, 415–420. [CrossRef]

58. Pérez-Gimeno, G.; Rupérez, A.I.; Vázquez-Cobela, R.; Herráiz-Gastesi, G.; Gil-Campos, M.; Aguilera, C.M.; Moreno, L.A.; Leis Trabazo, M.R.; Bueno-Lozano, G. Energy Dense Salty Food Consumption Frequency Is Associated with Diastolic Hypertension in Spanish Children. *Nutrients* **2020**, *12*, 1027. [CrossRef]

59. Da Costa, L.A.; Badawi, A.; El-Sohemy, A. Nutrigenetics and modulation of oxidative stress. *Ann. Nutr. Metab.* **2012**, *60* (Suppl. 3), 27–36. [CrossRef]

60. Rupérez, A.I.; Mesa, M.D.; Anguita-Ruiz, A.; González-Gil, E.M.; Vázquez-Cobela, R.; Moreno, L.A.; Gil, Á.; Gil-Campos, M.; Leis, R.; Bueno, G.; et al. Antioxidants and Oxidative Stress in Children: Influence of Puberty and Metabolically Unhealthy Status. *Antioxidants* **2020**, *9*, 618. [CrossRef]

61. González-Gil, E.M.; Tognon, G.; Lissner, L.; Intemann, T.; Pala, V.; Galli, C.; Wolters, M.; Siani, A.; Veidebaum, T.; Michels, N.; et al. Prospective associations between dietary patterns and high sensitivity C-reactive protein in European children: The IDEFICS study. *Eur. J. Nutr.* **2018**, *57*, 1397–1407. [CrossRef]

62. Antonopoulos, A.S.; Tousoulis, D. The molecular mechanisms of obesity paradox. *Cardiovasc. Res* **2017**, *113*, 1074–1086. [CrossRef]

63. Codoñer-Franch, P.; Valls-Bellés, V.; Arilla-Codoñer, A.; Alonso-Iglesias, E. Oxidant mechanisms in childhood obesity: The link between inflammation and oxidative stress. *Transl. Res.* **2011**, *158*, 369–384. [CrossRef]

64. Bulló, M.; Casas-Agustench, P.; Amigó-Correig, P.; Aranceta, J.; Salas-Salvadó, J. Inflammation, obesity and comorbidities: The role of diet. *Public Health Nutr.* **2007**, *10*, 1164–1172. [CrossRef]

65. Galland, L. Diet and inflammation. *Nutr. Clin. Pract.* **2010**, *25*, 634–640. [CrossRef]

66. Calder, P.C.; Ahluwalia, N.; Brouns, F.; Buetler, T.; Clement, K.; Cunningham, K.; Esposito, K.; Jönsson, L.S.; Kolb, H.; Lansink, M.; et al. Dietary factors and low-grade inflammation in relation to overweight and obesity. *Br. J. Nutr.* **2011**, *106* (Suppl. 3), S5–S78. [CrossRef]

2

Mothers' Vegetable Consumption Behaviors and Preferences as Factors Limiting the Possibility of Increasing Vegetable Consumption in Children in a National Sample of Polish and Romanian Respondents

Barbara Groele [1], Dominika Głąbska [1,*], Krystyna Gutkowska [2] and Dominika Guzek [2]

[1]   Department of Dietetics, Faculty of Human Nutrition and Consumer Sciences, Warsaw University of Life Sciences (SGGW-WULS), 159C Nowoursynowska Street, 02-787 Warsaw, Poland; barbara_groele@sggw.pl
[2]   Department of Organization and Consumption Economics, Faculty of Human Nutrition and Consumer Sciences, Warsaw University of Life Sciences (SGGW-WULS), 159C Nowoursynowska Street, 02-787 Warsaw, Poland; krystyna_gutkowska@sggw.pl (K.G.); dominika_guzek@sggw.pl (D.G.)
*   Correspondence: dominika_glabska@sggw.pl

2

Mothers' Vegetable Consumption Behaviors and Preferences as Factors Limiting the Possibility of Increasing Vegetable Consumption in Children in a National Sample of Polish and Romanian Respondents

Barbara Groele [1], Dominika Głąbska [1,*], Krystyna Gutkowska [2] and Dominika Guzek [2]

[1]   Department of Dietetics, Faculty of Human Nutrition and Consumer Sciences, Warsaw University of Life Sciences (SGGW-WULS), 159C Nowoursynowska Street, 02-787 Warsaw, Poland; barbara_groele@sggw.pl
[2]   Department of Organization and Consumption Economics, Faculty of Human Nutrition and Consumer Sciences, Warsaw University of Life Sciences (SGGW-WULS), 159C Nowoursynowska Street, 02-787 Warsaw, Poland; krystyna_gutkowska@sggw.pl (K.G.); dominika_guzek@sggw.pl (D.G.)
*   Correspondence: dominika_glabska@sggw.pl

Abstract: Increasing the insufficient intake of vegetables in children may be difficult, due to the influence of parents and at-home accessibility. The aim of this study was to analyze the association between self-reported vegetable consumption behaviors and preferences of mothers and the behaviors and preferences of their children, as declared by them. The nationally representative Polish ($n = 1200$) and Romanian ($n = 1157$) samples of mothers of children aged 3–10 were obtained using the random quota sampling method, and interviewed for their and their children's general frequency of consumption and preferences of vegetables in years 2012–2014. A 24 h dietary recall of vegetable consumption was conducted for mothers and their children. Associations were observed for general number of servings consumed per day by mother–child pairs ($p < 0.0001$; $R = 0.6522$, $R = 0.6573$ for Polish and Romanian samples, respectively) and number of types indicated as preferred ($p < 0.0001$; $R = 0.5418$, $R = 0.5433$). The share of children consuming specific vegetables was 33.1–75.3% and 42.6–75.7% while their mothers also consumed, but 0.1–43.2% and 1.2–22.9% while their mothers did not. The share of children preferring specific vegetables was 16.7–74.1% and 15.2–100% when their mother shared the preference, but 1.3–46.9% and 0–38.3% when their mother did not. The mothers' vegetable consumption behaviors and preferences may be a factor limiting the possibility of increasing vegetable consumption in their children.

Keywords: children; mothers; vegetable intake; consumption behaviors; choice; preferences

1. Introduction

The World Health Organization (WHO) advocates regular consumption of vegetables and fruits as an important element of a child's diet, not only in order to prevent non-communicable diet-related diseases, but also to create beneficial dietary patterns that are commonly predictive of their adolescence and adulthood patterns [1]. It is especially stated that vegetable intake patterns and preferences remain stable during childhood and adolescence [2].

Insufficient intake of vegetables and fruits is common worldwide, and the WHO has flagged it as being among the top ten determinants of global mortality [3]. At the same time, in the systematic review and meta-analysis of Touyz et al. [4], it was indicated that children more often meet the nutritional recommendations for fruits than for vegetables, so it is especially important to conduct interventions targeted at vegetables in order to increase their intake.

The '5-a-day' campaign has been carried out in a number of countries in order to increase the vegetable and fruit intake of children and adults, however, both the quantity and the variety consumed are still not adequate [5]. Also, the Cochrane systematic review by Hodder et al. [6] indicated that some interventions may increase the intake of vegetables and fruits by children. However, the observed evidence was stated to be low-quality and the observed increase was stated to be minor, so future research is required [6]. Based on the analysis of consumption trends in 33 countries, it has been observed that the intake of vegetables and fruits is increasing in many countries [7]. However, the trend is not stable, as the Health Survey for England indicated an important decrease in the frequency of meeting the '5-a-day' recommendation for children, from 20% to 17% between 2011 and 2013, even though an increase had been noted earlier [8].

Increasing the intake of vegetables in children may be hindered by a number of barriers associated with both internal and external factors [9,10] associated with sensory attributes, perception, preferences, knowledge, price, convenience, availability and accessibility, and parental, peer, and media influence. One of the most important barriers is low accessibility, which may result from seasonality [11], place of residence [12], and relatively high prices compared to other food products [13]. The other group of barriers results from preferences associated with the sensory attributes of vegetables [14], parental food consumption patterns [15], and food neophobia [16].

In general, a child is dependent on a diet that is prepared at home, being an element of the family environment and under general parental influence, until other influencing factors, such as peers and media, become more prominent [17]. As a result, the diets of children and parents are similar, as was observed in the systematic review and meta-analysis of Yee et al. [18], who concluded that a number of consumption behaviors of parents and their children were correlated.

For a number of the indicated barriers, the influence of parents and at-home accessibility may be crucial to reducing the children's intake of vegetables. Such reduction of intake may be observed in spite of the fact that, in general, parents know that intake of vegetables is important for their children and believe that it will influence their health and vitality [19]. It has already been observed that in order to increase the intake of fruits by children, it is necessary to influence the fruit consumption preferences and behaviors of their mothers [20], but this has not been analyzed for vegetables so far. Taking this into account, the aim of the present study was to analyze the association between self-reported vegetable consumption behaviors and preferences of mothers and the vegetable consumption behaviors and preferences of their children, as reported by them in national samples of Polish and Romanian respondents.

2. Materials and Methods

2.1. Ethical Statement

The study was conducted on a national sample of Polish and Romanian respondents according to the guidelines laid down in the Declaration of Helsinki, and all procedures involving human subjects were approved by the Ethics Committee of the Faculty of Human Nutrition and Consumer Sciences of the Warsaw University of Life Sciences. All participants provided informed consent.

2.2. Studied Sample

The study was conducted on Polish and Romanian subjects, who were recruited using the same procedure and inclusion/exclusion criteria as previously described [20]. The study itself was conducted in Poland and Romania according to the same methodology, with identical questions being asked in the respondent's native language. The data gathering was financed by the National Polish Promotion Fund for Fruits and Vegetables Consumption and Polish Association of Juices Producers within funds of the 5xVFJ (5 Portions of Vegetables, Fruit or Juice) national campaign, as an element of policy development in order to obtain the aim of increasing vegetables and fruits consumption in children.

One thousand and two hundred Polish and 1200 Romanian mothers of children aged 3–10 were planned to be recruited as respondents. The random quota sampling procedure was applied and informed consent was obtained from each respondent. Due to some missing data in the questionnaires obtained in the Romanian sample, 43 recruited respondents (3.6%), who were included in interviewing but did not complete it, were excluded. Finally, 1200 representative Polish respondents and 1157 Romanian respondents were included in years 2012–2014.

Recruitment was done in cooperation with a professional international agency that assesses public opinion and perception, and the agency was responsible for carrying out the random quota sampling. The planned quotas were determined for age, education, and residence (region and size of the city) in order to obtain representative Polish and Romanian samples of mothers of children aged 3–10.

The applied inclusion criteria were as follows: women, mother of child/children aged 3–10, inhabitant of Poland/Romania, aged 25–45. The applied exclusion criteria were as follows: lack of informed consent to participate, any missing data in the questionnaire.

2.3. Methods

The Computer-Assisted Telephone Interviewing (CATI) was done in cooperation with a professional international agency that assesses public opinion and perception, and the agency was hired as a partner responsible for data gathering, as in the previously described study [20]. Women aged 25–45 were randomly recruited while using the national database—they were invited to participate in the study during a telephone call and, if agreeing, they were verified for inclusion/exclusion criteria, as well as quota sampling being applied. The participation was compensated by a low value digital gift voucher code, according to commonly applied standards [21].

The assessment of vegetable consumption behaviors and preferences was conducted using questions that were asked about the mother's own behaviors and preferences (self-reported) and, in separate questions, about the behaviors and preferences of her child (as reported by the mother). A mother who declared she had more than one child aged 3–10 was asked to choose one of them arbitrarily and, afterwards, to inform about vegetable consumption behaviors and preferences of only this child during the whole interview.

In spite of the fact that while parents report the intake of their children, there may be important bias associated with proxy-reporting, there is also a bias associated with self-reporting by children, as it is indicated that they are able to self-report their intake from the age of 8 [22]. As a result, it would not be effective to assess the intake self-reported by children, as in the present study, the nutritional habits of children aged 3–10 were to be assessed. In general, for younger children mothers commonly report their intake [23]. In order to not apply various methodology (proxy-reporting for younger children and self-reporting for older ones), it was decided to assess the behaviors and preferences of children as reported by mothers in all cases, as for mothers.

In addition to the questions that were planned to be analyzed, respondents were also asked additional 'dummy questions'. They were associated with consumed vegetables, but not directly with behaviors and preferences of mothers and their children, as they were related to issues such as the place where vegetables are consumed, applied techniques of preparation of vegetables, known campaigns that promote vegetables consumption, and advantages and disadvantages of increased vegetable consumption. They were applied between main questions, in order to avoid interruptions of answers by the previous questions and answers. Respondents were also informed about the typical serving size (80 g, as defined by Food and Agriculture Organization of the United Nations (FAO) and WHO [24]) that was defined using a few examples of typical household measures for fresh and processed vegetables.

The vegetable consumption behaviors and preferences of mothers were assessed as follows:

- The general frequency of consumption of vegetables—based on the answer to the open-ended question about the number of servings of raw and processed vegetables consumed by them per day (self-reported);

- The previous day's frequency of consumption of vegetables—based on the 24 h dietary recall of the mothers' vegetable intake (self-reported);
- Preferred vegetables—based on the answer to the open-ended question to list the vegetables most preferred by them (self-reported);
- Consumed vegetables—based on the 24 h dietary recall of the mothers' vegetable intake (self-reported).

The vegetable consumption behaviors and preferences of children were assessed as follows:

- The general frequency of consumption of vegetables—based on the answer to the open-ended question about the number of servings of raw and processed vegetables consumed per day by their children (reported by the mothers);
- The previous day's frequency of consumption of vegetables—based on the 24 h dietary recall of the vegetable intake of the children (reported by the mothers);
- Preferred vegetables—based on the answer to the open-ended question to list the vegetables most preferred by their children (reported by the mothers);
- Consumed vegetables—based on the 24 h dietary recall of vegetable intake by children (reported by the mothers).

During the interview, the respondents were instructed to exclude potatoes and dry pulses from the declared number of servings of consumed vegetables. In the case of the 24 h dietary recall of vegetable intake and the list of most preferred vegetables, potatoes, dry pulses, and corn were excluded during analysis if they had been included.

2.4. Statistical Analysis

The normality of the distribution was verified using the Kolmogorov–Smirnov test and, afterwards, an analysis of correlation was carried out using Spearman's rank correlation coefficient due to the non-parametric distribution. The shares of the groups were compared using the chi^2 test and afterwards the obtained results were controlled for the false discovery results (FDR) using the Benjamini–Hochberg procedure.

$P \leq 0.05$ was considered significant. Statistical analysis was conducted using the following software packages: Statgraphics Plus for Windows 5.1 (Statgraphics Technologies Inc., The Plains, VA, USA), Statistica software version 8.0 (StatSoft Inc., Tulsa, OK, USA), and the Benjamini–Hochberg procedure spreadsheet by McDonalds [25].

3. Results

3.1. Analysis of the Association between the Quantity of Vegetables Consumed and Preferred by Mothers and Their Children

An analysis of the correlation between the daily frequency of vegetable consumption of the mothers and their children in nationally representative samples of Polish and Romanian mother–child pairs is presented in Table 1.

Table 1. Analysis of the correlation between the daily frequency of vegetables consumption of mothers and of their children in nationally representative samples of Polish ($n = 1200$) and Romanian ($n = 1157$) mother–child pairs.

Analyzed Correlation		p-Value [a]	R
Polish mother–child pairs ($n = 1200$)	general daily frequency	<0.0001	0.6522
	previous day frequency	<0.0001	0.4172
Romanian mother–child pairs ($n = 1157$)	general daily frequency	<0.0001	0.6573
	previous day frequency	<0.0001	0.3897

[a] Spearman's rank correlation coefficient.

The median for the open-ended question about general number of servings of vegetables consumed by mothers in both Polish and Romanian samples was two servings a day, and it ranged from not consuming at all to five servings a day. Similarly, for their children it was also two servings a day, and it ranged from not consuming at all (for the Polish sample) or consuming less than once a week (for the Romanian sample) to five servings a day. For both the Polish and Romanian samples, a significant correlation was observed between the number of servings consumed in general by the mothers and their children ($p < 0.0001$; $R = 0.6522$ for the Polish sample, $R = 0.6573$ for the Romanian sample).

In order to verify the association, the number of servings of vegetables consumed the previous day was analyzed, based on a 24 h dietary recall of vegetable consumption. The median for the number of servings of vegetables consumed the previous day for both mothers and their children in both Polish and Romanian samples was four servings a day, and it varied from not consuming at all to five servings a day. For both Polish and Romanian samples, a significant correlation was observed between the number of servings consumed the previous day by the mothers and their children ($p < 0.0001$; $R = 0.4172$ for the Polish sample, $R = 0.3897$ for the Romanian sample).

An analysis of the correlation between the number of types of vegetables indicated as consumed and preferred by mothers and their children in nationally representative samples of Polish and Romanian mother–child pairs is presented in Table 2.

Table 2. Analysis of the correlation between the number of types of vegetables indicated as consumed and preferred by mothers and by their children in nationally representative samples of Polish ($n = 1200$) and Romanian ($n = 1157$) mother–child pairs.

Analyzed Correlation		p-Value [a]	R
Polish mother–child pairs ($n = 1200$)	number of vegetables indicated as consumed	<0.0001	0.5418
	number of vegetables indicated as preferred	<0.0001	0.2872
Romanian mother–child pairs ($n = 1157$)	number of vegetables indicated as consumed	<0.0001	0.5433
	number of vegetables indicated as preferred	<0.0001	0.3878

[a] Spearman's rank correlation coefficient.

The median for the general number of types of vegetables indicated as consumed by the mothers in both Polish and Romanian samples was two, and it varied from a lack of types consumed to nine types. Similarly, for the children it was also two types, and it varied from a lack of types consumed to seven types (for the Polish sample) or nine types (for the Romanian sample). For both the Polish and Romanian samples, a significant correlation was observed between the number of types of vegetables indicated as consumed by mothers and their children ($p < 0.0001$; $R = 0.5418$ for the Polish sample, $R = 0.5433$ for the Romanian sample).

The median for the general number of types of vegetables indicated as preferred for both mothers and children in the Polish sample was three, and it ranged from a lack of types preferred to 19 types (for mothers) or 17 types (for children). The median for the general number of types of vegetables indicated as preferred for both mothers and children in the Romanian sample was two, and it ranged from a lack of types preferred to 17 types (for mothers) or 15 types (for children). For both the Polish and Romanian samples, a significant correlation was observed between the number of types of vegetables indicated as preferred by mothers and children ($p < 0.0001$; $R = 0.2772$ for the Polish sample, R = 0.3878 for the Romanian sample).

3.2. Analysis of the Association between the Variety of Vegetables Consumed and Preferred by Mothers and Their Children

An analysis of the association between the vegetable consumption behaviors self-reported by mothers and reported by them for their children in a nationally representative sample of Polish mother–child pairs is presented in Table 3. For all the vegetables that were declared by the mothers as consumed, there was a statistically significant association ($p < 0.0001$ for chi^2 test; $p < 0.0001$ after controlling for the FDR using a Benjamini–Hochberg procedure)—types consumed by the mothers were also consumed by their children, as compared to types not consumed by the mothers. For the specific types consumed by the mothers, the consumption by the children ranged from 33.1% (for peppers) to 75.3% (for carrots), while for types not consumed by the mothers, the consumption by the children ranged from 0.1% (for eggplant) to 43.2% (for tomatoes).

Table 3. Analysis of the association between the vegetable consumption behaviors self-reported by the mothers and reported by them for their children in a nationally representative sample of Polish mother–child pairs ($n = 1200$).

Vegetable [a]	Mothers Consuming the Specified Vegetable [b]		Mothers not Consuming the Specified Vegetable [b]		p-Value [c]
	Reporting their Children as also Consuming	Reporting their Children as not Consuming	Reporting their Children as Consuming	Reporting their Children as also not Consuming	
Carrot ($n = 592; n = 608$)	446 (75.3%)	146 (24.7%)	141 (23.2%)	467 (76.8%)	<0.0001
Tomato ($n = 393; n = 807$)	231 (58.8%)	162 (41.2%)	349 (43.2%)	458 (56.8%)	<0.0001
Cucumber ($n = 325; n = 875$)	196 (60.3%)	129 (39.7%)	330 (37.7%)	545 (62.3%)	<0.0001
Cabbage ($n = 167; n = 1033$)	90 (53.9%)	77 (46.1%)	64 (6.2%)	969 (93.8%)	<0.0001
Pepper ($n = 133; n = 1067$)	44 (33.1%)	89 (66.9%)	32 (3.0%)	1035 (97.0%)	<0.0001
Lettuce ($n = 120; n = 1080$)	48 (40.0%)	72 (60.0%)	48 (4.4%)	1032 (95.6%)	<0.0001
Celery ($n = 103; n = 1097$)	40 (38.8%)	63 (61.2%)	25 (2.3%)	1072 (97.7%)	<0.0001
Beetroot ($n = 103; n = 1097$)	73 (70.9%)	30 (29.1%)	52 (4.7%)	1045 (95.3%)	<0.0001
Onion ($n = 97; n = 1103$)	47 (48.5%)	50 (51.5%)	34 (3.1%)	1069 (96.9%)	<0.0001
Broccoli ($n = 88; n = 1112$)	38 (43.2%)	50 (56.8%)	16 (1.4%)	1096 (98.6%)	<0.0001
Cauliflower ($n = 66; n = 1134$)	34 (51.5%)	32 (48.5%)	32 (2.8%)	1102 (97.2%)	<0.0001
Chinese cabbage ($n = 45; n = 1155$)	20 (44.4%)	25 (55.6%)	15 (1.3%)	1140 (98.7%)	<0.0001
Green peas ($n = 38; n = 1162$)	18 (47.4%)	20 (52.6%)	19 (1.6%)	1143 (98.4%)	<0.0001
Beans ($n = 27; n = 1173$)	11 (40.7%)	16 (59.3%)	12 (1%)	1161 (99%)	<0.0001
Zucchini ($n = 23; n = 1177$)	13 (56.5%)	10 (43.5%)	2 (0.2%)	1175 (99.8%)	<0.0001
Eggplant ($n = 5; n = 1195$)	3 (60.0%)	2 (40.0%)	1 (0.1%)	1194 (99.9%)	<0.0001

[a] the number of mothers consuming the specific vegetable, followed by the number of mothers non-consuming the specific vegetable; [b] assessed based on the previous day's vegetable consumption behaviors; [c] chi^2 test.

An analysis of the association between the vegetable consumption behaviors self-reported by the mothers and reported by them for their children in a nationally representative sample of Romanian mother–child pairs is presented in Table 4. There was a statistically significant association ($p < 0.0001$ for chi^2 test; $p < 0.0001$ after controlling for the FDR using a Benjamini–Hochberg procedure) for all vegetables that were declared by the mothers as consumed—types consumed by the mothers were also consumed by their children, as compared to types not consumed by the mothers. For the types consumed by the mothers, the consumption by the children ranged from 42.6% (for eggplant) to 75.7% (for carrots), while for types not consumed by the mothers, the consumption by the children ranged from 1.2% (for broccoli) to 22.9% (for carrots).

Table 4. Analysis of the association between the vegetable consumption behaviors self-reported by the mothers and reported by them for their children, in a nationally representative sample of Romanian mother–child pairs ($n = 1157$).

Vegetable [a]	Mothers Consuming the Specified Vegetable [b]		Mothers not Consuming the Specified Vegetable [b]		p-Value [c]
	Reporting their Children as also Consuming	Reporting their Children as not Consuming	Reporting their Children as Consuming	Reporting their Children as also not Consuming	
Carrot ($n = 568$; $n = 589$)	430 (75.7%)	138 (24.3%)	135 (22.9%)	454 (77.1%)	<0.0001
Pepper ($n = 429$; $n = 728$)	254 (59.2%)	175 (40.8%)	102 (14.0%)	626 (86.0%)	<0.0001
Tomato ($n = 406$; $n = 751$)	243 (59.9%)	163 (40.1%)	93 (12.4%)	658 (87.6%)	<0.0001
Onion ($n = 324$; $n = 833$)	177 (54.6%)	147 (45.4%)	73 (8.8%)	760 (91.2%)	<0.0001
Cucumber ($n = 200$; $n = 957$)	116 (58.0%)	84 (42.0%)	81 (8.5%)	876 (91.5%)	<0.0001
Celery ($n = 191$; $n = 966$)	104 (54.5%)	87 (45.5%)	60 (6.2%)	906 (93.8%)	<0.0001
Cabbage ($n = 103$; $n = 1054$)	56 (54.4%)	47 (45.6%)	44 (4.2%)	1010 (95.8%)	<0.0001
Beans ($n = 91$; $n = 1066$)	44 (48.4%)	47 (51.6%)	26 (2.4%)	1040 (97.6%)	<0.0001
Green peas ($n = 63$; $n = 1094$)	42 (66.7%)	21 (33.3%)	27 (2.5%)	1067 (97.5%)	<0.0001
Eggplant ($n = 61$; $n = 1096$)	26 (42.6%)	35 (57.4%)	17 (1.6%)	1079 (98.4%)	<0.0001
Zucchini ($n = 49$; $n = 1108$)	23 (46.9%)	26 (53.1%)	27 (2.4%)	1081 (97.6%)	<0.0001
Lettuce ($n = 51$; $n = 1106$)	18 (35.3%)	33 (64.7%)	20 (1.8%)	1086 (98.2%)	<0.0001
Cauliflower ($n = 35$; $n = 1122$)	16 (45.7%)	19 (54.3%)	16 (1.4%)	1106 (98.6%)	<0.0001
Broccoli ($n = 27$; $n = 1130$)	17 (63.0%)	10 (37.0%)	13 (1.2%)	1117 (98.8%)	<0.0001
Beetroot ($n = 22$; $n = 1135$)	15 (68.2%)	7 (31.8%)	17 (1.5%)	1118 (98.5%)	<0.0001

[a] the number of mothers consuming the specific vegetable followed by the number of mothers non-consuming the specific vegetable; [b] assessed based on the previous day's vegetable consumption behaviors; [c] chi^2 test.

An analysis of the association between the vegetable preferences self-reported by the mothers and reported by them for their children in a nationally representative sample of Polish mother-child pairs is presented in Table 5. There was a statistically significant association ($p < 0.002$ for chi^2 test; $p < 0.002$ after controlling for the FDR using a Benjamini-Hochberg procedure) for all vegetables that were declared by the mothers as preferred—types preferred by the mothers were also preferred by their children, as compared to types not preferred by the mothers. For specific types preferred by the mothers, children's preferences varied from 16.7% (for eggplant) to 74.1% (for carrots), while for types not preferred by the mothers, children's preferences ranged from 1.3% (for eggplant) to 46.9% (for carrots).

Table 5. Analysis of the association between the vegetable preferences self-reported by the mothers and reported by them for their children in a national representative sample of Polish mother–child pairs ($n = 1200$).

Vegetable [a]	Mothers Indicating the Specified Vegetable as the Most Preferred		Mothers not Indicating the Specified Vegetable as the Most Preferred		p-Value [b]
	Reporting their Children as also Preferring	Reporting their Children as not Preferring	Reporting their Children as Preferring	Reporting their Children as also not Preferring	
Carrot ($n = 665$; $n = 535$)	493 (74.1%)	172 (25.9%)	251 (46.9%)	284 (53.1%)	<0.0001
Tomato ($n = 576$; $n = 624$)	342 (59.4%)	234 (40.6%)	222 (35.6%)	402 (64.4%)	<0.0001
Cucumber ($n = 433$; $n = 767$)	313 (72.3%)	120 (27.7%)	345 (45.0%)	422 (55.0%)	<0.0001
Broccoli ($n = 279$; $n = 921$)	97 (34.8%)	182 (65.2%)	112 (12.2%)	809 (87.8%)	<0.0001
Cauliflower ($n = 269$; $n = 931$)	123 (45.7%)	146 (54.3%)	192 (20.6%)	739 (79.4%)	<0.0001
Beetroot ($n = 205$; $n = 995$)	88 (42.9%)	117 (57.1%)	236 (23.7%)	759 (76.3%)	<0.0001
Cabbage ($n = 191$; $n = 1009$)	71 (37.2%)	120 (62.8%)	154 (15.3%)	855 (84.7%)	<0.0001
Lettuce ($n = 181$; $n = 1010$)	58 (32.0%)	123 (68%)	166 (16.3%)	853 (83.7%)	<0.0001
Pepper ($n = 153$; $n = 1047$)	56 (36.6%)	97 (63.4%)	143 (13.7%)	904 (86.3%)	<0.0001
Beans ($n = 92$; $n = 1108$)	41 (44.6%)	51 (55.4%)	133 (12.0%)	975 (88.0%)	<0.0001
Chinese cabbage ($n = 77$; $n = 1123$)	21 (27.3%)	56 (72.7%)	147 (13.1%)	976 (86.9%)	0.0010
Celery ($n = 77$; $n = 1123$)	15 (19.5%)	62 (80.5%)	48 (4.3%)	1075 (95.7%)	<0.0001
Onion ($n = 71$; $n = 1129$)	14 (19.7%)	57 (80.3%)	79 (7.0%)	1050 (93.0%)	0.0003
Zucchini ($n = 62$; $n = 1138$)	12 (19.4%)	50 (80.6%)	86 (7.6%)	1052 (92.4%)	0.0022
Green peas ($n = 48$; $n = 1152$)	21 (43.8%)	27 (56.3%)	146 (12.7%)	1006 (87.3%)	<0.0001
Eggplant ($n = 24$; $n = 1176$)	4 (16.7%)	20 (83.3%)	15 (1.3%)	1161 (98.7%)	<0.0001

[a] the number of mothers preferring the specific vegetable followed by the number of mothers non-preferring the specific vegetable; [b] chi^2 test.

An analysis of the association between vegetable preferences self-reported by the mothers and reported by them for their children in a nationally representative sample of Romanian mother–child pairs is presented in Table 6. There was a statistically significant association ($p < 0.0001$ for chi^2 test; $p < 0.0001$ after controlling for the FDR using a Benjamini–Hochberg procedure) for all vegetables that were declared by the mothers as preferred—types preferred by the mothers were also preferred by their children as compared to types not preferred by the mothers. For specific types preferred by the mothers, children's preferences varied from 15.2% (for cauliflower) to 100.0% (for Chinese cabbage), while for types not preferred by the mothers, children's preferences ranged from 0.0% (for Chinese cabbage) to 38.3% (for carrot).

Table 6. Analysis of the association between the vegetable preferences self-reported by the mothers and reported by them for their children in a nationally representative sample of Romanian mother–child pairs ($n = 1157$).

Vegetable [a]	Mothers Indicating the Specified Vegetable as the Most Preferred		Mothers not Indicating the Specified Vegetable as the Most Preferred		p-Value [b]
	Reporting their Children as also Preferring	Reporting their Children as not Preferring	Reporting their Children as Preferring	Reporting their Children as also not Preferring	
Tomato ($n = 571$; $n = 586$)	289 (50.6%)	282 (49.4%)	108 (18.4%)	478 (81.6%)	<0.0001
Carrot ($n = 447$; $n = 710$)	328 (73.4%)	119 (26.6%)	272 (38.3%)	438 (61.7%)	<0.0001
Pepper ($n = 378$; $n = 779$)	136 (36.0%)	242 (64.0%)	111 (14.2%)	668 (85.8%)	<0.0001
Cucumber ($n = 341$; $n = 816$)	191 (56.0%)	150 (44.0%)	184 (22.5%)	632 (77.5%)	<0.0001
Cabbage ($n = 157$; $n = 1000$)	60 (38.2%)	97 (61.8%)	81 (8.1%)	919 (91.9%)	<0.0001
Eggplant ($n = 140$; $n = 1017$)	32 (22.9%)	108 (77.1%)	34 (3.3%)	983 (96.7%)	<0.0001
Onion ($n = 130$; $n = 1027$)	30 (23.1%)	100 (76.9%)	43 (4.2%)	984 (95.8%)	<0.0001
Cauliflower ($n = 105$; $n = 1052$)	16 (15.2%)	89 (84.8%)	29 (2.8%)	1023 (97.2%)	<0.0001
Beans ($n = 91$; $n = 1066$)	24 (26.4%)	67 (73.6%)	32 (3%)	1034 (97%)	<0.0001
Lettuce ($n = 87$; $n = 1070$)	17 (19.5%)	70 (80.5%)	25 (2.3%)	1045 (97.7%)	<0.0001
Celery ($n = 87$; $n = 1070$)	14 (16.1%)	73 (83.9%)	14 (1.3%)	1056 (98.7%)	<0.0001
Green peas ($n = 69$; $n = 1088$)	24 (34.8%)	45 (65.2%)	33 (3%)	1055 (97%)	<0.0001
Zucchini ($n = 64$; $n = 1093$)	20 (31.3%)	44 (68.8%)	23 (2.1%)	1070 (97.9%)	<0.0001
Broccoli ($n = 63$; $n = 1094$)	20 (31.7%)	43 (68.3%)	14 (1.3%)	1080 (98.7%)	<0.0001
Beetroot ($n = 35$; $n = 1122$)	7 (20.0%)	28 (80.0%)	16 (1.4%)	1106 (98.6%)	<0.0001
Chinese cabbage ($n = 1$; $n = 1156$)	1 (100.0%)	0 (0.0%)	0 (0.0%)	1156 (100.0%)	<0.0001

[a] the number of mothers preferring the specific vegetable followed by the number of mothers non-preferring the specific vegetable; [b] chi^2 test.

4. Discussion

The strong associations between vegetable consumption preferences and behaviors of mothers and their children were observed both for Polish and Romanian samples. Moreover, they were observed both for assessed quantity and variety of vegetables consumed. This corresponds with the previously observed associations for fruit consumption preferences and behaviors [20], in spite of the fact that for children, fruit and vegetable preferences and exposure commonly differ [26]. As indicated by Korinek et al. [26], this is associated with children's preference for the sweet taste and pleasant texture of fruits, and because of this, parents offer them fruits rather than vegetables, resulting in not only a higher amount, but also in a wider variety of consumed fruits as compared to vegetables.

It is stated that repeated exposure may change the preferences, but this is more effective for fruits than vegetables [27]. Moreover, other stimuli are also more effective in increasing the intake of fruits than vegetables [28]. As a result, when comparing vegetables and fruits it may be said that, for children, fruits are not only more preferred over vegetables and a higher amount and variety is consumed, but they are also more frequently offered by parents and their intake is also easier to adopt. So, in order to assess the intake of vegetables, two domains must be analyzed—not only the consumption behaviors, but also consumption preferences, as they may be crucial for correcting nutritional behaviors.

Despite the fact that changing the preferences of vegetables may be more difficult than for fruits, it is still possible, as was proven in a number of intervention studies [29–32]. All the indicated above studies [29–32] allow us to conclude that, for children, it is possible to increase not only vegetable consumption but also preferences for the disliked ones when the exposure is applied at home. This is also confirmed by Cooke's [33] review, which showed that both laboratory studies and interventions conducted so far for assessing the efficacy of exposure confirmed that opportunities to taste unfamiliar food products results in increased consumption and preferences. However, no national-scale studies have been conducted so far, in Poland or Romania, to analyze the association between vegetable consumption behaviors and preferences of mothers and of their children. Such observations would give broader perspective, not only to make a conclusion based on small studies of various stimuli to increase vegetable intake, but also to observe associations in real conditions.

The results of our own study indicate a significant barrier for increasing vegetable exposure at home, as the vegetable consumption behaviors of mothers determine the consumption behaviors of their children. A similar association was observed for vegetable preferences. It may be concluded that, in spite of a number of studies having proven the possibility of increasing the consumption of vegetables, our own study indicates that if mother does not like a vegetable and does not consume it, the exposure of her child to this vegetable does not exist, and this, consequently, results in lack of preference in her child.

Johnson et al. [34] classified the determinants of the size of the serving consumed by a child into child-centered (including individual preferences and general consumption behaviors of the child as well as the previous meals) and mother-centered (including their opinions about the nutritional value of products and the need to avoid wastage of money and time). Such mother-centered determinants are associated not only with child's feeding and cooking for family members but also with her individual diet, and are observed by the child during the process of learning preferences at home [35]. However, for feeding a child there are additional factors, such as maternal feeding self-efficacy, that influence the kind and amount of products offered to the child and the child's final eating behaviors [36].

The association between eating behaviors of mothers and their children that was observed in the conducted study is confirmed by the results of another Polish study, as a similar strong association between eating behaviors of mothers and their adolescent daughters was observed [37], and it also contributed to similar excessive body mass risk [38] and similarities in other health-related consequences [39]. This may be important, as an excessive body mass of children was commonly observed in a recent study of Polish adolescents [40]. However, a mother may also transfer her dislikes to her child and create their preferences similar to her own [41]. This may be associated with the fact that children mimic their parents in a number of behaviors, including nutritional ones [42].

Parents commonly declare that food product preferences of their children are influenced by the marketing of food, and some of them state that they make choices of food products available at home based on those preferences [43]. However, the availability of unhealthy food products at home is associated with the children's choice of such products and the consumption of such products [44], and so if a child prefers unhealthy food products and the mother provides it, the child will consume it. At the same time, a number of parents believe that they provide such products to overcome the negative food product preferences of their children and promote a healthy diet [45]. But the question is, are they really are able to do it if their own preferences set in. A systematic review by Pearson et al. [46] indicated that vegetable and fruit consumption of children is associated not only with at home accessibility, family rules, and parental encouragement, but also with parental intake, and so parents may promote a healthy diet not by just providing it to their children but only if they also have such a diet.

The choice of food products and purchase decisions are influenced by a number of factors, including those related to health [47], nutritional knowledge [48], and the place where the product is purchased [49], but convenience and preferences may be the crucial ones [50]. This was confirmed by the results of a study by Horning et al. [51], where it was observed that the common reasons for choosing pre-packed processed meals instead of non-processed ones are preferences and time. So, even if parents declare that they want to promote healthy food decisions by their children through their own choices, other factors may interfere.

In general, when a child asks the parent for a specific vegetable or fruit, they tend to comply with this request [52]. But for children aged 2–5 years, it was observed that food product choices based on their desire may decrease their preference for healthy food products, including vegetables, as they would rather ask about products other than vegetables [53]. As a result, parents cannot wait for their child to ask for a specific product but should provide at home accessibility. Moreover, in order to provide effective exposure, parents should not only purchase vegetables but also include them in their own diet, in order to influence their child through the role-modeling mechanism, in addition to healthy products being provided in schools and childcare institutions.

In spite of the fact that the presented study was conducted in the nationally representative samples of Polish and Romanian respondents, some limitations must be indicated. The main limitations are associated with the proxy-reporting, due to the fact that the consumption preferences and behaviors of children were declared by their mothers. Moreover, there were the different participation rates in the Polish and Romanian samples, with some missing data in the Romanian sample. It must also be indicated that the mother was able to arbitrarily choose which of her children to discuss, with no randomization. Moreover, the 24 h dietary recall of vegetable consumption turned out to be a tool that over reported the intake, so results of general declared intake rather than the previous day's intake should be taken into account. All the indicated issues may result in some bias and must be taken into account in the further studies.

5. Conclusions

In Polish and Romanian representative samples of mother–child pairs, it was observed that vegetable consumption preferences and behaviors of mothers and their children were associated, both for the quantity and variety of consumed vegetables. A mother's lack of preference for specific vegetables may cause a lack of at-home accessibility (namely, lack of exposure for their children) and a resultant lack of preference of their children. In order to increase the vegetable intake in a child's diet, effective exposure should be provided, not only by purchasing the products and by at home accessibility (exposure), but also by including them in the diet of parents (role-modeling).

Author Contributions: B.G. and D.G. (Dominika Głąbska) made study conception and design; B.G. performed the research; B.G., D.G. (Dominika Głąbska) and D.G. (Dominika Guzek) analyzed the data; B.G., D.G. (Dominika Głąbska) and D.G. (Dominika Guzek) interpreted the data; B.G., D.G. (Dominika Głąbska), K.G. and D.G. (Dominika Guzek) wrote the paper. All authors read and approved the final manuscript.

Acknowledgments: Nothing to declare.

References

1. World Health Organization (WHO). *Increasing Fruit and Vegetable Consumption to Reduce the Risk of Noncommunicable Diseases*; WHO: Geneva, Switzerland, 2014.
2. Albani, V.; Butler, L.T.; Traill, W.B.; Kennedy, O.B. Fruit and vegetable intake: Change with age across childhood and adolescence. *Br. J. Nutr.* **2017**, *117*, 759–765. [CrossRef] [PubMed]
3. World Health Organization (WHO). *Fruit and Vegetable Promotion Initiative—A Meeting Report*; WHO: Geneva, Switzerland, 2003.

4. Touyz, L.M.; Wakefield, C.E.; Grech, A.M.; Quinn, V.F.; Costa, D.S.J.; Zhang, F.F.; Cohn, R.J.; Sajeev, M.; Cohen, J. Parent-targeted home-based interventions for increasing fruit and vegetable intake in children: A systematic review and meta-analysis. *Nutr. Rev.* **2018**, *76*, 154–173. [CrossRef] [PubMed]

5. Pem, D.; Jeewon, R. Fruit and Vegetable Intake: Benefits and Progress of Nutrition Education Interventions-Narrative Review Article. *Iran. J. Public Health* **2015**, *44*, 1309–1321. [PubMed]

6. Hodder, R.K.; O'Brien, K.M.; Stacey, F.G.; Wyse, R.J.; Clinton-McHarg, T.; Tzelepis, F.; James, E.L.; Bartlem, K.M.; Nathan, N.K.; Sutherland, R.; et al. Interventions for increasing fruit and vegetable consumption in children aged five years and under. *Cochrane Database Sys. Rev.* **2018**, *5*, sCD008552. [CrossRef]

7. Vereecken, C.; Pedersen, T.P.; Ojala, K.; Krølner, R.; Dzielska, A.; Ahluwalia, N.; Giacchi, M.; Kelly, C. Fruit and vegetable consumption trends among adolescents from 2002 to 2010 in 33 countries. *Eur. J. Public Health* **2015**, *25*, 16–19. [CrossRef] [PubMed]

8. Roberts, C. Chapter 7: Fruit and vegetable consumption. In *Health Survey for England 2013*, 1st ed.; Craig, R., Mindell, J., Eds.; NHS Digital: Leeds, UK, 2013. Available online: http://content.digital.nhs.uk/catalogue/PUB16076/HSE2013-Ch7-fru-veg-com.pdf (accessed on 1 March 2019).

9. Rasmussen, M.; Krølner, R.; Klepp, K.I.; Lytle, L.; Brug, J.; Bere, E.; Due, P. Determinants of fruit and vegetable consumption among children and adolescents: A review of the literature. Part I: Quantitative studies. *Int. J. Behav. Nutr. Phys. Act.* **2006**, *3*, 22. [CrossRef] [PubMed]

10. Krølner, R.; Rasmussen, M.; Brug, J.; Klepp, K.I.; Wind, M.; Due, P. Determinants of fruit and vegetable consumption among children and adolescents: A review of the literature. Part II: Qualitative studies. *Int. J. Behav. Nutr. Phys. Act.* **2011**, *8*, 112. [CrossRef]

11. Lautenschlager, L.; Smith, C. Beliefs, knowledge, and values held by inner-city youth about gardening, nutrition, and cooking. *Agric. Hum. Values* **2007**, *24*, 245–258. [CrossRef]

12. Thurber, K.A.; Banwell, C.; Neeman, T.; Dobbins, T.; Pescud, M.; Lovett, R.; Banks, E. Understanding barriers to fruit and vegetable intake in the Australian Longitudinal Study of Indigenous Children: A mixed-methods approach. *Public Health Nutr.* **2016**, *20*, 832–847. [CrossRef]

13. Ard, J.D.; Fitzpatrick, S.; Desmond, R.A.; Sutton, B.S.; Pisu, M.; Allison, D.B.; Franklin, F.; Baskin, M.L. The impact of cost on the availability of fruits and vegetables in the homes of schoolchildren in Birmingham, Alabama. *Am. J. Public Health* **2007**, *97*, 367–372. [CrossRef]

14. Zeinstra, G.G.; Koelen, M.A.; Kok, F.J.; de Graaf, C. Cognitive development and children's perceptions of fruit and vegetables; a qualitative study. *Int. J. Behav. Nutr. Phys. Act.* **2007**, *4*, 30. [CrossRef]

15. Draxten, M.; Fulkerson, J.A.; Friend, S.; Flattum, C.F.; Schow, R. Parental role modeling of fruits and vegetables at meals and snacks is associated with children's adequate consumption. *Appetite* **2014**, *78*, 1–7. [CrossRef]

16. Guzek, D.; Głąbska, D.; Lange, E.; Jezewska-Zychowicz, M. A Polish Study on the Influence of Food Neophobia in Children (10–12 Years Old) on the Intake of Vegetables and Fruits. *Nutrients* **2017**, *9*, 563. [CrossRef]

17. Scaglioni, S.; De Cosmi, V.; Ciappolino, V.; Parazzini, F.; Brambilla, P.; Agostoni, C. Factors Influencing Children's Eating Behaviours. *Nutrients* **2018**, *10*, 706. [CrossRef]

18. Yee, A.Z.; Lwin, M.O.; Ho, S.S. The influence of parental practices on child promotive and preventive food consumption behaviors: A systematic review and meta-analysis. *Int. J. Behav. Nutr. Phys. Act.* **2017**, *14*, 47. [CrossRef]

19. Hingle, M.; Beltran, A.; O'Connor, T.; Thompson, D.; Baranowski, J.; Baranowski, T. A model of goal directed vegetable parenting practices. *Appetite* **2011**, *58*, 444–449. [CrossRef]

20. Groele, B.; Głąbska, D.; Gutkowska, K.; Guzek, D. Mother's Fruit Preferences and Consumption Support Similar Attitudes and Behaviors in Their Children. *Int. J. Environ. Res. Public Health* **2018**, *15*, 2833. [CrossRef]

21. Cheff, R.; Roche, B. *Considerations for Compensating Research Participants Fairly & Equitably*; Wellesley Institute: Toronto, ON, Canada, 2018; pp. 1–11.

22. Livingstone, M.B.; Robson, P.J. Measurement of dietary intake in children. *Proc. Nutr. Soc.* **2000**, *59*, 279–293. [CrossRef]

23. Oliveria, S.A.; Ellison, R.C.; Moore, L.L.; Gillman, M.W.; Garrahie, E.J.; Singer, M.R. Parent-child relationships in nutrient intake: The Framingham Children's Study. *Am. J. Clin. Nutr.* **1992**, *56*, 593–598. [CrossRef]

24. World Health Organization (WHO). *Diet, Nutrition and the Prevention of Chronic Diseases*; Report of a Joint FAO/WHO Expert Consultation; Technical Report Series, No. 916; WHO: Geneva, Switzerland, 2003.

25. McDonald, J.H. *Handbook of Biological Statistics*, 3rd ed.; Sparky House Publishing: Baltimore, MD, USA, 2014; pp. 254–260.

26. Korinek, E.V.; Bartholomew, J.B.; Jowers, E.M.; Latimer, L.A. Fruit and vegetable exposure in children is linked to the selection of a wider variety of healthy foods at school. *Mater. Child. Nutr.* **2013**, *11*, 999–1010. [CrossRef]

27. Chung, L.M.Y.; Fong, S.S.M. Appearance alteration of fruits and vegetables to increase their appeal to and consumption by school-age children: A pilot study. *Health Psychol. Open* **2018**, *5*. [CrossRef]

28. Guzek, D.; Głąbska, D.; Mellová, B.; Zadka, K.; Żywczyk, K.; Gutkowska, K. Influence of Food Neophobia Level on Fruit and Vegetable Intake and Its Association with Urban Area of Residence and Physical Activity in a Nationwide Case-Control Study of Polish Adolescents. *Nutrients* **2018**, *10*, 897. [CrossRef]

29. Fildes, A.; van Jaarsveld, C.H.; Wardle, J.; Cooke, L. Parent-administered exposure to increase children's vegetable acceptance: A randomized controlled trial. *J. Acad. Nutr. Diet.* **2014**, *114*, 881–888. [CrossRef]

30. Remington, A.; Añez, E.; Croker, H.; Wardle, J.; Cooke, L. Increasing food acceptance in the home setting: A randomized controlled trial of parent-administered taste exposure with incentives. *Am. J. Clin. Nutr.* **2012**, *95*, 72–77. [CrossRef]

31. Holley, C.E.; Haycraft, E.; Farrow, C. 'Why don't you try it again?' A comparison of parent led, home based interventions aimed at increasing children's consumption of a disliked vegetable. *Appetite* **2015**, *87*, 215–222. [CrossRef] [PubMed]

32. Corsini, N.; Slater, A.; Harrison, A.; Cooke, L.; Cox, D.N. Rewards can be used effectively with repeated exposure to increase liking of vegetables in 4–6-year-old children. *Public Health Nutr.* **2013**, *16*, 942–951. [CrossRef]

33. Cooke, L. The importance of exposure for healthy eating in childhood: A review. *J. Hum. Nutr. Diet.* **2007**, *20*, 294–301. [CrossRef]

34. Johnson, S.L.; Goodell, L.S.; Williams, K.; Power, T.G.; Hughes, S.O. Getting my child to eat the right amount. Mothers' considerations when deciding how much food to offer their child at a meal. *Appetite* **2015**, *88*, 24–32. [CrossRef] [PubMed]

35. Savage, J.S.; Fisher, J.O.; Birch, L.L. Parental influence on eating behavior: Conception to adolescence. *J. Law Med. Ethics* **2007**, *35*, 22–34. [CrossRef]

36. Koh, G.A.; Scott, J.A.; Woodman, R.J.; Kim, S.W.; Daniels, L.A.; Magarey, A.M. Maternal feeding self-efficacy and fruit and vegetable intakes in infants. Results from the SAIDI study. *Appetite* **2014**, *81*, 44–51. [CrossRef] [PubMed]

37. Wadolowska, L.; Slowinska, M.A.; Pabjan-Adach, K.; Przybylowicz, K.; Niedzwiedzka, E. The Comparison of Food Eating Models of Mothers and Their Daughters. *Pak. J. Nutr.* **2007**, *6*, 381–386. [CrossRef]

38. Wadolowska, L.; Ulewicz, N.; Sobas, K.; Wuenstel, J.W.; Slowinska, M.A.; Niedzwiedzka, E.; Czlapka-Matyasik, M. Dairy-Related Dietary Patterns, Dietary Calcium, Body Weight and Composition: A Study of Obesity in Polish Mothers and Daughters, the MODAF Project. *Nutrients* **2018**, *10*, 90. [CrossRef]

39. Sobas, K.; Wadolowska, L.; Slowinska, M.A.; Czlapka-Matyasik, M.; Wuenstel, J.; Niedzwiedzka, E. Like Mother, Like Daughter? Dietary and Non-Dietary Bone Fracture Risk Factors in Mothers and Their Daughters. *Iran. J. Public Health* **2015**, *44*, 939–952. [PubMed]

40. Głąbska, D.; Guzek, D.; Mellová, B.; Zadka, K.; Żywczyk, K.; Gutkowska, K. The National After-School Athletics Program Participation as a Tool to Reduce the Risk of Obesity in Adolescents after One Year of Intervention: A Nationwide Study. *Int. J. Environ. Res. Public Health* **2019**, *16*, 405. [CrossRef] [PubMed]

41. Osera, T.; Tsutie, S.; Kobayashi, M.; Kurihara, N. Relationship of Mothers' Food Preferences and Attitudes with Children's Preferences. *Food Nutr. Sci.* **2012**, *3*, 1–6. [CrossRef]

42. Sutherland, L.A.; Beavers, D.P.; Kupper, L.L.; Bernhardt, A.M.; Heatherton, T.; Dalton, M.A. Like parent, like child: Child food and beverage choices during role playing. *Arch. Pediatr. Adolesc. Med.* **2008**, *162*, 1063–1069. [CrossRef]

43. Campbell, K.J.; Crawford, D.A.; Hesketh, K.D. Australian parents' views on their 5–6-year-old children's food choices. *Health Promot. Int.* **2007**, *22*, 11–18. [CrossRef]

44. Campbell, K.J.; Crawford, D.A.; Salmon, J.; Carver, A.; Garnett, S.P.; Baur, L.A. Associations between the home food environment and obesity-promoting eating behaviors in adolescence. *Obesity* **2007**, *15*, 719–730. [CrossRef]

45. Nepper, M.J.; Chai, W. Parents' barriers and strategies to promote healthy eating among school-age children. *Appetite* **2016**, *103*, 157–164. [CrossRef]

46. Pearson, N.; Biddle, S.J.; Gorely, T. Family correlates of fruit and vegetable consumption in children and adolescents: A systematic review. *Public Health Nutr.* **2009**, *12*, 267–283. [CrossRef]

47. Zysk, W.; Głąbska, D.; Guzek, D. Role of Front-of-Package Gluten-Free Product Labeling in a Pair-Matched Study in Women with and without Celiac Disease on a Gluten-Free Diet. *Nutrients* **2019**, *11*, 398. [CrossRef]

48. Gutkowska, K.; Czarnecki, J.; Głąbska, D.; Guzek, D.; Batóg, A. Consumer perception of health properties and of other attributes of beef as determinants of consumption and purchase decisions. *Rocz. Panstw. Zakl. Hig.* **2018**, *69*, 413–419. [CrossRef]

49. Olewnik-Mikołajewska, A.; Guzek, D.; Głąbska, D.; Gutkowska, K. Consumer behaviors towards novel functional and convenient meat products in Poland. *J. Sens. Stud.* **2016**, *31*, 193–205. [CrossRef]

50. Castro, I.A.; Majmundar, A.; Williams, C.B.; Baquero, B. Customer Purchase Intentions and Choice in Food Retail Environments: A Scoping Review. *Int. J. Environ. Res. Public Health* **2018**, *15*, 2493. [CrossRef]

51. Horning, M.L.; Fulkerson, J.A.; Friend, S.E.; Story, M. Reasons Parents Buy Prepackaged, Processed Meals: It Is More Complicated Than "I Don't Have Time". *J. Nutr. Educ. Behav.* **2016**, *49*, 60–66. [CrossRef]

52. Beltran, A.; O'Connor, T.M.; Hughes, S.O.; Thompson, D.; Baranowski, J.; Nicklas, T.A.; Baranowski, T. Parents' Qualitative Perspectives on Child Asking for Fruit and Vegetables. *Nutrients* **2017**, *9*, 575. [CrossRef]

53. Russell, C.G.; Worsley, A.; Liem, D.G. Parents' food choice motives and their associations with children's food preferences. *Public Health Nutr.* **2015**, *18*, 1018–1027. [CrossRef] [PubMed]

3

Dietary Patterns among Vietnamese and Hispanic Immigrant Elementary School Children Participating in an After School Program

Megan A. McCrory [1,*], **Charles L. Jaret** [2], **Jung Ha Kim** [2] and **Donald C. Reitzes** [2]

1   Department of Health Sciences, Programs in Nutrition, Sargent College of Health
    and Rehabilitation Sciences, Boston University, Boston, MA 02215, USA
2   Department of Sociology, College of Arts and Sciences, Georgia State University, Atlanta, GA 30302, USA;
    cjaret@gsu.edu (C.L.J.); jhkim@gsu.edu (J.H.K.); dreitzes@gsu.edu (D.C.R.)
*   Correspondence: mamccr@bu.edu

Abstract: Immigrants in the U.S. may encounter challenges of acculturation, including dietary habits, as they adapt to new surroundings. We examined Vietnamese and Hispanic immigrant children's American food consumption patterns in a convenience sample of 63 Vietnamese and Hispanic children in grades four to six who were attending an after school program. Children indicated the number of times they consumed each of 54 different American foods in the past week using a food frequency questionnaire. We ranked each food according to frequency of consumption, compared the intake of foods to the USDA Healthy Eating Pattern, and performed dietary pattern analysis. Since the data were not normally distributed we used two nonparametric tests to evaluate statistical significance: the Kruskal–Wallis tested for significant gender and ethnicity differences and the Wilcoxon signed-rank test evaluated the food consumption of children compared with the USDA recommended amounts. We found that among USDA categories, discretionary food was most commonly consumed, followed by fruit. The sample as a whole ate significantly less than the recommended amount of grains, protein foods, and dairy, but met the recommended amount of fruit. Boys ate significantly more grains, proteins, and fruits than did girls. Dietary pattern analysis showed a very high sweet snack consumption among all children, while boys ate more fast food and fruit than girls. Foods most commonly consumed were cereal, apples, oranges, and yogurt. Ethnicity differences in food selection were not significant. The high intake of discretionary/snack foods and fruit, with low intake of grains, vegetables, protein, and dairy in our sample suggests Vietnamese and Hispanic immigrant children may benefit from programs to improve diet quality.

Keywords: food preferences; food habits; diet/standards; gender factors; acculturation

1. Introduction

Immigrants in the U.S. may encounter challenges of acculturation, including dietary habits, as they adapt to new surroundings in the host country [1]. Studies show a health paradox in that early in their arrival, immigrants may be healthier than their U.S. counterparts, but later go on to develop health risks as they adapt to a more Western lifestyle [2]. In general, a higher level of acculturation is associated with greater risk for chronic diseases [3,4]. The impact of acculturation may in part be responsible for the large disparities in rates of obesity and chronic disease among U.S. minority immigrants [5]. In the U.S., African Americans and Hispanics are at higher risk for obesity, diabetes [6], and heart disease [7] than Caucasians. Few studies have been conducted among Asian Americans. A recent U.S. national survey showed that although non-Hispanic Asians generally are not as unhealthy as other U.S. adults, there was great diversity in the health of different Asian American groups [8].

In particular, 16.8% of Vietnamese adults were considered to be in fair or poor health, compared to 8.1–12.2% for other Asian American groups and 12.4% for all U.S. adults [8].

Dietary choices during childhood are important for health during childhood and later life [9,10]. Therefore, the dietary intake of immigrant children is important for their health as adults. Relatively few studies have been conducted on the dietary intake of immigrant children. As reviewed recently [11], Asian American youth as a whole have high intakes of fruits, vegetables, and white rice, as well as high fat and high sugar foods, and as a result of acculturation their diets consist of both traditional Asian foods and American foods. "Asian Americans" include many different Asian cultures, each having different diets, but relatively few studies have been done on specific Asian subgroups so it is difficult to make firm conclusions about each. In one study of Vietnamese, Hispanic, African American and Caucasian adolescents residing in Worcester, Massachusetts, Vietnamese youth had higher fruit and vegetable intake and lower dairy intake compared to Caucasians, while Hispanic youth had a lower intake of fruits and vegetables, but dairy did not differ from that of Caucasians [12]. In another study of California youth, Mexican and other Hispanic children did not differ substantially in dietary practices, whereas among seven Asian American subgroups, Filipino, Korean, Vietnamese, and Japanese children were more likely to consume fast food than Chinese children [13]. Yet, Vietnamese, Koreans, and Filipinos were also likely to consume more vegetables than the Chinese. In the same study, there was no significant gender difference in consumption among Hispanic youth, but among Asian Americans, girls had significantly lower vegetable intake, and non-significantly lower fruits, fruit juice, and fast food intake. In a study of Korean Americans, there was a shift away from Korean foods to more American foods, but the quality of diet did not vary by acculturation status [14]. However, a study of South Asian immigrants in Canada showed a mix of positive and negative outcomes: the more acculturated ate more fruits and vegetables and less deep fried food, but also more convenience food, red meat, and high-sugar foods [15].

The purposes of this study were to examine the quality of food selection in a convenience sample of school-aged immigrant Vietnamese and Hispanic girls and boys based on their answers on a simple food intake questionnaire, and to test for differences by gender and ethnicity. We defined the quality of food selection in two ways: (1) consistency with the USDA Healthy Eating Pattern [16]; and (2) dietary pattern analysis to determine which foods listed on the questionnaire were eaten in similar patterns (e.g., if children who ate a lot of chocolate candy also frequently ate cookies and cake; or if those who rarely ate apples also did not eat other fruits).

2. Materials and Methods

2.1. Study Design

The data used in this study were from a survey, "My Food Choices," conducted by the Asian American Community Research Institute of the Center for Pan Asian Community Services, Inc. (CPACS) in Atlanta, GA, USA. We obtained the data with permission from CPACS. CPACS is the oldest and largest grassroots community organization in the Southeast serving Asian immigrant and refugee families and their descendants [17]. A considerable number of Hispanic children also participate in its after-school programs. As of December 2015, over 40 percent of all children and youth programs participants at CPACS were Hispanic [18,19].

2.2. Participants and Recruitment

The survey was conducted at three of CPACS's after-school program sites in January and February of 2012. CPACS's purpose in conducting the survey was to determine the types of foods and beverages readily available and consumed by the children attending its after-school programs. The children participating in these programs were either Vietnamese or Hispanics living in a low-income immigrant community. All children who participated in the survey were fourth, fifth, and sixth graders, eligible for free lunch at school and had at least one immigrant or refugee parent/guardian.

Because the survey targeted young children, CPACS sent a bi-lingual letter to each child's parents to obtain informed consent for their child's participation in the survey. Data were collected from only the children with parental approval to participate in the survey. A total of 63 children (approximately 90% of those who were eligible) completed the survey. On-site teachers or tutors recorded site information and assigned a unique identification number to all collected surveys. The present research team obtained the questionnaires in Fall 2015. Because the questionnaires were de-identified, the Institutional Review Board at Georgia State University determined the project was not human subjects research as per U.S. Dept. of Health and Human Services.

2.3. Instruments

The "My Food Choices" questionnaire was designed by CPACS staff. The questionnaire consisted of 54 questions, each asking about the frequency of consumption of a type or class of food, e.g., "carrots," "fried chicken or nuggets," or "yogurt." The foods and beverages included on the questionnaire were typical American foods that may be consumed by children at home, school, or restaurants, and represented examples from all food groups (fruits, vegetables, dairy, meat and beans, cereals, sweets). Many of the foods on the questionnaire were often served to the children at CPACS, or in their school cafeteria. A sample question is shown in Appendix A (Figure A1). Next to the name of each food type was a small photo of a serving of the food or a package containing it. For each food type the questionnaire asked: "In the last week, how many times did you eat/drink?". The possible responses were: zero, one, two, three, four, five, six, and seven or more times. The children read and completed the questionnaire without assistance from CPACS staff or parents. Children took approximately 15–20 min to complete the questionnaire.

2.4. Data Analysis

The data were analyzed using SPSS, version 20 (IBM, Armonk, NY, USA). Prior to analysis, a number of steps were taken. First, missing data were filled in when possible using multiple regression analysis and discriminant analysis as described below. Variables were also examined for normality. None of the variables were normally distributed (based on the Shapiro-Wilk statistic and on skewness and kurtosis), therefore the data are described by reporting the median and interquartile range (Q1, Q3), and further analyses were carried out using nonparametric procedures. In addition, while the original 54-item questionnaire had water as one of the food items, this item was excluded from analysis (except to describe consumption frequency) because water, although a required nutrient, does not fit into one of the U.S. Department of Agriculture's (USDA) food groups [16].

We used the nonparametric Wilcoxon signed-rank test to determine whether there was a statistically significant difference between their actual food consumption and the USDA recommended amounts. Although we were interested in testing for differences by gender within each ethnicity, the small number of Vietnamese ($n = 15$) compared to Hispanic ($n = 48$) children in our sample made it statistically impractical to examine a gender by ethnicity interaction effect. Therefore, our main focus was to test for gender and ethnicity differences. The nonparametric Kruskal–Wallis test was performed to test for differences in food intake between boys and girls. In supplemental analyses, we tested the independent associations of gender and ethnicity with food intake by using ANOVA with gender as a fixed factor and ethnicity as a covariate, modeling only the main effects and not the interaction effects. The results of these analyses were not qualitatively different from those generated by the nonparametric tests. For all analyses, statistical significance was set at $\alpha = 0.05$.

2.4.1. Response Rate and Procedures for Filling in Missing Data

Overall, children's response rate on questionnaire was very good, with only 50 of the 3402 potential responses (1.5%) to the food items left unanswered. Where possible, we obtained an estimated value to replace a missing value by utilizing a multiple regression equation to predict how frequently a child ate that food item. A multiple regression model for a food item on which there was missing data was created by using other food items to predict the frequency of consumption of the food item in question. If the best multiple regression model could predict actual consumption of that food item with a high degree of accuracy (i.e., R^2 of 0.60 or higher and low standard error), then it was used to predict the child's food consumption for that item. If the multiple regression equation was of lessor quality or if the child had more than five missing values on food consumption items, then no estimate was made and a "missing value" code in the data analysis of that food item was retained.

In three cases, data on the child's gender was missing and in one case the child's ethnicity was missing. In these cases, discriminant analysis proved highly accurate in distinguishing boys from girls and Vietnamese from Hispanics. Specifically, by identifying a small subset of food items on which consumption levels of boys (or Hispanics) were very different than girls (or Vietnamese), discriminant analysis was able to correctly classify 86.2% of known boys (25 out of 29) boys and 89.7% of known girls (26 out of 29). This discriminant analysis classified two children with missing data on gender as female, while the third case retained a missing value code because it had too much missing data on food consumption items used in the discriminant analysis. Discriminant analysis also correctly classified 83.3% of known Vietnamese children (10 out of 12) and 87.2% of known Hispanic (41 out of 47), and that analysis led to a classification of "Hispanic" for the one case with missing data on ethnicity. Thus, the demographic composition of this sample was: 26 Hispanic boys, 22 Hispanic girls, 5 Vietnamese boys, and 9 Vietnamese girls (one Vietnamese child had missing data for his/her gender).

2.4.2. Determination of Adherence to the USDA Dietary Guidelines for Americans

We categorized each of the food items according to USDA food groups (Table 1). Note that the categorization was not mutually exclusive, i.e., a food could appear in one or more of the groups (e.g., macaroni and cheese was assigned to both the grains and the dairy categories). This is because many foods contain components that belong to different food groups, as described by the USDA [20]. We then compared the actual number of servings per week of vegetables, fruits, grains, dairy, and proteins food groups, as well as oils and discretionary foods consumed by the children with the USDA recommended number of servings for 10-year-old children (which we estimated to be the average age of the children in our sample) based on the USDA Healthy Eating Pattern [16]. To perform this analysis, we assumed that the portion of each food consumed was equivalent to one serving. We calculated the recommended number of servings per week in each food group by multiplying the daily number of recommended servings by seven days per week.

Table 1. Classification of food frequency questionnaire items into USDA food groups.

Food Group	Food Items
Fruits	fruit juice, bananas, apples, grapes, pears, oranges, raisins, mixed fruit, peaches
Vegetables	green beans, other beans, carrots, greens, broccoli, sweet potatoes, French fries or tater tots, other potatoes, corn, tossed salad, yellow squash, tomatoes, vegetable soup
Grains	cereal, honey buns, pretzels, spaghetti, macaroni and cheese, fried rice, other rice, rice and gravy, hamburger, pizza, cookies, snack cake, cake
Protein Foods	peanut butter, hot chicken wings, chicken not fried, fried chicken or chicken nuggets, fish sticks, hamburger, cheese-burger, pizza
Dairy	low fat milk, whole milk, yogurt, cheese, macaroni and cheese, cheeseburger, pizza, ice cream
Oils	chips, hot chicken wings, fried chicken or chicken nuggets, fish sticks, fried rice, French fries or tater tots, salad, mayonnaise
Discretionary	fruit-flavored drinks, soda, cereal, honey buns, chips, yogurt, rice and gravy, mayonnaise, ice cream, cookies, snack cake, chocolate candy, cake, jam, jelly or syrup

2.4.3. Factor Analysis to Determine Dietary Patterns

We performed factor analysis on the 53 food items (excluding water) with quartimax rotation. We used quartimax rather than varimax rotation because we were more interested in learning which foods load most strongly on a factor (quartimax rotation) than minimizing the number of foods associated with each factor (varimax rotation). Thirteen factors with eigenvalues over 1.00 were produced (accounting for 80.1% of the variance), but the most substantively interesting were the first five factors (which account for 58.1% of total variance). These five factors are shown in Table 2. Factor loadings for food items used to compute each factor score are shown in bold.

Table 2. Dietary patterns based on factor analysis of Vietnamese and Latino children's food selections ($n = 63$).

	Veggies Plus	Sweet Snacks	Fruit	Fast Food	Other Veggies
fish sticks	**0.797**	0.162	0.050	0.094	−0.072
broccoli	**0.784**	0.112	0.124	0.062	0.228
carrots	**0.770**	0.081	0.309	0.138	−0.002
other beans	**0.747**	0.044	0.145	0.077	−0.027
green beans	**0.709**	0.136	−0.069	0.046	0.158
sweet potatoes	**0.681**	0.212	−0.091	0.181	0.321
rice & gravy	**0.657**	0.249	−0.143	0.198	−0.039
pretzels	**0.653**	0.087	0.437	0.135	0.107
spaghetti	**0.599**	0.335	0.147	0.171	0.117
snack cakes	0.169	**0.824**	0.102	0.199	−0.032
cookies	0.292	**0.789**	0.220	0.087	−0.113
mayonnaise	0.163	**0.781**	0.034	0.056	0.067
chocolate candy	0.102	**0.768**	0.117	0.280	0.003
ice cream	0.184	**0.734**	0.120	0.373	−0.145
cake	0.178	**0.653**	0.139	0.091	0.364
jam, jelly, syrup	−0.022	**0.647**	0.141	−0.108	0.325
chips	−0.050	**0.625**	0.270	0.199	0.034
popcorn	0.210	**0.584**	0.115	0.169	0.060
fruit-flavored drink	−0.103	**0.570**	0.034	0.231	−0.129
oranges	0.016	0.221	**0.816**	0.107	0.030
apples	0.156	0.363	**0.728**	0.075	0.001
bananas	0.217	0.419	**0.726**	0.070	0.063
fruit juice	0.236	0.004	**0.622**	−0.133	−0.202
grapes	0.360	0.340	**0.589**	−0.054	−0.052
peaches	0.522	−0.062	**0.575**	0.283	−0.055
hamburgers	0.216	0.303	0.142	**0.816**	0.064
pizza	0.253	0.371	0.049	**0.782**	−0.013
hot wings	0.284	0.296	−0.005	**0.701**	−0.112
french fries/tater tots	0.216	0.165	−0.013	**0.680**	−0.036
fried chicken/nuggets	0.196	0.355	0.125	**0.641**	0.114
yellow squash	0.374	0.226	0.036	0.002	**0.761**
tomatoes	0.341	0.020	−0.003	0.008	**0.711**
tossed salad	0.208	−0.010	−0.104	−0.004	**0.618**
greens	0.502	−0.081	−0.001	−0.081	**0.350**
Eigenvalue	15.86	5.60	3.82	3.09	2.40
%Variance	29.93	10.57	7.21	5.83	4.53

The factor loadings used to compute each factor score are shown in boldface type.

3. Results

On the first factor ("Veggies Plus"), foods with the highest factor loadings were mainly vegetables (beans, carrots, broccoli, sweet potatoes) plus rice with gravy and three unexpected foods: fish sticks, spaghetti, and pretzels. Children who ranked high on the Veggies Plus factor ate a relatively healthy diet, with low consumption of soda, fruit-flavored drinks, and chips. Factor 2 ("Sweet Snacks") reflected the least healthy foods, with items like snack cakes, cookies, chips, and ice cream loading strongly on this factor. Children with high scores on the Sweet Snacks factor ate very little greens, peaches, salad, and pears. Factor 3 ("Fruit") represented fruit consumption, with items like oranges, bananas, apples, and fruit juice having the highest factor scores. Those with high scores on the Fruits factor ate little vegetable soup, salad, or hot wings, and do not drink soda. The foods loading strongest on factor 4 ("Fast Food") were hamburgers, pizza, hot wings, French fries or tater tots, and fried chicken/nuggets. Those who were high on the Fast Food factor also often ate cheeseburgers and ice cream and infrequently ate fruit, cereal, and vegetables other than corn. The less often eaten vegetables (yellow squash, vegetable soup, tossed salad, and greens) comprised factor 5 ("Other Veggies"), and it partially reflected a healthy diet, since children scoring high on this factor ate little ice cream or cookies, but they also ate little chicken, fruit, and cereal. To produce an index for each of these factors, we summed children's scores on the food items specified in boldface type in Table 2. The reliability of these indexes is quite good, as Cronbach's alphas are: factor 1 (vegetables plus) = 0.91; factor 2 (sweets) = 0.91; factor 3 (fruits) = 0.87; factor 4 (fast food) = 0.89; and factor 5 (less popular veggies) = 0.79.

In general, this sample of immigrant children's food consumption responses clustered at the low end of the range (Table 3). For 17 of the 54 foods listed, 16 had a median of 0 and one had a median of 1, while 20 other items (including carrots, hamburgers, fried chicken or nuggets, and other beans) were eaten only once per week. Cereal was the most often eaten food (its median was four times per week, as was milk for low-fat and whole milk combined). Certain fruits (e.g., apples, oranges, grapes, bananas) were eaten fairly often, but other fruits (pears, peaches, and raisins) were infrequently eaten by most immigrant children. Most protein sources like hamburgers, fried chicken, peanut butter, and chicken were each consumed one or fewer times per week. Concerning beverages, water was most often consumed, followed by fruit-flavored drinks, fruit juice, low fat milk and whole milk, and sodas were consumed the least often. Snack foods like chips, cookies, and ice cream were among the most commonly consumed items at twice per week each, while others of these types of snack foods including snack cakes, cake, pretzels, and honey buns were consumed fairly infrequently.

Table 3. Food consumption frequency (per week) for a sample of Vietnamese and Hispanic immigrant children ($n = 63$).

Food	Median (Times/Week)	Interquartile Range	Type of Food	Median (Times/Week)	Interquartile Range
water	>6	4–7	popcorn	1.0	0–3
cereal	4.0	2–7	fried chicken or nuggets	1.0	0–3
apples	3.0	2–7	hot chicken wings	1.0	0–3
oranges	3.0	2–5	peanut butter	1.0	0–3
yogurt	3.0	0–5	macaroni & cheese	1.0	0–3
grapes	2.0	1–6	other beans	1.0	0–3
bananas	2.0	1–5	fried rice	1.0	0–3
chips	2.0	1–5	other rice	1.0	0–3
fruit-flavored drinks	2.0	1–5	cheese	1.0	0–2
pizza	2.0	1–4	other potatoes	1.0	0–2
cookies	2.0	0–5	mayonnaise	0.5	0–3
fruit juice	2.0	0–4	peaches	0.0	0–4
ice cream	2.0	0–5	greens	0.0	0–2
low fat milk	2.0	0–4	cheeseburger	0.0	0–2
mixed fruit	2.0	0–5	green beans	0.0	0–3
broccoli	2.0	0–4	pretzels	0.0	0–2
whole milk	2.0	0–4	jam, jelly, or syrup	0.0	0–2
chocolate candy	1.0	0–5	chicken not fried	0.0	0–2
French fries or tater tots	1.0	0–4	honey buns	0.0	0–2
carrots	1.0	0–4	tomatoes	0.0	0–2
hamburgers	1.0	0–3	tossed salad	0.0	0–2
snack cakes	1.0	0–4	raisins	0.0	0–1
spaghetti	1.0	0–4	sweet potatoes	0.0	0–1
soda	1.0	0–3	vegetable soup	0.0	0–2
pears	1.0	0–3	fish sticks	0.0	0–1
corn	1.0	0–3	yellow squash	0.0	0–1
cake	1.0	0–3	rice with gravy	0.0	0–1

3.1. Consumed vs. Recommended Number of Servings in USDA Food Groups

Figure 1 shows the median and interquartile range for consumption per week of foods grouped into USDA categories compared with the recommended number of servings per week, arranged in descending order of the recommendation for all children, boys, girls, Vietnamese, and Hispanic children. The sample as a whole ate significantly less than the recommended amount of grains, protein foods, and dairy, but met the recommended amount of fruit. Examining USDA food group consumption by gender, while the median consumption was higher in boys than in girls for all food groups, the differences were significant for grains, protein foods, and fruits (all $p < 0.05$), and marginally nonsignificant for dairy, oils, and discretionary foods (p-values ranged from 0.056 to 0.09). Results were similar when analyzed by ANOVA, controlling for ethnicity (Table S1). In addition, compared with the recommended number of servings, boys' median consumption was significantly lower for grains and protein foods, and significantly higher for fruits, while girls' median consumption was significantly lower for grains, protein foods, and dairy, and significantly higher for fruits. For both boys and girls, the highest number of servings came from discretionary foods, followed by grains and fruits. Of the food groups, fruit consumption was relatively high, with 67% of the sample reaching the recommended value (75% of boys and 58% of girls). A relatively high number of boys also reached the recommended number of servings for dairy (58%) and vegetables (50%), while only 31% and 20% of boys reached the recommended number of servings for grains and protein foods, respectively. Only 35% of girls reached the recommended number of servings for vegetables, and 23, 10, and 6% of girls consumed the recommended number of dairy, grain, and protein servings, respectively.

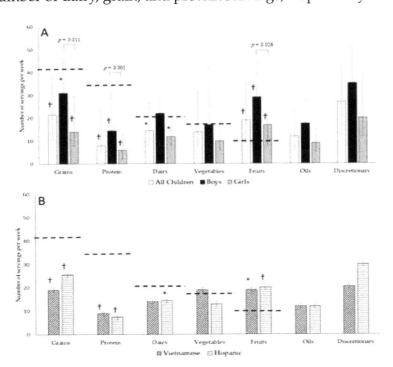

Figure 1. Reported median number of servings per week consumed in USDA food groups versus recommended values in a sample of fourth, fifth, and sixth grade Vietnamese and Hispanic immigrant children ($n = 63$) for (**A**) all children, boys, and girls; and (**B**) Vietnamese and Hispanic children. Error bars show interquartile range (25th and 75th percentiles). Dotted horizontal lines represent USDA recommended number of servings per week for 10-year-old boys and girls [16]. Symbol next to vertical bar indicates significant difference between number of servings consumed compared with the USDA recommendation (* for $p < 0.05$; † for $p < 0.01$). p-values are shown for Kruskal–Wallis test for significant differences between boys and girls; p-values for gender differences in consumption of other food groups were 0.058 for dairy, 0.117 for vegetables, 0.056 for oils, and 0.09 for discretionary. Differences by ethnicity were not significant (p-values ranged from 0.398 to 0.993).

In contrast, the figure also shows that there were no significant differences in food group intake by ethnicity. Results were similar when analyzed by ANOVA, controlling for gender (Table S1). While a majority of Vietnamese and Hispanic children met or exceeded the recommended number of servings of fruits ($p < 0.05$ and $p < 0.01$, respectively), they consumed a significantly lower number of servings of grains and protein foods ($p < 0.01$). In fact, only 8% and 14% of Vietnamese children met or exceeded the recommended amount of grains and proteins, respectively; while only 23% and 13% of Hispanic children ate the recommended amount of grains and protein foods. Most Vietnamese and Hispanic children also consumed a lower number of dairy servings compared with the recommendation, but this difference was significant only for Hispanic children ($p < 0.05$). The recommended number of vegetable servings was met by 62% of Vietnamese but only 38% of Hispanic children.

3.2. Dietary Patterns Discerned by Factor Analysis

Dietary patterns from factor analysis for all of the children in our sample, as well as by ethnicity and gender, are shown in Table 4. For all children, foods in the Sweet Snacks and Fruits factors were most frequently consumed, followed by foods in the Veggies Plus factor, then the Fast Food and Other Veggies Factors. Dietary patterns did not differ significantly by ethnicity, although Hispanic children consumed foods in Sweet Snacks much more frequently and Other Veggies much less frequently than did Vietnamese children. When examined by gender, however, frequency of consumption in each factor was higher for boys than for girls. This gender difference reached statistical significance for Fruits and Fast Food factors, and was marginally nonsignificant for the Veggies Plus factor.

Table 4. Median (Q1, Q3) consumption frequency per week of factor analysis-derived dietary patterns for a sample of Vietnamese and Hispanic immigrant children ($n = 63$).

	All Children	Ethnicity Analysis			Gender Analysis		
		Vietnamese ($n = 15$)	Hispanic ($n = 48$)	Kruskal–Wallis p-Value [1]	Boys ($n = 31$)	Girls ($n = 31$)	Kruskal–Wallis p-Value [1]
Sweet Snacks	19.0 (7, 34)	12.5 (7, 20)	22.0 (7, 39)	0.160	23.0 (8, 39)	13.0 (7, 26)	0.157
Fruits	15.0 (8, 26)	13.0 (7, 22)	15.5 (8, 29)	0.262	21.0 (9, 33)	13.0 (7, 22)	0.043
Veggies Plus	7.0 (4, 20)	7.0 (4, 13)	7.5 (4, 21)	0.951	11.0 (5, 37)	6.0 (3, 15)	0.069
Fast Food	6.0 (3, 16)	8.0 (3, 15)	6.0 (2, 21)	0.853	9.5 (4, 23)	4.0 (2, 14)	0.029
Other Veggies	2.0 (0, 8)	7.5 (1, 10)	2.0 (0, 7)	0.185	2.0 (0, 14)	2.0 (0, 8)	0.648

[1] Probabilities are statistical significance of Kruskal–Wallis test for differences in consumption of foods in each factor by ethnicity and gender. One Vietnamese child whose gender was unknown was not included in the gender analysis.

4. Discussion

We examined dietary patterns based on USDA food groups and dietary pattern analysis (factor analysis) in a convenience sample of Vietnamese and Hispanic school-aged immigrant children attending after-school programs. Several findings are especially interesting. On the positive side, most children in this sample ate the recommended number of servings per week of fruit, and approximately half of the boys ate the recommended number of servings of vegetables and dairy foods. Also, given the concern that many children drink too much soda, another positive finding was that the frequency of soda consumption was low (median was only once per week and interquartile range was 0 to 3). On the negative side, many of the children in our sample reported that for several food groups, their diets were below the recommended number of servings. Indeed, 87% of the sample was below the weekly amount in protein foods, 80% below in grains, 60% below in dairy, and 57% below the recommended weekly servings of vegetables. In addition, we found high levels of consumption of sweet snacks and fast food. Differences between the two ethnicities were not significant, but boys consumed significantly more servings per week of grains, protein, and fruits than girls. These findings suggest a generally unhealthy diet in these immigrant children, and that they may benefit from programs and interventions to improve diet quality.

Our finding of relatively high fruit consumption and low consumption of vegetables and diary is consistent with previous studies that find immigrants' adoption of American diets and eating patterns is typically not a wholly healthy change [21–23] and it may put them at risk of unhealthy outcomes [24–26]. In particular, our results in Vietnamese children which showed high consumption frequencies of fruit and vegetables and a low consumption frequency of dairy are in general agreement with previous studies [12,13,27], but there is some disagreement on consumption of meat (which falls into the protein foods group) between our study and another [27]. In addition, the findings of previous studies in Hispanic children with regard to these food groups are mixed [12,13], making comparisons with our results difficult and also mixed. Both ethnicities in our study had a relatively high intake of discretionary foods, which was not high in Vietnamese children in previous research [12] but was high in another study in Hispanic children [13]. Comparison of our data with previous studies must be done with caution due to methodological variations across the studies including differences in sample size, age groups, family income, acculturation status, and secular trends in U.S. food supply since the data across studies were collected from 1986 to 2013. Potentially, the generally unhealthy diet of children in our sample might be attributable to low family incomes (given that all the children qualified for free school lunches) and/or that traditional Vietnamese and Hispanic diets may be lower in protein and dairy foods than Western diets. We note that this survey was not a full inventory of all American foods eaten (nor did it cover traditional Vietnamese or Latin American foods), so it did not include some potential sources of protein (e.g., eggs, pork, or fish other than fish sticks). Therefore, it is possible that the low intake of protein foods is not as severe as these data imply. Nonetheless, the apparent low consumption of protein and other healthy foods found here merits further research. Taken together, our findings highlight the need for extensive investigation of the dietary practices of immigrant groups in general and children in particular. We need to discover whether continued eating of traditional foods by immigrants or their children can alleviate deficits in consumption of healthy food categories, or if they can shift to healthier choices of American foods. Also, we need to investigate how low income, the spatial location of good grocery stores, and the cultural meanings of traditional and American foods affect immigrants' food choices.

Further, we found interesting differences in food consumption by gender. For most food groups, especially proteins, grains, and fruits, boys reported more servings than girls. Several factors may account for this gender difference in food consumption. First, although within this age group, the recommedations for energy intake and the recommended number of servings in each food group do not differ between boys and girls [16], in US national survey data, boys report a higher energy intake than girls [28]. Therefore, it may be expected that the boys in our sample would report consuming more servings of any or all of the food groups than girls. In addition, there may be some behavioral and cultural factors that potentially contributed to the gender differences in intake observed in our study. Specifically, here may be traditional cultural gender norms that favor boys and place higher value on the good health of boys and men over girls and women [29]. In addition, studies show that immigrant parents allow sons more freedom to explore and adopt American cultural behaviors but often discourage or prohibit it for daughters, preferring that they maintain traditional customs [30,31]. This could help explain the more frequent consumption of American food by boys in our sample. It is also possible that gender norms encourage boys to be more assertive in interpersonal interactions [32] and therefore encourage boys to ask for and expect more servings of food than girls. Similarly, greater food consumption may be perceived as more masculine and as a means of confirming a male masculine identity, as well as a sense of personal empowerment [33]. In stark contrast, traditional gender norms may highlight petite body images for girls and associate positive self-meanings to girls who eat less and are slim in appearance [34,35]. The gender difference in our study may suggest the need for more in-depth study of the relationship between gender norms and the gender-related meanings assigned to food, both within Western culture and the traditional cultures of immigrant groups.

There are several limitations to this study. Beginning with the sample, the respondents were not randomly selected. However, we took advantage of the data which had been collected by CPACS as an opportunity to quantify the diet quality of immigrant children, a population whose diet and health have been understudied. A larger number of Vietnamese respondents would have enabled us to more directly investigate ethnic and cultural differences in food selection. In addition, about 10% of the children who were eligible to complete the survey did not participate, and there could have been differences between children who participated and those who did not, including age, grade level, and family income differences. Concerning the latter, however, any income differences were small, and unlikely to have created bias in the sample since all children were from families whose income was below the U.S. poverty line. Similarly, a question on the survey asking the respondent's age would have allowed us to control for age differences in our analysis of gender and independently investigate possible age effects. Another limitation is that while we have data on the number of times a child ate each pictured food, we do not know the actual amount of food consumed per serving. Further, the food items pictured in the questionnaire were all typically American and did not include traditional ethnic foods. The 54 foods included on the questionnaire were a subset of all of the actual (or potential) foods that the children in this sample may eat. Although many of the foods listed on the questionnaire were served to the children in their after school programs at CPACS and thus were believed to have been appropriately included, it is possible that a questionnaire containing a longer or different list of foods could have produced results that differed from our findings. In addition, the food consumption data were self-reported (rather than a precise measurement of the volume of food eaten) and therefore are subject to social desirability bias. The study was conducted in January and February, and did not take into account potential effects of seasonality on the results. The study is also limited by its lack of data on children's families and other demographic information. While all the children in this study were eligible for free lunch at school and had at least one parent/guardian who is an immigrant or refugee, a more complete analysis would have included variables such as total family income, English-speaking ability, parents' and children's immigration status, and their length of time in the United States. These limitations mean that we must be cautious in drawing conclusions from our findings. Nevertheless, this research may be a useful initial step in learning about the nutritional status of these two important groups of immigrant children, and can inform future, more in-depth studies on this topic.

5. Conclusions

While our sample size was relatively small and non-random, the results of the present study suggest that further study of the diets and food consumption of immigrant and refugee children is an important direction for continued research. First and foremost, the link between food consumption and health outcomes needs to be directly investigated with more comprehensive measures of the children's diets, health status, and health risks. Further studies should also compare children from different racial and ethnic groups, as well as the possible independent effects of immigration status and social background factors on food selection and health outcomes. The results also may have implications for helping Hispanic, Vietnamese, and other immigrant children. Educational and outreach programs in partnership with community organizations and religious institutions should focus on encouraging families to serve healthful traditional foods, especially those that increase portions of grains and proteins. In this regard, the food consumption of boys and girls may need to be recognized as different with special efforts to offer girls more servings of nutritious foods, and for boys to moderate their consumption of discretionary food such as candy and other high calorie snacks.

Acknowledgments: The study was not funded by outside sources. We thank CPACS for the use of the survey data, and Zoe Elizabeth Fawcett for technical assistance.

Author Contributions: J.H.K. conceived and designed the study; J.H.K. administered the questionnaire; C.L.J. analyzed the data; M.A.M., C.L.J. and D.C.R. wrote and edited the paper; J.H.K. edited the paper. All authors interpreted the results, provided substantive comments, and read and approved the final manuscript.

Appendix A

In the last week, how many times did you eat oranges?

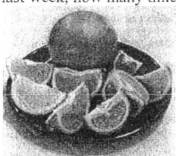

a.   0 times last week

b.   1 time last week

c.   2 times last week

d.   3 times last week

e.   4 times last week

f.   5 times last week

g.   6 times last week

h.   7 or more times last week

Figure A1. Sample question from 54 item food frequency questionnaire. The full questionnaire is available from the authors upon request.

References

1.   Wang, Y.; Min, J.; Harris, K.; Khuri, J.; Anderson, L.M. A systematic examination of food intake and adaptation to the food environment by refugees settled in the United States. *Adv. Nutr.* **2016**, *7*, 1066–1079. [CrossRef] [PubMed]

2.   Rosas, L.G.; Guendelman, S.; Harley, K.; Fernald, L.C.; Neufeld, L.; Mejia, F.; Eskenazi, B. Factors associated with overweight and obesity among children of Mexican descent: Results of a binational study. *J. Immigr. Minor. Health* **2011**, *13*, 169–180. [CrossRef] [PubMed]

3.   Kobel, S.; Lammle, C.; Wartha, O.; Kesztyus, D.; Wirt, T.; Steinacker, J.M. Effects of a randomised controlled school-based health promotion intervention on obesity related behavioural outcomes of children with migration background. *J. Immigr. Minor. Health* **2017**, *19*, 254–262. [CrossRef] [PubMed]

4.   Wang, S.; Quan, J.; Kanaya, A.M.; Fernandez, A. Asian Americans and obesity in California: A protective effect of biculturalism. *J. Immigr. Minor. Health* **2011**, *13*, 276–283. [CrossRef] [PubMed]

5.   Wang, M.C. Obesity and Asian Americans: Prevalence, risk factors, and future research directions. In *Handbook of Asian American Health*; Yoo, G.J., Le, M.-N., Oda, A.Y., Eds.; Springer: New York, NY, USA, 2013.

6.   Goran, M.I.; Ball, G.D.; Cruz, M.L. Obesity and risk of type 2 diabetes and cardiovascular disease in children and adolescents. *J. Clin. Endocrinol. Metab.* **2003**, *88*, 1417–1427. [CrossRef] [PubMed]

7.   Chen, J.L.; Weiss, S.; Heyman, M.B.; Lustig, R. Risk factors for obesity and high blood pressure in Chinese American children: Maternal acculturation and children's food choices. *J. Immigr. Minor. Health* **2011**, *13*, 268–275. [CrossRef] [PubMed]

8.   Bloom, B.; Black, L.I. Health of non-Hispanic Asian adults: United States, 2010–2014. *NCHS Data Brief* **2016**, *247*, 1–8.

9. Kelder, S.H.; Perry, C.L.; Klepp, K.I.; Lytle, L.L. Longitudinal tracking of adolescent smoking, physical activity, and food choice behaviors. *Am. J. Public Health* **1994**, *84*, 1121–1126. [CrossRef] [PubMed]

10. Qi, Y.; Niu, J. Does childhood nutrition predict health outcomes during adulthood? Evidence from a population-based study in China. *J. Biosoc. Sci.* **2015**, *47*, 650–666. [CrossRef] [PubMed]

11. Diep, C.S.; Foster, M.J.; McKyer, E.L.; Goodson, P.; Guidry, J.J.; Liew, J. What are Asian-American youth consuming? A systematic literature review. *J. Immigr. Minor. Health* **2015**, *17*, 591–604. [CrossRef] [PubMed]

12. Wiecha, J.M.; Fink, A.K.; Wiecha, J.; Hebert, J. Differences in dietary patterns of Vietnamese, White, African-American, and Hispanic adolescents in Worcester, Mass. *J. Am. Diet. Assoc.* **2001**, *101*, 248–251. [CrossRef]

13. Guerrero, A.D.; Ponce, N.A.; Chung, P.J. Obesogenic dietary practices of Latino and Asian subgroups of children in California: An analysis of the California Health Interview Survey, 2007–2012. *Am. J. Public Health* **2015**, *105*, e105–e112. [CrossRef] [PubMed]

14. Lee, S.K.; Sobal, J.; Frongillo, E.A., Jr. Acculturation and dietary practices among Korean Americans. *J. Am. Diet. Assoc.* **1999**, *99*, 1084–1089. [CrossRef]

15. Lesser, I.A.; Gasevic, D.; Lear, S.A. The association between acculturation and dietary patterns of South Asian immigrants. *PLoS ONE* **2014**, *9*, e88495. [CrossRef] [PubMed]

16. U.S. Department of Health and Human Services; U.S. Department of Agriculture. *2015–2020 Dietary Guidelines for Americans*, 8th ed.; USDA: Washington, DC, USA, 2015.

17. Center for Pan Asian Community Services. Available online: http://www.cpacs.org (accessed on 29 December 2016).

18. Center for Pan Asian Community Services. *2013–2014 Annual Report*; CPACS: Atlanta, GA, USA, 2014.

19. Center for Pan Asian Community Services. *2014–2015 Annual Report*; CPACS: Atlanta, GA, USA, 2015.

20. Bowman, S.A.; Clemens, J.C.; Friday, J.E.; Theorig, R.C.; Mosfegh, A.J. *Food Patterns Equivalents Database 2011–12: Methodology and User Guide*; U.S. Department of Agriculture, Agricultural Research Service, Beltsville Human Nutrition Research Center, Food Surveys Research Group: Beltsville, MD, USA, 2014.

21. Creighton, M.J.; Goldman, N.; Pebley, A.R.; Chung, C.Y. Durational and generational differences in Mexican immigrant obesity: Is acculturation the explanation? *Soc. Sci. Med.* **2012**, *75*, 300–310. [CrossRef] [PubMed]

22. Lara, M.; Gamboa, C.; Kahramanian, M.I.; Morales, L.S.; Bautista, D.E. Acculturation and Latino health in the United States: A review of the literature and its sociopolitical context. *Annu. Rev. Public Health* **2005**, *26*, 367–397. [CrossRef] [PubMed]

23. Park, S.Y.; Murphy, S.P.; Sharma, S.; Kolonel, L.N. Dietary intakes and health-related behaviours of Korean American women born in the USA and Korea: The Multiethnic Cohort Study. *Public Health Nutr.* **2005**, *8*, 904–911. [CrossRef] [PubMed]

24. Cho, Y.; Frisbie, W.P.; Hummer, R.A.; Rogers, R.G. Nativity, duration of residence, and health of Hispanic adults in the United States. *Int. J. Migr. Rev.* **2004**, *38*, 184–211. [CrossRef]

25. Jasti, S.; Lee, C.H.; Doak, C. Gender, acculturation, food patterns, and overweight in Korean immigrants. *Am. J. Health Behav.* **2011**, *35*, 734–745. [CrossRef] [PubMed]

26. Yang, E.J.; Chung, H.K.; Kim, W.Y.; Bianchi, L.; Song, W.O. Chronic diseases and dietary changes in relation to Korean Americans' length of residence in the United States. *J. Am. Diet. Assoc.* **2007**, *107*, 942–950. [CrossRef] [PubMed]

27. Betts, N.M.; Weidenbenner, A. Dietary intakes, iron status, and growth status of Southeast Asian refugee children. *Nutr. Res.* **1986**, *6*, 509–515. [CrossRef]

28. U.S. Department of Agriculture, Agricultural Research Service. *What We Eat in America, NHANES 2013–2014, Individuals 2 Years and over (Excluding Breastfed Children), Day 1*; USDA: Washington, DC, USA, 2016.

29. Vlassoff, C. Gender differences in determinants and consequences of health and illness. *J. Health Popul. Nutr.* **2007**, *25*, 47–61. [PubMed]

30. Espiritu, Y.L. *We Don't Sleep around Like White Girls Do: Family, Culture, and Gender in Filipina American Lives*; University of California Press: Berkeley, CA, USA, 2003.

31. Zhou, M.; Bankston, C.L. *Growing Up American: How Vietnamese Children Adapt to Life in the United States*; Russel Sage: New York, NY, USA, 1998.

32. Costa, P.T., Jr.; Terracciano, A.; McCrae, R.R. Gender differences in personality traits across cultures: Robust and surprising findings. *J. Personal. Soc. Psychol.* **2001**, *81*, 322–331. [CrossRef]

33. Turner, K.; Ferguson, S.; Craig, J.; Jeffries, A.; Beaton, S. Gendered identity negotiations through food consumption. *Young Consum.* **2013**, *14*, 280–288. [CrossRef]
34. Wardle, J.; Robb, K.A.; Johnson, F.; Griffith, J.; Brunner, E.; Power, C.; Tovee, M. Socioeconomic variation in attitudes to eating and weight in female adolescents. *Health Psychol.* **2004**, *23*, 275–282. [CrossRef] [PubMed]
35. McGinnis, J.M.; Gootman, J.A.; Kraak, V.I. *Food Marketing to Children and Youth: Threat or Opportunity*; National Academies Press: Washington, DC, USA, 2006; pp. 91–132.

4

Micronutrient-Fortified Milk and Academic Performance among Chinese Middle School Students: A Cluster-Randomized Controlled Trial

Xiaoqin Wang [1],*, Zhaozhao Hui [1], Xiaoling Dai [2], Paul D. Terry [3], Yue Zhang [1], Mei Ma [1], Mingxu Wang [1], Fu Deng [4], Wei Gu [1], Shuangyan Lei [1], Ling Li [1], Mingyue Ma [1] and Bin Zhang [1]

[1] Department of Public Health, Xi'an Jiaotong University Health Science Center, Xi'an 710061, China; huizhaozhao93@163.com (Z.H.); zymoon95@126.com (Y.Z.); wysun201314195@163.com (M.M.); wangmx601@mail.xjtu.edu.cn (M.W.); 232guwei@mail.xjtu.edu.cn (W.G.); shuangyan724@163.com (S.L.); liling-ch@163.com (L.L.); mamingyue66@163.com (M.M.); zhbin@mail.xjtu.edu.cn (B.Z.)

[2] Department of Nursing, Shaanxi Provincial Tumor Hospital, Xi'an 710061, China; Daixling113@126.com

[3] Department of Medicine, University of Tennessee Medical Center, Knoxville, TN 37996, USA; pdterry@utk.edu

[4] Xi'an Tie Yi High School, Xi'an 710000, China; dengfu01@126.com

* Correspondence: wangxiaoqin@mail.xjtu.edu.cn

Abstract: Many children suffer from nutritional deficiencies that may negatively affect their academic performance. This cluster-randomized controlled trial aimed to test the effects of micronutrient-fortified milk in Chinese students. Participants received either micronutrient-fortified ($n = 177$) or unfortified ($n = 183$) milk for six months. Academic performance, motivation, and learning strategies were estimated by end-of-term tests and the Motivated Strategies for Learning Questionnaire. Blood samples were analyzed for micronutrients. In total, 296 students (82.2%) completed this study. Compared with the control group, students in the intervention group reported higher scores in several academic subjects ($p < 0.05$), including languages, mathematics, ethics, and physical performance at the end of follow-up. Students in the intervention group showed greater self-efficacy and use of cognitive strategies in learning, and reported less test anxiety ($p < 0.001$). Moreover, vitamin B_2 deficiency (odds ratio (OR) = 0.18, 95% confidence interval (CI): 0.11~0.30) and iron deficiency (OR = 0.34, 95% CI: 0.14~0.81) were less likely in the students of the intervention group, whereas vitamin D, vitamin B_{12}, and selenium deficiencies were not significantly different. "Cognitive strategy" had a partial mediating effect on the test scores of English (95% CI: 1.26~3.79) and Chinese (95% CI: 0.53~2.21). Our findings suggest that micronutrient-fortified milk may improve students' academic performance, motivation, and learning strategies.

Keywords: fortified milk; micronutrient; middle school students; academic performance; motivated strategies for learning

1. Introduction

More than 2 billion people suffer from micronutrient deficiencies worldwide, including many school-aged children and adolescents in developing countries [1]. A recent systematic review reported that China has a high prevalence of micronutrient deficiencies, and that 55.7%, 45.2%, and 84.7% of children have insufficient iron, vitamin D, and selenium, respectively [2]. For instance, iron deficiency can have a detrimental effect on physical performance in children and adolescents [3]. Vitamin D deficiency in early life may negatively affect neuronal differentiation, axonal connectivity, dopamine ontogeny, and brain structure and function [4]. Retinoic acid, the active metabolite of vitamin A, is tied to processes of neural plasticity, and may influence memory [5,6]. Micronutrient deficiencies have been linked to damaging physical performance [3], impaired cognitive functioning [7], suboptimal learning [8], and poor academic performance [9]. These endpoints, in turn, may lead to an increased risk of adulthood obesity [10,11], living in poverty [12], depression [13], and other psychiatric disorders [14]. Hence, there is a need to identify and evaluate safe, tolerable, and cost-effective nutritional interventions in school children and adolescents.

Food fortification has been an effective public health strategy to decrease micronutrient deficiencies [15,16], but the effect of micronutrient-fortified food on academic performance remains unclear [17,18]. A 2012 literature review [17] identified four studies, none of which showed a positive effect of micronutrient supplementations on school examination grades. On the other hand, a systematic review of randomized controlled trials (RCTs) in 2016 [18] reported a lack of consistency in school performance among students receiving micronutrient interventions. In the latter review, 8 of 19 trials incorporated assessment of academic performance, and one reported significant improvements in mathematics, while no improvement was observed in other academic subjects. Several factors might influence the effect of fortified food on academic performance, such as motivation and learning strategies, which also play important roles in the process of learning and have significant influences on academic performance [19]. In a cross-sectional study, milk intake showed significant positive correlations with testing technique and learning strategy in Korean male high school students [20]. However, there have been few studies investigating the effect of fortified food on both motivated strategies for learning and academic performance.

China has a considerable number of school-aged children and adolescents who would benefit from an integrated nutrition improvement policy approach. In 2011, the General Office of the State Council launched the Nutrition Improvement Program for Rural Compulsory Education Students (NIPRCES), which allots children undergoing compulsory education a daily container of milk and a chicken egg [21]. Although NIPRCES has been implemented for several years, it has not yet been utilized fully in many urban areas, and has yet to be studied for potential effects on school performance. Given this dearth of knowledge, we hypothesized that milk fortified with micronutrients would go further than regular milk in improving micronutrient status, and would positively influence academic performance, motivation, and use of effective studying strategies.

2. Materials and Methods

2.1. Study Design and Participants

We conducted a cluster-randomized controlled trial among healthy Chinese middle school students, aged 12 to 14 years between June 2015 and January 2016. This study was carried out according to the guidelines laid down in the Declaration of Helsinki and all procedures involving human subjects were approved by the Biomedical Ethics Committee of Xi'an Jiaotong University Health Science Center (Project identification code: 2015-356). Prior to the data collection, written informed consent was obtained from a parent or guardian of all participating students along with verbal assent from each student. The exclusion criteria for children included moderately/severely undernourished children (Body Mass Index (BMI) for age z-score < -2 SD) [22], severe anemia (Hemoglobin (Hb) < 8 g/dL), infection (White Blood Cell (WBC) $> 10.0 * 10^9$/L), history of food allergies, children consuming nutritional supplements, and those participating in another nutritional program.

A total of 681 students were recruited from Xi'an Middle School. After excluding 321 students (47.1%) who missed the screening examination, declined to participate, or were deemed ineligible, 360 students were enrolled in the present study. Participating children were allocated to either an intervention group ($n = 177$) or a control group ($n = 183$) with random number table by the research staff, considering each class as a cluster, such that each student in the class, if eligible, would be included. The schematic flow of the participants in the present study is shown in Figure 1. Subjects of the intervention group were given 250 mL micronutrient-fortified milk (Future Star, Mengniu Dairy Company Limited, Hohhot, China) per day for six months; students of the control group were provided pure milk with approximately the same caloric value of the fortified milk (Milk Deluxe, China Mengniu Dairy Company Limited, Hohhot, China) (Table 1). The milk was given to each student by the research assistants, and its consumption was supervised by the students' teachers. Academic performance, motivation, and learning strategies, and micronutrient status were all assessed at baseline and at the end of follow-up. Children, study investigators, and the data analyst were not blinded to treatment allocation.

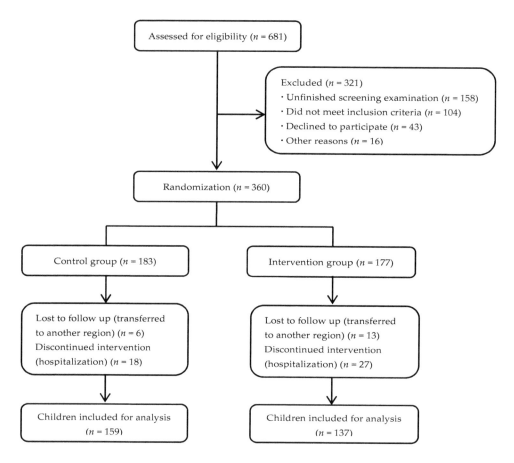

Figure 1. Schematic flow of the participants.

Table 1. Nutrient composition of the micronutrient fortified milk and pure milk in the present study.

Nutrients	Units	Fortified Milk per 100 mL	Pure Milk per 100 mL	FAO/WHO RNI for 10–18 Years [a]	Chinese DRIs EER/RNI/AI/EAR for 11–14 Years [b]
Energy	KJ	332	309	—	7530/8580 [c]
Protein	g	3.1	3.6	—	55/60
Fat	g	3.6	4.4	—	<60
Carbohydrate	g	8.6	5.0	—	150
Sodium	mg	58	65	—	1400
Vitamin A	μg RE	78	0	600	630/670 [c]
Vitamin D	μg	1.5	0	5	10
Vitamin E	mg α-TE	2.0	0	7.5/10.0 [c]	13
Vitamin B$_2$	mg	0.09	0	1.0/1.3 [c]	1.1/1.3 [c]
Pantothenic acid	mg	0.2	0	5.0	4.5
Phosphorus	mg	70	0	—	640
Calcium	mg	100	120	1300	1200
Zinc	mg	0.34	0	7.2/8.6 [c]	9.0/10.0 [c]

RNI: Recommended Nutrient Intake; DRIs: Dietary Reference Intakes; EER: Estimated Energy Requirement; AI: Adequate Intake; EAR: Estimated Average Requirement; RE: Retinol Equivalent; α-TE: α-Tocopherol Equivalent; [a] Food and Agriculture Organization of the United Nations (FAO) and World Health Organization (WHO), 2004. Vitamins and Mineral Requirements in Human Nutrition. Second Edition; [b] Chinese Nutrition Society, 2013. Chinese Dietary Reference Intakes; [c] Female/Male.

2.2. Screening Examination

The screening examination included anthropometric measurements and routine blood tests. Body height and weight were measured by trained personnel using standard anthropometric techniques. Subjects removed their shoes, emptied their pockets, and wore indoor clothing. Weight was recorded to the nearest 0.1 kg using a digital weighing scale. Height was measured to the nearest 0.1 cm using a stadiometer from head to foot. The weight and height of each participant were measured twice by study personnel. A third height and/or weight measurement was taken in the rare event that the first two measurements were not in agreement. BMI was derived from weight and height (kg/m^2), and thereafter BMI z-scores were calculated based on growth reference algorithms developed by the World Health Organization (WHO) for children and youth [23].

Hb and WBC counts were also assessed before the intervention to exclude children with severe anemia and infection. Non-fasting venous blood samples were collected in tubes containing anticoagulant (EDTA–K2). Blood samples were stored at 4 °C and analyzed within 4 hours. Hb and WBC counts were measured with an automatic hematology analyzer (XFA6100, PERLONG, Nanjing, China).

2.3. Academic Performance

Academic performance was measured using age- and gender-standardized end-of-term test scores retrieved from the school administration system. Academic tests were designed and administered by the Education Bureau of Xi'an, and scores obtained before the intervention were compared with those obtained at the end of follow-up. Test scores were analyzed using a percentage grading system, with 100 as the maximum grade and 60 percent as the minimum passing grade. The subjects of Chinese, mathematics, English, physics, social science, ethics, and physical performance were evaluated in the present study. Physical performance was assessed by a Physical Fitness Test, which includes a 1000-metre race for boys/800-metre race for girls, a 50-metre race, a standing long jump, sit-and-reach exercises, and pull-ups for boys/sit-ups for girls. Performance on the Physical Fitness Test was converted to a percentile score based on the national standard.

2.4. Motivation and Learning Strategies

Motivation and learning strategies were assessed by the Motivated Strategies for Learning Questionnaire (MSLQ) [24]. The MSLQ is a 44-item self-reported instrument consisting of three motivational belief subscales (Self-Efficacy, Intrinsic Value, and Test Anxiety), the Cognitive Strategy subscale and the Self-regulation subscale. The Self-Efficacy subscale is constructed by adding the scores of the students' responses to nine items regarding perceived competence and confidence in performance of class work. The Intrinsic Value subscale consists of nine items concerning intrinsic interest, perceived importance of course work, as well as preference for "challenge" and mastery of goals. Four items concerning worry about, and cognitive interference on, academic tests were used in the Test Anxiety subscale. The Cognitive Strategy Use subscale consists of 13 items pertaining to the use of rehearsal strategies, elaboration strategies, and organizational strategies. A Self-Regulation subscale was constructed from nine metacognitive and effort management items. Scores for each subscale were computed by summing the scores of specific items. Several items within the MSLQ are negatively worded and must be reversed before the respective score is calculated. Prior to the present study, the psychometric properties of the MSLQ were examined by a questionnaire survey with 30 subjects who did not participate in the present study, indicating a sound reliability (Cronbach's alpha = 0.79).

2.5. Micronutrient Status

Non-fasting venous blood specimens were collected by professional phlebotomist. Serum and plasma samples were separated within 4 hours of collection and stored at $-80\ °C$ until analysis. Micronutrient status was measured at baseline and at the end of follow-up for serum ferritin (SF), soluble transferrin receptor (sTfR), vitamin D, vitamin B_2, vitamin B_{12}, and selenium. SF, vitamin D, and vitamin B_{12} were measured with electrochemiluminescence technique (Elecsys 2010, Roche Diagnostics, Mannheim, Germany). sTfR was measured using immunoturbidimetry (IMMAGE 800, Beckman Coulter, Carlsbad, America). Vitamin B_2 was measured by the Erythrocyte Glutathione Reductase Activity Coefficient method using UV-VIS 1800 spectrophotometer by the modified ascorbic acid methodology [25]. The serum selenium levels were determined by atomic fluorescence spectrometry (RGF-8780, Bohui, Beijing, China). All biochemical analyses were carried out at the Micronutrient Laboratory, Division of Nutrition, Xi'an Jiaotong University Health Science Center. SF less than 15 mg/L or sTfR greater than 8.5 mg/L was considered to be a sign of iron deficiency. Deficiencies of vitamin D, vitamin B_2, vitamin B_{12}, and selenium were defined as vitamin D less than 11 ng/mL, the activity coefficient of vitamin B_2 greater than 1.2 AC, vitamin B_{12} less than 203 pg/mL, and body selenium less than 84.9 mg/mL, respectively. Body iron was calculated as Body Iron (mg/kg) $= -[\log (R/F\ ratio) - 2.8229]/0.1207$ where R/F ratio = sTfR/SF [26].

2.6. Statistical Analysis

Data management and data analysis were performed using Epidata (The Epidata Association, Odense, Denmark) and SPSS (Statistical Package for the Social Sciences for Windows, IBM, Armonk, NY, USA) version 23.0. The nominal variables are presented as frequency and proportion. The distribution normality of the quantitative variables was tested by One-Sample Kolmogorov-Smirnov test. The normally distributed variables are presented as mean $\pm$ standard deviation (SD). Student's t-tests were performed to analyze the differences in anthropometric parameters such as age, height, weight, and BMI, whereas gender difference and the prevalence of micronutrient deficiencies at baseline between the two groups were tested using Chi-square tests. For categories with small numbers (theoretical frequency < 5), the Fisher's exact test was used. After the intervention, the prevalence of micronutrient deficiencies was analyzed with logistic regression models. Analysis of covariance (ANCOVA) was used to test differences in academic performance, motivation and learning strategies while adjusting for baseline measures of independent variance. The mediating effects of motivation and learning strategies on academic performance in micronutrients were analyzed with nonparametric Bootstrap methods [27]. Statistical significance was set at $p < 0.05$; all tests were two-sided.

3. Results

3.1. Demographic and Anthropometric Characteristics of Subjects

The demographic and anthropometric characteristics of the subjects in this study are shown in Table 2. Overall, 137 students in the intervention group (77.4%) and 159 students in the control group (86.9%) completed this study. The mean age of the students at the time of enrollment was 13.2 ± 1.0 years and 13.4 ± 0.9 years in the intervention group and the control group, respectively. The study sample included more girls than boys, although the proportions did not differ significantly by intervention group ($p = 0.894$). There were also no significant differences in age ($p = 0.071$), height ($p = 0.283$), weight ($p = 0.100$), BMI ($p = 0.252$), or BMI z-scores ($p = 0.509$) between the two groups.

Table 2. Demographic and anthropometric characteristics of subjects in the intervention and control groups.

Variables	Intervention (n = 137)	Control (n = 159)	t/X^2	p
Age (years)	13.2 ± 1.0	13.4 ± 0.9	1.811	0.071
Gender			0.018	0.894
Male (n (%))	38 (27.7)	43 (27.0)		
Female (n (%))	99 (72.3)	116 (73.0)		
Height (cm)	163.9 ± 1.7	163.7 ± 1.5	1.075	0.283
Weight (kg)	58.8 ± 4.1	58.1 ± 3.2	1.648	0.100
BMI (kg/m^2)	21.2 ± 0.8	21.1 ± 0.7	1.147	0.252
BMI z-scores	0.1 ± 1.3	0.2 ± 1.3	0.660	0.509

BMI: Body Mass Index.

3.2. Micronutrient Deficiencies

Micronutrient deficiencies in students were comparable between the intervention group and the control group at baseline (Table 3). The effects of micronutrient-fortified milk consumption on iron, vitamin D, vitamin B$_2$, vitamin B$_{12}$, and selenium deficiencies analyzed with logistic regression models are shown in Table 4. After six months, students in the intervention group were less likely to be iron deficient (odds ratio (OR) = 0.34, 95% confidence interval (CI): 0.14~0.81) and vitamin B$_2$ deficient (OR = 0.18, 95% CI: 0.11~0.30) when compared with the control group. However, there was no statistically significant difference in the prevalence of vitamin D, vitamin B$_{12}$, and selenium deficiencies between the two groups.

Table 3. Prevalence of iron, vitamin D, vitamin B$_2$, vitamin B$_{12}$, and selenium deficiencies in subjects at baseline between the intervention and control group.

Micronutrients	Intervention (n = 137)	Control (n = 159)	X^2	p
Iron deficiency	10 (7.3)	13 (8.3)	0.079	0.779
Vitamin D deficiency	5 (3.6)	5 (3.1)		0.999 *
Vitamin B$_2$ deficiency	127 (92.7)	145 (91.2)	0.224	0.636
Vitamin B$_{12}$ deficiency	12 (8.8)	15 (9.4)	0.040	0.841
Selenium deficiency	68 (49.6)	77 (48.4)	0.043	0.836

* p value was compared using Fisher's exact test.

Table 4. The effects of micronutrient-fortified milk on the prevalence of iron, vitamin D, vitamin B$_2$, vitamin B$_{12}$, and selenium deficiencies.

Micronutrients	Intervention (n = 137)	Control (n = 159)	Adjusted OR	95% CI	p
Iron deficiency	7 (5.1)	22 (13.8)	0.34 [a]	0.14~0.81	0.012
Vitamin D deficiency	6 (4.4)	8 (5.0)	0.87 [b]	0.29~2.56	0.792
Vitamin B$_2$ deficiency	31 (22.6)	99 (62.3)	0.18 [c]	0.11~0.30	0.000
Vitamin B$_{12}$ deficiency	4 (2.9)	3 (1.9)	1.56 [d]	0.34~7.11	0.708
Selenium deficiency	53 (38.7)	59 (37.1)	1.07 [e]	0.67~1.71	0.780

OR: Odds Ratio; CI: Confidence Interval; [a] Adjusted by gender, age, BMI, vitamin D, vitamin B$_2$, vitamin B$_{12}$, selenium; [b] Adjusted by gender, age, BMI, iron, vitamin B$_2$, vitamin B$_{12}$, selenium; [c] Adjusted by gender, age, BMI, iron, vitamin D, vitamin B$_{12}$, selenium; [d] Adjusted by gender, age, BMI, iron, vitamin D, vitamin B$_2$, selenium; [e] Adjusted by gender, age, BMI, iron, vitamin D, vitamin B$_2$, vitamin B$_{12}$.

3.3. Academic Performance

The academic scores of trial participants are shown in Table 5. The academic performance of the subjects was comparable between the intervention group and the control group at baseline (p > 0.05). Compared with students receiving unfortified milk, students receiving micronutrient-fortified milk showed significantly higher scores in the subjects of Chinese, mathematics, English, ethics, and physical performance ($p < 0.05$), whereas the scores for physics were higher but not statistically significant ($p = 0.224$). No significant difference was observed in social science scores ($p = 0.428$). When modeled as independent variables, both iron and vitamin B_2 were associated with improved performance in the subjects of Chinese, mathematics, English, ethics, and physical performance ($p < 0.05$).

Table 5. Academic scores of the end-of-term tests between the control and intervention group in middle school students.

Subjects	Intervention (n = 137)		Control (n = 159)		F	p	F′	p′
	Baseline	Post-Trial	Baseline	Post-Trial				
Chinese	72.1 ± 2.0	81.2 ± 2.2	72.3 ± 2.1	78.5 ± 2.0	127.852	0.000	127.395	0.000
Mathematics	82.8 ± 2.0	86.1 ± 2.1	82.4 ± 2.0	85.6 ± 2.0	9.416	0.002	8.013	0.005
English	73.0 ± 2.0	84.1 ± 1.9	72.6 ± 2.0	79.3 ± 2.0	497.398	0.000	483.216	0.000
Physics	62.6 ± 2.1	70.0 ± 2.0	62.2 ± 2.2	69.5 ± 2.4	1.766	0.185	1.484	0.224
Social science	81.3 ± 2.1	84.9 ± 2.0	80.9 ± 1.8	85.2 ± 2.2	0.591	0.443	0.629	0.428
Ethics	72.6 ± 1.9	77.8 ± 2.1	72.4 ± 2.1	74.9 ± 2.0	127.497	0.000	127.637	0.000
Physical performance	68.7 ± 3.7	83.3 ± 4.7	69.3 ± 3.4	78.5 ± 4.4	79.162	0.000	59.090	0.000

F′: Adjusted by gender, age, BMI, iron, vitamin D, vitamin B_2, vitamin B_{12}, selenium, self-efficacy, intrinsic value, test anxiety, cognitive strategy, and self-regulation. The effect sizes (Eta Square) are 0.303, 0.027, 0.623, 0.005, 0.002, 0.004, and 0.168 for Chinese, mathematics, English, physics, social science, ethics, and physical performance, respectively.

3.4. Motivation and Learning Strategies

Baseline motivation and learning strategy scores were comparable between the intervention groups for self-efficacy, intrinsic value, test anxiety, cognitive strategy, and self-regulation (Table 6). After the intervention, students in the fortified milk group showed higher scores for self-efficacy ($p < 0.001$), and lower scores for test anxiety ($p < 0.001$), than those in the control group. There was no significant difference in scores for "intrinsic value". Regarding use of learning strategies, students who consumed fortified milk were more likely to incorporate cognitive strategies into their study routines ($p < 0.001$). However, no significant difference was observed in "self-regulation" between the two groups. In addition, the use of cognitive strategies had a partial mediating effect on academic scores in relation to iron and vitamin B_2, accounting for 29.3% (95% CI: 1.26~3.79) of the improved performance in English and 14.7% (95% CI: 0.53~2.21) for Chinese.

Table 6. Motivation and learning strategy scores between the control and intervention group in middle school students.

Dimensions	Score				F	p	F′	p′
	Intervention (n = 137)		Control (n = 159)					
	Baseline	Post-Trial	Baseline	Post-Trial				
Self-efficacy	50.3 ± 2.7	52.5 ± 0.9	49.9 ± 2.0	51.9 ± 0.7	19.497	0.000	17.621	0.000
Intrinsic value	50.8 ± 3.3	53.0 ± 2.9	51.3 ± 2.5	52.6 ± 2.7	0.375	0.541	0.285	0.594
Test anxiety	22.0 ± 5.5	20.1 ± 4.3	21.4 ± 4.3	22.8 ± 3.7	41.278	0.000	40.905	0.000
Cognitive strategy	58.2 ± 2.8	61.1 ± 3.1	57.7 ± 2.6	60.1 ± 2.7	15.885	0.000	15.730	0.000
Self-regulation	47.6 ± 3.2	47.5 ± 1.7	48.0 ± 2.5	47.6 ± 2.1	0.987	0.321	1.174	0.279

F′: Adjusted by gender, age, BMI, iron, vitamin D, vitamin B_2, vitamin B_{12}, and selenium. The effect sizes (Eta Square) are 0.057, 0.001, 0.123, 0.051, and 0.004 for self-efficacy, intrinsic value, test anxiety, cognitive strategy, and self-regulation, respectively.

4. Discussion

We conducted a cluster-randomized, controlled feeding intervention study to determine the effect of micronutrient-fortified milk versus unfortified milk on academic performance among Chinese middle school students aged 12 to 14 years. The micronutrient-fortified milk intervention raised blood vitamin B_2 and iron levels, and appeared to increase academic performance, physical performance, learning motivation, and the successful use of study strategies.

Children in our study who consumed micronutrient-fortified milk had significantly higher academic performance than those who consumed unfortified milk, not entirely consistent with findings in previous studies [9,17,28,29]. A recent literature review found that there was a correlation between micronutrients and the academic performance in school children [9]. However, another systematic review concluded no positive effect of multiple micronutrient supplementations on school examination grades [17]. For specific micronutrients, one cross-sectional study showed that iron insufficiency was related to disadvantages in learning, and insufficient serum iron concentration was correlated with significantly lower mathematic scores in female students (r = 0.628) [27]. Another interventional study suggested that improving iron status through fortified rice can enhance school performance ($p = 0.022$) [29]. In addition, a systematic review concluded that serum vitamin B_{12} levels were associated with cognitive function [30], which may further influence academic performance in school children [31]. Moreover, Babur demonstrated the negative effect of selenium deficiency on learning and memory in adult rats [32].

The beneficial effect on academic performance in the present study can be attributed to improved vitamin B_2 and iron status. Students who consumed fortified milk showed less iron deficiency, although iron was not added to the milk. The reason for this finding is unclear, although vitamin B_2 may influence iron status, possibly at the level of iron absorption [33]. Micronutrient levels have been linked in Indian school children to improved cognitive and physical performance [34]. Iron may alter the intracellular signaling pathways and electrophysiology of the developing hippocampus, the brain region responsible for recognition, learning, and memory [35]. In addition, we found that students in the intervention group had significantly higher physical performance than what was observed in controls. This may be attributed to improved iron status and oxygen carrying capacity in hemoglobin [36].

Another possible mechanism contributing to the improved academic performance might be the mediating role of learning strategies [37]. The present study found that students in the intervention group were more self-efficacious and had less test anxiety, and were also more likely to use cognitive strategies in the process of learning. Students' perception of self-efficacy and the evaluation of their own competence were significantly and positively related to academic achievement [38,39]. In a study of Finnish upper secondary school students [40], a statistically significant correlation was found between test anxiety levels and academic performance. Abdollahpour [41] also revealed that using cognitive strategies were positively correlated particularly with math achievement among male high school freshmen. Similarly, Zahrou [42] found that the consumption of fortified milk has a favorable effect on cognitive ability. Our data suggest that use of cognitive strategies may mediate the association between nutrient status and academic performance. Taken together with the results of these previous studies, our findings suggest a potentially long-term benefit to school-aged children from a relatively inexpensive intervention.

There are two strengths in the present study. Firstly, we not only examined the effect of fortified milk on students' nutritional status, but also on their academic performance, motivation, and use of learning strategies. Secondly, the cluster-randomized controlled trial design allows control of both measured and unmeasured confounding factors. Furthermore, the cluster-randomized design minimizes the possibility of contamination between the intervention and control group [43], because there is less opportunity to exchange the milk product for the participating students.

Several limitations of our study must be considered. Information on dietary factors other than nutritional supplements during the intervention period was not collected. Therefore, we cannot be certain that our results were not influenced by unmeasured dietary factors. Similarly, we did not account for factors such as "self-concept" [44], physical fitness [45], and cell phone use [46], which have been found to affect academic achievement. Lastly, the six-month follow-up period precluded the examination of longer-term effects of micronutrient-fortified milk on academic outcomes.

5. Conclusions

In conclusion, the results of the present study suggest that the consumption of micronutrient-fortified milk may improve academic performance, motivation, and learning strategies in Chinese school children. If our results are confirmed in future studies, additional studies will be needed to elucidate the underlying mechanisms and to identify subgroups of undernourished student populations that are most likely to benefit from this intervention.

Acknowledgments: We especially thank the teachers and administrators of Xi'an High School and gratefully acknowledge the students and their parents for their participation in the present study. This work was financially supported by a grant (Grant No. 81101333) from the National Natural Science Foundation of China and a grant (Grant No. 13-168-201608) from China Medical Board. The funders had no role in the design, analysis, or writing of this article.

Author Contributions: Xiaoqin Wang and Paul D. Terry conceived and designed the experiments; Xiaoling Dai, Mingxu Wang, Shuangyan Lei, Mingyue Ma, Ling Li, Fu Deng, Wei Gu, and Bin Zhang performed the experiments; Yue Zhang and Mei Ma analyzed the data; Zhaozhao Hui wrote the paper. Xiaoqin Wang and Paul D. Terry had primary responsibility for final content. All authors read and approved the final manuscript.

Abbreviations

The following abbreviations are used in this manuscript:

MSLQ	Motivated Strategies for Learning Questionnaire
EAR	Estimated Average Requirement
NIPRCES	Nutrition Improvement Program for Rural Compulsory Education Students
BMI	Body Mass Index
Hb	Hemoglobin
WBC	White Blood Cell
RNI	Recommended Nutrient Intake
DRIs	Chinese Dietary Reference Intakes
EER	Estimated Energy Requirement
AI	Adequate Intake
SF	Serum Ferritin
STfR	Soluble Transferrin Receptor
SPSS	Statistical Package for the Social Sciences
SD	Standard Deviation

References

1. Allen, L.; Benoist, B.D.; Dary, O.; Hurrell, R. *Guidelines on Food Fortification with Micronutrients*; World Health Organization and Food and Agriculture Organization: Geneva, Switzerland, 2006.
2. Wong, A.Y.; Chan, E.W.; Chui, C.S.; Sutcliffe, A.G.; Wong, I.C. The phenomenon of micronutrient deficiency among children in China: A systematic review of the literature. *Public Health Nutr.* **2014**, *17*, 2605–2618. [CrossRef] [PubMed]
3. Gera, T.; Sachdev, H.P.; Nestel, P. Effect of iron supplementation on physical performance in children and adolescents: Systematic review of randomized controlled trials. *Indian Pediatr.* **2007**, *44*, 15–24. [PubMed]
4. Eyles, D.W.; Burne, T.H.; McGrath, J.J. Vitamin D, effects on brain development, adult brain function and the links between low levels of vitamin D and neuropsychiatric disease. *Front. Neuroendocrinol.* **2013**, *34*, 47–64. [CrossRef] [PubMed]
5. Shearer, K.D.; Stoney, P.N.; Morgan, P.J.; McCaffery, P.J. A vitamin for the brain. *Trends Neurosci.* **2012**, *35*, 733–741. [CrossRef] [PubMed]
6. Ormerod, A.D.; Thind, C.K.; Rice, S.A.; Reid, I.C.; Williams, J.H.; McCaffery, P.J. Influence of isotretinoin on hippocampal based learning in human subjects. *Psychopharmacology* **2012**, *221*, 667–674. [CrossRef] [PubMed]
7. Black, M.M. Micronutrient deficiencies and cognitive functioning. *J. Nutr.* **2003**, *133*, 3927S–3931S. [PubMed]

8. Osendarp, S.J.; Baghurst, K.I.; Bryan, J.; Calvaresi, E.; Hughes, D.; Hussaini, M.; Karyadi, S.J.; van Klinken, B.J.; van der Knaap, H.C.; Lukito, W.; et al. Effect of a 12-mo micronutrient intervention on learning and memory in well-nourished and marginally nourished school-aged children: 2 parallel, randomized, placebo-controlled studies in Australia and Indonesia. *Am. J. Clin. Nutr.* **2007**, *86*, 1082–1093. [PubMed]

9. Syam, A.; Palutturi, S.; Djafar, N.; Astuti, N.; Thaha, A.R. Micronutrients, Academic Performance and Concentration of Study: A Literature Review. 2016. Available online: http://repository.unhas.ac.id/bitstream/handle/123456789/20833/IJABER?sequence = 1 (accessed on 13 January 2016).

10. Alatupa, S.; Pulkki-Råback, L.; Hintsanen, M.; Ravaja, N.; Raitakari, O.T.; Telama, R.; Viikari, J.S.; Keltikangas-Järvinen, L. School performance as a predictor of adulthood obesity: A 21-year follow-up study. *Eur. J. Epidemiol.* **2010**, *25*, 267–274. [CrossRef] [PubMed]

11. Sobol-Goldberg, S.; Rabinowitz, J. Association of childhood and teen school performance and obesity in young adulthood in the US National Longitudinal Survey of Youth. *Prev. Med.* **2016**, *89*, 57–63. [CrossRef] [PubMed]

12. Hoddinott, J.; Behrman, J.R.; Maluccio, J.A.; Melgar, P.; Quisumbing, A.R.; Ramirezzea, M.; Stein, A.D.; Yount, K.M.; Martorell, R. Adult consequences of growth failure in early childhood. *Am. J. Clin. Nutr.* **2013**, *98*, 1170–1178. [CrossRef] [PubMed]

13. Lehtinen, H.; Raikkonen, K.; Heinonen, K.; Raitakari, O.T.; Keltikangas-Jarvinen, L. School performance in childhood and adolescence as a predictor of depressive symptoms in adulthood. *Sch. Psychol. Int.* **2006**, *27*, 281–295. [CrossRef]

14. Bjorkenstam, E.; Dalman, C.; Vinnerljung, B.; Weitoft, G.R.; Walder, D.J.; Burstrom, B. Childhood household dysfunction, school performance and psychiatric care utilisation in young adults: A register study of 96 399 individuals in stockholm county. *J. Epidemiol. Community Health* **2016**, *70*, 473–480. [CrossRef] [PubMed]

15. Nga, T.T.; Winichagoon, P.; Dijkhuizen, M.A.; Khan, N.C.; Wasantwisut, E.; Furr, H.; Wieringa, F.T. Multi-micronutrient-fortified biscuits decreased prevalence of anemia and improved micronutrient status and effectiveness of deworming in rural Vietnamese school children. *J. Nutr.* **2009**, *139*, 1013–1021. [CrossRef] [PubMed]

16. Goyle, A.; Prakash, S. Effect of supplementation of micronutrient fortified biscuits on haemoglobin and serum iron levels of adolescent girls from Jaipur city, India. *Nutr. Food Sci.* **2010**, *40*, 477–484. [CrossRef]

17. Eilander, A.; Gera, T.; Sachdev, H.S.; Transler, C.; van der Knaap, H.C.; Kok, F.J.; Osendarp, S.J. Multiple micronutrient supplementation for improving cognitive performance in children: Systematic review of randomized controlled trials. *Am. J. Clin. Nutr.* **2010**, *91*, 115–130. [CrossRef] [PubMed]

18. Long, F.L.; Lawlis, T.R. Feeding the brain-The effects of micronutrient interventions on cognitive performance among school-aged children: A systematic review of randomized controlled trials. *Clin. Nutr.* **2016**, *2016*, 1–8. [CrossRef]

19. Pintrich, P.R.; De Groot, E.V. Motivation and self regulated learning components of academic performance. In Proceedings of the 39th EUCEN Conference, Rovaniemi, Finland, 27–29 May 2010.

20. Kim, S.H.; Kim, W.K.; Kang, M.H. Relationships between milk consumption and academic performance, learning motivation and strategy, and personality in Korean adolescents. *Nutr. Res. Pract.* **2016**, *10*, 198–205. [CrossRef] [PubMed]

21. Zhang, F.; Hu, X.; Tian, Z.; Ma, G. Literature research of the Nutrition Improvement Programme for Rural Compulsory Education Students in China. *Public Health Nutr.* **2014**, *18*, 1–8. [CrossRef] [PubMed]

22. WHO Multicentre Growth Reference Study Group. WHO Child Growth Standards based on length/height, weight and age. *Acta Paediatr. Suppl.* **2006**, *450*, 76–85.

23. de Onis, M.; Onyango, A.W.; Borghi, E.; Siyam, A.; Nishida, C.; Siekmann, J. Development of a WHO growth reference for school-aged children and adolescents. *Bull. World Health Organ.* **2007**, *85*, 660–667. [CrossRef] [PubMed]

24. Pintrich, P.R.; de Groot, E.V. Motivational and self-regulated learning components of classroom academic performance. *J. Educ. Psychol.* **1990**, *82*, 33–40. [CrossRef]

25. Dror, Y.; Stern, F.; Komarnitsky, M. Optimal and stable conditions for the determination of erythrocyte glutathione reductase activation coefficient to evaluate riboflavin status. *Int. J. Vitam. Nutr. Res.* **1994**, *64*, 257–262. [PubMed]

26. Cook, J.D.; Flowers, C.H.; Skikne, B.S. The quantitative assessment of body iron. *Blood* **2003**, *101*, 3359–3364. [CrossRef] [PubMed]

27. Hayes, A.F. Introduction to mediation, moderation, and conditional process analysis: A regression-based approach. *J. Educ. Meas.* **2013**, *51*, 335–337.

28. Soleimani, N.; Abbaszadeh, N. Relationship between anaemia, caused from the iron deficiency, and academic achievement among third grade high school female students. *Procedia-Soc. Behav. Sci.* **2011**, *29*, 1877–1884. [CrossRef]

29. Fiorentino, M.; Perignon, M.; Kuong, K.; Burja, K.; Kong, K.; Parker, M.; Berger, J.; Wieringa, F.T. Rice fortified with iron in school meals improves cognitive performance in Cambodian school children. In Proceedings of the Micronutrient Forum Global Conference, Addis Ababa, Ethiopia, 2–6 July 2014.

30. Vogel, T.; Dali-Youcef, N.; Kaltenbach, G.; Andres, E. Homocysteine, vitamin B12, folate and cognitive functions: A systematic and critical review of the literature. *Int. J. Clin. Pract.* **2009**, *63*, 1061–1067. [CrossRef] [PubMed]

31. Haile, D.; Nigatu, D.; Gashaw, K.; Demelash, H. Height for age z score and cognitive function are associated with academic performance among school children aged 8–11 years old. *Arch. Public Health* **2016**, *74*, 17. [CrossRef] [PubMed]

32. Babur, E.; Bakkaloglu, U.; Erol, E.; Dursun, N.; Suer, C. The effect of selenium deficiency on learning and memory in adult rats. *Acta Physiol.* **2015**, *215*, 42.

33. Powers, H.J. Riboflavin (vitamin B-2) and health. *Am. J. Clin. Nutr.* **2003**, *77*, 1352–1360. [PubMed]

34. Swaminathan, S.; Edward, B.S.; Kurpad, A.V. Micronutrient deficiency and cognitive and physical performance in Indian children. *Eur. J. Clin. Nutr.* **2013**, *67*, 467–474. [CrossRef] [PubMed]

35. Fretham, S.J.; Carlson, E.S.; Georgieff, M.K. The role of iron in learning and memory. *Adv. Nutr.* **2011**, *2*, 112–121. [CrossRef] [PubMed]

36. Waldvogel-Abramowski, S.; Waeber, G.; Gassner, C.; Buser, A.; Frey, B.M.; Favrat, B.; Tissot, J.D. Physiology of iron metabolism. *Transfus. Med. Hemother.* **2014**, *41*, 213–221. [CrossRef] [PubMed]

37. Ning, H.K.; Downing, K. Influence of student learning experience on academic performance: The mediator and moderator effects of self-regulation and motivation. *Br. Educ. Res. J.* **2012**, *38*, 219–237. [CrossRef]

38. Mothabeng, D.J. The relationship between the self-efficacy, academic performance and clinical performance. In Proceedings of the World Confederation for Physical Therapy Congress, Singapore, 1–4 May 2015.

39. Tenaw, Y.A. Relationship between self-efficacy, academic achievement and gender in analytical chemistry at Debre Markos College of teacher education. *Afr. J. Chem. Educ.* **2013**, *3*, 3–28.

40. Green, E. Test Anxiety, Coping, Gender and Academic Performance in English Exams: A Study of Finnish upper Secondary School Students. 2016. Available online: http://www.doria.fi/handle/10024/124720 (accessed on 15 August 2016).

41. Abdollahpour, M.A.; Kadivar, P.; Abdollahi, M.H. Relationships between cognitive styles, cognitive and meta-cognitive strategies with academic achievement. *Psychol. Res.* **2006**, *8*, 30–44.

42. Zahrou, F.E.; Azlaf, M.; El Menchawy, I.; El Mzibri, M.; El Kari, K.; El Hamdouchi, A.; Mouzouni, F.Z.; Barkat, A.; Aguenaou, H. Fortified iodine milk improves iodine status and cognitive abilities in schoolchildren aged 7–9 years living in a rural mountainous area of Morocco. *J. Nutr. Metab.* **2016**, *2016*, 8468594. [CrossRef] [PubMed]

43. Chenot, J.F. Cluster randomised trials: An important method in primary care research. *Z. Evidenz Fortbild. Qual. Gesundhwes.* **2009**, *103*, 475–480. [CrossRef]

44. Pottebaum, S.M.; Keith, T.Z.; Ehly, S.W. Is there a causal relation between self-concept and academic achievement? *J. Educ. Res.* **2015**, *79*, 140–144. [CrossRef]

45. Torrijos-Niño, C.; Martínez-Vizcaíno, V.; Pardo-Guijarro, M.J.; García-Prieto, J.C.; Arias-Palencia, N.M.; Sánchez-López, M. Physical fitness, obesity, and academic achievement in schoolchildren. *J. Pediatr.* **2014**, *165*, 104–109. [CrossRef] [PubMed]

46. Lepp, A.; Barkley, J.E.; Karpinski, A.C. The relationship between cell phone use, academic performance, anxiety, and satisfaction with life in college students. *Comput. Hum. Behav.* **2014**, *31*, 343–350. [CrossRef]

5

Pediatric-Adapted Liking Survey (PALS): A Diet and Activity Screener in Pediatric Care

Kayla Vosburgh [1], Sharon R. Smith [2], Samantha Oldman [1], Tania Huedo-Medina [1] and Valerie B. Duffy [1,*]

[1]   Department of Allied Health Sciences, University of Connecticut, Storrs, CT 06269, USA
[2]   CT Children's Medical Center, University of Connecticut School of Medicine, Hartford, CT 06106 2, USA
*   Correspondence: valerie.duffy@uconn.edu

Abstract: Clinical settings need rapid yet useful methods to screen for diet and activity behaviors for brief interventions and to guide obesity prevention efforts. In an urban pediatric emergency department, these behaviors were screened in children and parents with the 33-item Pediatric-Adapted Liking Survey (PALS) to assess the reliability and validity of a Healthy Behavior Index (HBI) generated from the PALS responses. The PALS was completed by 925 children (average age = 11 ± 4 years, 55% publicly insured, 37% overweight/obese by Body Mass Index Percentile, BMI-P) and 925 parents. Child–parent dyads differed most in liking of vegetables, sweets, sweet drinks, and screen time. Across the sample, child and parent HBIs were variable, normally distributed with adequate internal reliability and construct validity, revealing two dimensions (less healthy—sweet drinks, sweets, sedentary behaviors; healthy—vegetables, fruits, proteins). The HBI showed criterion validity, detecting healthier indexes in parents vs. children, females vs. males, privately- vs. publicly-health insured, and residence in higher- vs. lower-income communities. Parent's HBI explained some variability in child BMI percentile. Greater liking of sweets/carbohydrates partially mediated the association between low family income and higher BMI percentile. These findings support the utility of PALS as a dietary behavior and activity screener for children and their parents in a clinical setting.

Keywords: dietary screener; obesity prevention; sweet preference; children; diet quality

1. Introduction

The worldwide childhood overweight/obesity prevalence ranges from 22 to 24% [1]. Obesity in U.S. children is estimated at 17%, including 5.8% extreme obesity (BMI $\geq$ 120% of the 95th percentile) [2]. Obesity prevention requires a multi-sector approach [3], including screening, brief interventions and referrals between clinical and community sectors [4]. As the pediatric emergency department (PED) is utilized for non-urgent care [5], it should be part of this multi-sector approach [6–9] to reach low-income children who often have unhealthy dietary behaviors and lack access to primary care [6]. Brief obesity interventions have been successfully accomplished in the PED [7]. Clinicians need rapid, yet useful tools to screen behaviors for patient-centered interventions to promote healthy behaviors [10]. As parent involvement is critical [11], these tools should capture parent and child behaviors.

Conventional dietary assessment asks children or parents to recall food/beverage intake (e.g., 24-h recall,) or usual intake frequency [12,13], which is time intensive, often involves misreporting [14], and may cause defensive parent response and low-compliance in a clinical setting [15]. Screening usual consumption by asking likes/dislikes offers a feasible alternative. Recall of liking is quicker and cognitively simpler than behavioral recall with potentially less parent unease. Reported food liking correlates with reported intake [16–18], biomarkers of intake and/or adiposity in children [18] and adults [19–21]. The Pediatric-adapted Liking Survey (PALS) is fast, has a high response rate in the PED, with good-to-excellent clinical-to-home test–retest reliability [22]. Furthermore, results from an assessment of children's preference for food and physical activity (PA) can guide program planning [23]. Health promotion across the socio-ecological framework needs to develop healthy food and PA preferences in children [24].

The present study further develops PALS [22] to address needs in clinical settings. One need is to screen dietary behaviors in children and their parents (i.e., child–parent dyads) with comparable methods. The dietary patterns of children and parents can show weak-to-moderate resemblance [25].

The second is to assess dietary behaviors toward food/beverage groups and diet healthiness (i.e., diet quality). Few studies have examined diet quality in child–parent dyads [26]. We have shown that liking survey responses can form a reliable and valid diet quality index that explains significant variation in markers of nutritional status and health in preschoolers [18] and adults [21,27]. Diet quality indexes improve the understanding of diet-health relationships [28], inform interventions [29] and monitoring [30] in children. From analysis of three cycles of U.S. National Health and Nutrition Examination Survey (NHANES), diet quality among children is low, showing socio-economical and race/ethnic disparities [31]. The third need is to feasibly screen PA and sedentary behaviors in child–parent dyads. PA encouragement is key as children age, especially targeting those of economic disadvantage [32]. As questionnaires inform PA assessment [33], we enhanced the PALS [22] with physical and sedentary activities as well as additional foods.

Our specific objective was to screen both children's and parent's food and activity liking and to assess the reliability and validity of a Healthy Behavior Index (HBI) generated from the liking responses. Measures of reliability and validity followed that for the Healthy Eating Index [34], including the ability of the HBI to detect differences between child and parent, by the child's age and gender, proxies of the family's economic status, and the child's Body Mass Index Percentile (BMI-P). Finally, we examined models of interaction between income and food liking to explain variability in the child's BMI-P.

2. Materials and Methods

2.1. Participants

This observational study enrolled a convenience sample of 5 to 17-year-old children who sought medical care at the Connecticut Children's Medical Center's PED in Hartford, CT. The sample size was to capture diversity in the child to address the study aims and allow for multivariate analysis within a diverse sample. Children were excluded from participating if they had a history of severe behavioral/mental health conditions, were non-English speaking, or too ill to participate. Institutional Review Boards approved this study. To participate, parents/guardians signed informed consent, and children ages 7 and older signed an assent. Of those consenting to participate and meeting the inclusion criteria, 93% completed the protocol. The final sample, collected from March 2013 to April 2016, included 925 child–parent dyads who were diverse in child age, race/ethnicity, and family economic status (Table 1).

Table 1. Characteristics of children seeking medical care in a Pediatric Emergency Department.

	$n = 925$	%
Age (Avg. 10.9 years)		
5–<9 year	356	38
9–<13 year	257	28
13–17 year	312	34
Sex		
Male	463	50.1
Female	462	49.9
Race/Ethnicity		
Caucasian	357	38.6
Black	133	14.4
Hispanic	344	37.2
Other	91	9.8
Insurance		
Private	382	41.3
Public	507	54.8
Self pay	16	1.7
Other	20	2.2
Income Level *,a		
<$21,432	26	2.8
$21,433–41,186	288	31.1
$41,187–68,212	245	26.5
$68,213–112,262	313	33.8
≥$112,263	29	3.1
Food Insecurity *,b		
Greatest risk	574	62.1
Higher than average risk	102	11
Lower than average risk	134	14.5
Lowest risk	99	10.7

* Percentages ≠ 100 due to missing data (<3%); [a] Based on zip code analysis using U.S. Census Bureau data from the 2010–2014 American Community Survey 5-Year Estimates (U.S. Census Bureau. 2010–2014 American Community Survey 5-year estimates: Income in the past 12 months (in 2014 inflation-adjusted dollars)). American FactFinder: Community Facts Website. factfinder.census.gov/faces/nav/jsf/pages/index.xhtml. Accessed May 30, 2019.); [b] Based on data from the Zwick Center for Food and Resource Policy and the Cooperative Extension System at the University of Connecticut [35].

2.2. Study Procedure and Measures

Data collection took place in the patient's exam room. Research assistants enrolled patients, confirmed the inclusion/exclusion criteria, collected the child's address, age, gender, race/ethnicity, type of health insurance, and history of chronic medical condition (e.g., asthma, diabetes).

The community of family residence by zip code was reported by the parent/caregiver which served beyond type of health insurance as another proxy of family income and level of food insecurity. Median household income by zip code, reported by the U.S. Census Bureau, 2010–2014 American Community Survey 5-Year Estimates, was used to determine the family's income level. A Connecticut ranking of town food security (based on economic and social characteristics, access to food retailers, utilization of public food assistance) was used to assess participants' risk of food insecurity [35].

Pediatric-Adapted Liking Survey (PALS): Both child and parent/guardian were asked to complete the PALS, a food and activity liking/disliking survey, based on their own likes and dislikes (average completion time was <4 min). This three-page, paper/pencil PALS consisted of 33 food items and activities, represented with both pictures and words as described previously [22]. Participants reported their level of liking/disliking, marking a perpendicular line anywhere along the scale with seven faces labeled as "love it," "really like it," "like it," "it's ok," "dislike it," "really dislike it," and "hate it." Distance was measured from the scale center (0; "he/she thinks it's okay") to the participant's marking (±100; "he/she loves/hates it"). Children and parents/caregivers also could mark "never tried/done."

The Healthy Behavior Index (HBI) was conceptually constructed based on the 2015 Dietary Guidelines [36], with a single index similar to the Healthy Eating Index (HEI) and following our previously validated, liking-based diet quality indices [18,21] with the addition of PA and screen time (sedentary behavior). Foods and activities were sorted into conceptual groups and multiplied by weights consistent with the Dietary Guidelines [18,21,27]: vegetables (+3), fruits (+2), protein (+2), sweets (−3), sugary drinks (−3), fiber (+2), salty (−2), dairy (+2), PA (+2) and screen time (−3). The final HBI was the average of weighted groups that formed an internally reliable, normally distributed index: vegetables, fruits, protein, sweets, sugary drinks, and screen time. Higher indexes indicated healthier behaviors.

Measured and Self-Reported Adiposity: The child's height was measured by trained research assistants (cm; portable Stadiometer, Seca®) and weight was obtained from the electronic health record (kg; platform medical scale) to calculate Body Mass Index (BMI). Age-and-sex specific BMI-Ps were calculated with the with the online calculator [37], with the child's exact age (based on birth and measurement dates) and the U.S. Centers for Disease Control 2000 growth charts to assign underweight <5th, healthy weight 5th–<85th, overweight 85th–<95th, or obese ≥95th percentile [38]. Parents/caregivers and children self-reported the child's body size using a sex-specific, 7-point drawing [39] for categorization (underweight <2, healthy weight 2 to <5, overweight 5 to 6, obese ≥ 6).

2.3. Data Analysis

Data were analyzed using SPSS statistical software (version 22.0) with the Process v3.1 (afhayes@processmacro.org) with a significance criterion of $p < 0.05$. Descriptive statistics were used to compare BMI-P against national statistics and contrast measured versus self-rated body size. All variables were evaluated for distribution, normality and central tendency. Table 2 describes the assessment of reliability and validity of the HBI. Analysis of covariance included controlling for demographic variables (age, gender, race/ethnicity, income, as appropriate) as indicated in the results section. Direct relationships between parent and child HBI and adiposity were examined with standard multiple linear regression analysis while controlling for demographic variables and child's liking of PA. Additionally, multivariate modeling was used to assess associations between food liking, proxies of family income and food insecurity, and child BMI-P.

Table 2. Tests to assess the internal reliability and validity of the Healthy Behavior Index (HBI) [34].

Question	Test Statistic
Reliability	
How internally consistent is the total index?	Cronbach's Alpha
What are the relationships among the index components?	Pearson's r correlations between each component
Which components have the most influence on the total index?	Pearson's r correlations between each component and the total index
Construct and Concurrent Criterion Validity	
Does the index score foods and behaviors based on those recommended by the 2015 Dietary Guidelines?	Descriptive statistics
Does the index allow for sufficient variation in scores among individual?	Measures of central tendency, histogram, normality testing (Kolmogorov-Smirnov)
What is the underlying structure of the index (i.e., > 1 dimension)?	Principal component analysis and plot; derived factors to explain >50% of variance
Does the index distinguish between groups with known differences (i.e., concurrent criterion validity)?	Descriptive statistics, ANOVA with post-hoc analysis, ANCOVA, multiple regression analysis between demographic characteristics, PA liking and child's BMI-P

3. Results

Overall, 37.4% of children were classified as overweight or obese by BMI-P (Table 3), which was comparable to the U.S. average of 36.6% of children aged 5 to <18 years old [2]. Children ages 9 to 13 years old had higher rates of overweight (21%) and obesity (25.3%) than any other age group. Extreme obesity in children ages 6–11 and 12–19 years old was 7 and 9.5%, respectively, and exceeded U.S. averages of 4.3 and 9.1%, respectively [2]. Independent of age and gender, a higher BMI-P was seen in children covered by public health insurance (70.02 ± 1.26 SEM) than by private health insurance (62.64 ± 1.52) ($F(1,916) = 14.231$, $p < 0.001$). In similar analyses, higher BMI-P was seen in children from families who reported residency in communities with lower income (compressing the highest and low income levels ($F(2,894) = 5.583$, $p < 0.005$) and greater risk of food insecurity ($F(3,901) = 3.574$, $p = 0.014$). Among overweight children, nearly half of children (47.6%) and parents (49.7%) self-reported being a lower body size than measured; among obese children, most children (94.8%) and parents (84.4%) also self-reported being a lower body size than measured.

Table 3. Body Mass Index (BMI) percentiles by age and gender of children who were patients at a pediatric emergency department (PED).

	5–<18 Years		5–<9 Years		9–<13 Years		13–<18 Years	
	Count	% *	Count	% *	Count	% *	Count	% *
5th–<85th percentile								
Male	275	29.7	102	28.7	74	28.8	99	31.7
Female	277	29.9	110	30.9	59	23.0	108	34.6
Total	552	59.6	212	59.6	133	51.8	207	66.3
85th–<95th percentile								
Male	68	7.4	22	6.2	31	12.1	15	4.8
Female	82	8.9	27	7.6	23	8.9	32	10.3
Total	150	16.2	49	13.8	54	21.0	47	15.1
≥95th percentile								
Male	105	11.4	48	13.5	35	13.6	22	7.1
Female	91	9.8	28	7.9	30	11.7	33	10.6
Total	196	21.2	76	21.4	65	25.3	55	17.7

* Percentages ≠ 100 due to missing data (Percent of total sample size, $n = 925$; <2% missing). Underweight (<5th percentile) not shown due to small sample size ($n = 19$, avg. age = 9.7 years, mean BMI percentile = 1.52 and SD = 1.33).

3.1. Relative Comparison of Parent and Child Food and Activity Liking

Across the sample (Figure 1), parents averaged the highest preference for fruits and PA, while children reported the highest preference for sweets and screen time (e.g., watching TV, playing video games, listening to music). Children reported lower liking for fiber-rich foods and vegetables compared with parent reporting. Variance within food/activity groups was highest for children's liking of healthier groups (vegetables, fruit, proteins), and parental liking of the less healthy groups (sweets drinks and sweets) (Table 4). For children and parents, the least liked items had the highest variability in ratings. By effect sizes, the magnitude of difference between child–parent dyads was largest for vegetables, sweet drinks, screen time, and sweets.

Following our previous study [18], three groups of children were identified from the relative liking for sweets versus a pleasurable non-food: greater liking of screen time than sweets; equal liking; greater liking of sweets than screen time. From ANCOVA controlling for age and gender, children with higher affinity for screen time than sweets had significantly higher BMI-P [$F(2, 873) = 4.022$, $p < 0.05$] than children with higher affinity for sweets than screen time.

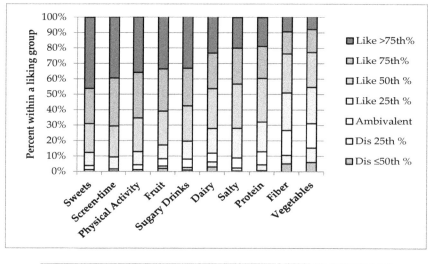

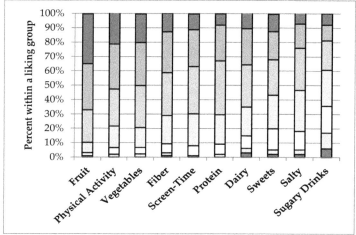

Figure 1. Liking of food/beverage and activity groups (left to right as most to least liked) in children (top graph) and parents (bottom graph), shown as percent within a food or activity group as liking (above the white neutral rating) and disliking (below the white neutral rating), with the darker the shading indicating stronger the liking or disliking.

Table 4. Variance and estimated effect sizes of child ($n = 925$) and parent ($n = 925$) survey-reported liking of foods and activities.

	Child			Parent			Effect Size
	Mean	SD	Variance	Mean	SD	Variance	Cohen's d
Vegetables	19.5	40.5	1636.6	48.4	30.6	938.3	0.8 *
Fruits	56.9	33.1	1098.0	60.5	27.4	749.7	0.1
Protein	40.9	35.3	1242.7	37.9	27.9	778.6	0.1
Sweet drinks	55.0	33.3	1108.7	14.1	39.6	1565.5	1.1 *
Screen time	64.3	26.5	701.6	39.9	27.7	768.0	0.9 *
Sweets	64.4	31.2	974.2	31.0	36.3	1317.7	1.0 *
Fiber	23.6	38.4	1476.7	41.6	30.6	936.4	0.5
Salty	44.1	32.1	1028.4	28.3	30.6	933.4	0.5
PA	59.5	29.8	888.1	49.3	30.7	940.4	0.3
Dairy	45.6	36.7	1346.3	35.5	34.6	1198.1	0.3

* Large effect size.

3.2. Internal Reliability of the HBI

The parent and child HBI approached acceptable internal reliability (α = 0.646 versus 0.613, respectively). Children and parents who reported high liking of sweets also reported significantly higher liking of screen time and sugary drinks, as well as lower liking (disliking) for vegetables (all Spearman's rho's, $p < 0.01$). Child and parent HBI were highly influenced by liking of vegetables, sugary drinks, and sweets (Pearson's r between ±0.47 and 0.71, $p < 0.01$).

3.3. Construct Validity of the HBI

The child and parent HBI were normally distributed (Figure 2), with the parent's distribution towards the higher indexes. Although weak, child and parent HBI were significantly correlated (r = 0.219, $p < 0.01$), with similar correlation across all groups making up the HBI.

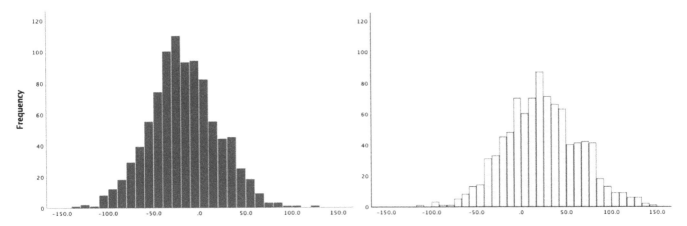

Figure 2. Histograms showing normal distributions of HBI in children (5–17 years old; left) and parents (right).

Principal component analysis (PCA) of the child HBI revealed two underlying dimensions—less healthy (screen time, sugary drinks, sweets) and healthy (vegetables, fruits, protein), which accounted for 57.2% of total variance. The PCA for the parents as well as child demographic and BMI-P categories (shown in Table 2) produced similar results for less healthy and healthy dimensions and >50% total variance explained, supporting a consistent underlying structure of the HBI.

3.4. Concurrent Criterion Validity of the HBI

The comparison of mean differences in child HBI via ANOVA, with post-hoc tests as appropriate, revealed significant effects of gender (males < females), health insurance type (public < private), race/ethnicity (Hispanic/Latino and Black/African American < White), income levels (determined through zip code analysis; low income < high income), and risk of food insecurity (high risk < low risk) (Table 5). Similar findings were seen for child or parent HBI. Greater age was correlated with healthier behaviors (r = 0.239, $p = 0.000$) as seen in females and males. In an income by race/ethnicity ANCOVA controlling for age and gender, income category was the sole significant contributor to child HBI ($p < 0.001$), with only a trend for an interaction with race/ethnicity ($p = 0.09$). In a gender by race ANCOVA, controlling for age, there were significant main effects on child HBI ($p = 0.008$ and 0.014, respectively), but no significant interaction effects. In summary, children who were older, white, female, covered by private insurance, and from communities with higher income and lower risk for food insecurity had the highest or healthiest HBI.

No significant differences in child HBI were found with BMI-P categories. However, a multiple linear regression model predicting child BMI-P from parent HBI, gender, insurance, and child liking for PA was significant among children of healthy weight (between 10th and 85th BMI-P). Significant predictors of higher child BMI-P were seen among lower parent HBI ($\beta = -0.11$, $p < 0.05$) and higher child liking of PA ($\beta = 0.15$, $p < 0.005$).

Table 5. Analysis of variance for mean child and parent Healthy Behavior Index (HBI) by child's demographics, community food environment, and adiposity.

Characteristic *	Child				Parent			
	Mean HBI	n	SD	p-Value	Mean HBI	n	SD	p-Value
Gender								
Male	−53.8	449	40.1	0.002 **	13.0	449	44.8	0.280
Female	−45.3	439	43.0		16.2	439	43.9	
Race/Ethnicity								
White	−41.1	341	42.3	0.000 **	23.0	341	43.1	<0.001 **
Af. Amer./Black	−55.2	129	39.3	0.006 †	10.1	129	43.3	0.023 †
Hispanic/Latino	−55.5	330	40.7	0.000 †	8.7	330	44.2	<0.001 †
Insurance Type								
Private	−44.0	364	40.4	0.001 **	23.7	364	41.3	<0.001 **
Public	−53.7	490	41.9		7.3	490	45.0	
Income Level								
$21,433–41,186	−58.9	277	40.9	0.000 **	4.8	277	45.2	<0.001 *
$41,187–68,212	−47.4	234	41.5	0.015 ᵃ	14.7	234	41.3	0.075
$68,213–112,262	−41.8	301	41.0	0.000 ᵃ	24.4	301	42.3	<0.001 ᵃ
Food Insecurity								
Greatest risk	−54.2	552	40.9	0.000 **	7.8	552	43.5	<0.001 **
>than avg. risk	−46.1	99	42.1	0.272	19.7	99	46.4	0.058
<than avg. risk	−40.7	125	39.0	0.005 ᵇ	27.9	125	39.9	<0.001 ᵇ
Lowest risk	−36.8	97	44.6	0.001 ᵇ	27.3	97	42.3	<0.001 ᵇ
BMI Percentile								
Normal weight	−49.6	523	40.7		14.8	523	44.3	
Overweight	−46.6	149	42.4	0.716 ˆ	12.0	149	40.7	0.767 ˆ
Obese	−49.0	189	42.7	0.984 ˆ	15.1	189	44.5	0.996 ˆ
Overall	−49.4	908	42.1	—	14.5	904	43.9	—

* Characteristics of child, not parent; the overall number is less than 925 due to missing data; ** Overall significant result, $p < 0.05$; † Significant result, $p < 0.05$, compared to white; a Significant result, $p < 0.05$, compared to lower income level ($21,43 3–41,186); b Significant result, $p < 0.05$, compared to those at greatest risk for food insecurity; ˆ p-value compared to normal weight.

Due to the interactions between health insurance (proxy of family income), parent liking and BMI-P, the possibility that parent-liking mediates the relationship between health insurance and child BMI-P was examined. Of several models tested, parent liking for carbohydrate-rich foods (average of salty, sweet drinks, fiber, sweets groups; Cronbach's $\alpha = 0.74$), was most explanatory, particularly in younger children (5 to 9 years old). Shown in Figure 3, higher parent liking of these foods explained some of the correlation between public insurance and higher child BMI-P ($Z = 1.954$, $p = 0.05$; bootstrap lower level confidence interval = 0.2239, bootstrap upper level confidence interval = 3.6938).

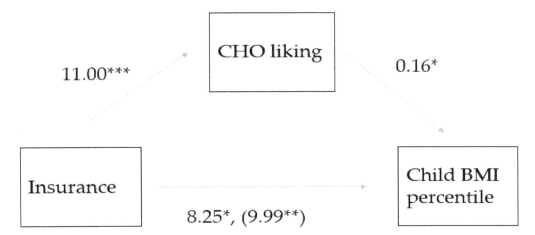

Figure 3. Model of the association between health insurance as a proxy of family income (dichotomous variable, where 1 = private; 2 = public) and the child's Body Mass Index Percentile (BMI-P), mediated by the parent's liking of carbohydrate-rich foods among 925 in children seen in an urban pediatric emergency department. * $p \leq 0.05$; ** $p \leq 0.01$; *** $p \leq 0.005$. The (coefficient in the parenthesis) represents the association between insurance and BMI-P before parent liking was added to the model, indicating that parent liking partially mediated the insurance and BMI-P relationship (indirect coefficient = 1.954, $p = 0.05$).

4. Discussion

Clinical settings need brief measures to screen children's behaviors in a method that is acceptable to families, has reasonable utility, can guide child and family-centered messages to encourage healthy behaviors, and can inform interventions for the prevention of obesity, particularly in at-risk groups. The present observational study recruited children and families from an urban, pediatric emergency department (PED) to assess children's and parents' liking of foods and activities with the Pediatric-Adapted Liking Survey (PALS) and test the reliability and validity of a Healthy Behavior Index (HBI), constructed from their PALS responses. The study sample of 925 child–parent dyads was diverse in race/ethnicity and >50% low-income, with children ranging in age from 5 to 17 years old, and with rates of overweight and obesity at or exceeding that for the U.S. The PALS is a novel diet and activity screener that showed good acceptability in this clinical setting and diverse sample. It was easily completed by children and parents and identified expected differences (children reporting a greater affinity for sugary foods/beverages and screen time, but lower affinity for vegetables than parents). The HBI neared adequate internal reliability and had normal distribution across both parents and children. For validity, the HBI measured two themes (healthy and less healthy), supporting its construct validity, and detected expected differences in healthy behaviors between groups, supporting its criterion validity. Healthier indexes were seen in females versus males, older versus younger children, parent versus child, families on private versus public insurance, and those living in higher income/food secure versus lower income/food insecure communities. For Body Mass Index Percentile (BMI-P), a higher parent-reported HBI was associated with lower percentiles across children who fell in the healthy range (between the 10th and 85th percentiles). In sub-analysis, part of the association between higher child BMI-P among families on public health insurance (i.e., lower income) was explained by greater parent liking of carbohydrate/sweet foods and beverages.

Simple indices with low participant and practitioner burden, such as the PALS and generated HBI, can be useful in a clinical setting [40] and to assess changes in response to interventions for children and families [30]. The indexes emphasize that positive health arises from moderating less healthy behaviors and encouraging those that are healthier. As the most effective obesity prevention programs for children involve the family [11], clinicians could begin conversations based on similarities and differences between child and parent dietary/activity likes and dislikes [41]. Parents influence the child's consumption of healthy and less healthy foods through controlling their availability, modeling consumption of these foods, and setting norms and attitudes toward healthy eating [42]. In the present study, child–parent dyads differed most for liking of sweets and sugary beverages. This agrees with a large multi-center study of families, which found stronger associations between parents and children for healthy rather than unhealthy foods [43]. Children prefer higher level of sweets than adults, linked to physical growth and energy need during development [44]. As higher added sugar consumption associates with poor diet quality and excess adiposity [45], families can look to healthier sweet options including fruit and fruit-based desserts. Parenting behaviors of restricting less healthy foods, using foods as a punishment or reward, or pressuring children to eat are ineffective at improving healthy eating behaviors [42]. Child–parent dyads also differed significantly in vegetable liking. Clinicians can encourage parents to show explicit liking of healthier foods [42], including tasting and consuming a variety of vegetables, involving children in cooking, supporting school meal participation, and family mealtime. Parents and children differed significantly in liking screen time yet were closer in liking for PA. Parent's liking and knowledge about screen time is significantly related to levels of screen time activity in children, which supports screen time interventions that target the child and the parent [46]. Parent modeling and support, including co-activity, can improve PA in children [47]. As preferences, attitudes and believes of parents are important predictors of PA that is performed with parents and children together [48], clinicians could probe beyond the PALS screening to identify which activities are enjoyed by both the child and parent and ways to facilitate and encourage family-based PA.

The indexes derived from the PALS showed good variability across the sample with acceptable internal reliability and validity. Although Cronbach's alpha for the HBI fell below the traditionally accepted value of $\alpha = 0.70$, this may be expected due to the complex nature of measuring diet quality, and therefore may not be a required characteristic [34]. Additionally, the child and parent HBI had a similar multi-dimensional structure of healthy (fruits, vegetables, protein) and less healthy (sweets, sweet drinks, and screen time) items. The HBI showed concurrent criterion validity through distinguishing between groups with known differences. Our results and others have found higher diet quality and health behavior indexes among females [49]. However, our findings that older children had higher diet quality and health behavior indexes differed from others, which found the opposite age relationship [50,51]. The present study found that white children reported higher diet quality and health behaviors than Hispanics/Latinos, consistent with an analysis of 2003–2004 U.S. NHANES [50], yet no significant difference was found between Blacks/African Americans and Hispanics/Latinos [50]. Finally, by using proxies of family income from community demographics, lower HBIs were found among children from families with lower income, receiving public medical insurance, and living in communities at high risk for food insecurity, consistent with multiple studies [50–52]. Our results are comparable to previous work that find healthier diet quality and behaviors among parents than their children [53].

The value of diet quality and health indexes is the ability to associate with health outcomes [40]. The present study found a significant but weak association between healthier parent HBI and lower BMI-P in healthy weight children. However, the child-reported HBI did not associate significantly with BMI-P. The association between indexes of diet quality or health behaviors and adiposity in recent scientific literature has been inconsistent. In cross-sectional studies, it has ranged from better diet quality and higher adiposities among children [54], to no significant association [55–57] or lack of consistent association [58], to healthier diet patterns in those who were overweight or obese [59]. Other studies only report demographic differences in diet quality in children and not the diet quality–adiposity association [60,61]. However, a large prospective study in children found significant associations with less healthy diet quality and increased adiposity over time [62]. Regarding activity, obese children have higher reported screen time and lower PA than do non-obese children from a systematic review, but the differences are small [63]. In the present study, the lack of significant association between the child-reported HBI and BMI-P may reflect a higher level of misreporting among overweight/obese children. Weight status has been shown to influence dietary reports by children, with heavier children being more likely to misreport due to social pressures and expectations [64]. It also may be important to examine dietary components to improve the diet quality and lower energy intakes, such as sugary beverages [65], fruits and vegetables [57] or, as in the present study, carbohydrate/sweet foods. Additionally, improvements in diet quality have been associated with improvements in body composition across an intensive diet and lifestyle intervention for overweight/obese adolescents [66]. According to a critical review, improvements in diet quality are required to improve cardiometabolic health, including obesity [67].

We found a positive association between child-reporting liking of PA and BMI-P, which is consistent with finding that obese children were more likely to report taking part in healthy behaviors [68]. Obese children are more likely to have been informed of their weight status by a physician [68], despite their perception of lower body size than what is measured in this study and others [69]. In the present study, children reported a high liking for screen time. Higher liking of screen time activities in children has been shown to associated with greater screen time behaviors [46]. Excessive screen time has been linked to lower diet quality [70], increased rates of obesity and negative health conditions [71]. When compared to liking for sweets, we found that children with a relatively higher affinity for screen time than sweets had significantly higher BMI-P than those who preferred sweets to screen time. Examining these relative rankings could help tailor messages to support healthy behavior and healthy weight. Parental encouragement has shown positive longitudinal effects on PA in adolescents [72].

Despite the findings of the present study, the question remains whether it is useful to ask parents and children to self-report their diet and PA behaviors. Furthermore, can asking likes or dislikes of foods/beverages and activities be reflective enough of usual behaviors to serve as a screener to guide a dialogue between health professionals, children and families? Screeners are short instruments to, for example, distinguish between healthier versus less healthy behaviors. Behavioral screeners need to be useful but not overly burdensome or cause families to become defensive [15]. All self-reported measures have the potential for reporting bias yet supply important information despite the emergence of dietary intake biomarkers [73]. If over time, for example, we eat what we like and avoid what we do not, reported liking reflects a pattern of what was consumed, but cannot capture total energy intake. Taste and food preference drive consumption. Food preference and intake are used interchangeably in nutrition literature [74,75] and food preference provides a proxy of consumption for examining health outcomes [76]. Survey-reported preference or liking correlates with self-reported intake in children [18,77] and adults [16,19,27,78–80], as well as with biomarkers of dietary intake and/or adiposity in children [18] and adults [19–21]. Similar to the present study, liking survey responses can be formed into an index of diet quality that explains variability in carotenoid status in preschoolers [18] and cardiovascular disease risk factors and BMI [21,27] in adults. However, food preference or liking can show marginal [19] or non-significant [81,82] associations with self-reported intake or BMI. Discrepancy in reported liking and intake does not imply that reported liking is inaccurate, and instead may reflect dietary restraint (intake is less than liking) in adults [19,27,83] and parents who are trying to limit their children's consumption of less healthy foods [18]. Conversely, individuals who are trying to improve their diet healthiness may consume a food that is not well liked [18,27].

Encounters between health professionals and families can motivate attention to and action towards improving a child's healthy behaviors for obesity prevention [84]. Improvements in the healthiness of a child's diet is promoted when both parents and children prefer the same food/beverage [85]. The PALS in the present study has previously identified patterns of food preferences that are associated with parent feeding practices [86]. Having children and parents self-evaluate their food and activity liking can act as a stepping stone to introduce a conversation regarding healthy behaviors and to identify goals and areas for change. Even if children are not overweight or obese at the time of the assessment, their behaviors may put them at future health risk. It is important to address and improve pleasure from healthy eating to achieve healthier dietary behaviors [17,87,88] and tailor nutrition education messages [89]. Preliminary work from our group has shown that doing the PALS online is acceptable in children and parents, is reported to stimulate self-reflection on diet and activity behaviors, can generate immediate tailored feedback on diet quality and healthy behaviors [90]. Preferences can change, including in response to marketing of unhealthy foods [91] as well as with interventions to improve preference for healthy foods [92–95] and decrease preference for less healthy foods [83,96].

This study had both strengths and weaknesses. The PED can be an acceptable setting to screen health behaviors related to obesity risk and for brief interventions, particularly because it provides health care to high-risk populations, such as low-income, minority families [6–9]. Additionally, this study utilized the PALS diet and activity screener, which was acceptable to both children and parents, with testing of reliability and validity using multiple statistical techniques and criteria [34,97]. The PALS was similar in structure and methods to our previous study in preschoolers, which was parent-reported, validated against reported dietary intake, a biomarker of carotenoid status and BMI-P [18,98]. As a limitation, only one measure of dietary behaviors was assessed without a more complete evaluation of PA behaviors. Since obesogenic dietary behaviors involve both hedonic responses to pleasurable foods and appetite, the PALS could be supplemented with constructs of appetite and satiety [99]. Previous work by our group has shown increased precision in making diet-health associations by combining the liking survey with multiple measures of dietary behaviors [18]. Because the intent was to screen for dietary and PA, the present study did not include a biomarker of nutritional status or a device to measure PA. Furthermore, the HBI did not explain BMI-P across children with lowest to highest percentiles, but only among children of healthy BMI-P. Detecting associations between child adiposity, dietary patterns and behaviors may require longitudinal study designs [100]. Further, BMI-P may not be the most useful measure of adiposity for a racially/ethnically diverse sample of children and adolescents [101].

5. Conclusions

Pediatric clinical and translational research settings need rapid yet useful ways to screen for health behaviors to inform brief interventions, referrals, and obesity prevention programs. A simple liking survey provides an acceptable and useful screener of diet and activity behaviors in child–parent dyads. The survey took less than 4 min to complete on average and had a high participation rate. Liking for foods and activities was formed into a healthy behavior index that had acceptable internal reliability and good variability across children and parents. Healthier behavior indexes were seen in children from income-disadvantaged families and those from less food secure communities. Liking for less healthy foods explained some of the association between low family income and higher child BMI percentile. Health care providers could use the liking survey responses to initiate conversations with children and parents and to encourage healthy diet and physical activity behaviors. The PALS can be performed as a paper/pencil survey, but for future direction, also can be performed online with theory-based health promotion messages delivered to the children and parents based on response algorithms [90,102]. PALS responses across groups of child–parent dyads can inform broader nutrition education programming and messages, such as in the nutrition education arm of the U.S. Supplemental Nutrition Assistance Program (SNAP-Ed) [103].

Author Contributions: S.R.S. and V.B.D. conceived and designed the study; K.V. and S.O. oversaw the experimental methods; K.V., S.O., T.H.-M. and V.B.D. conducted the statistical analyses; K.V., S.O., T.H.-M. and V.B.D. interpreted the data; K.V., S.O. and V.B.D. wrote the manuscript; all authors reviewed the manuscript.

References

1. Ng, M.; Fleming, T.; Robinson, M.; Thomson, B.; Graetz, N.; Margono, C.; Mullany, E.C.; Biryukov, S.; Abbafati, C.; Abera, S.F.; et al. Global, regional, and national prevalence of overweight and obesity in children and adults during 1980–2013: A systematic analysis for the Global Burden of Disease Study 2013. *Lancet* **2014**, *384*, 766–781. [CrossRef]

2. Ogden, C.L.; Carroll, M.D.; Lawman, H.G.; Fryar, C.D.; Kruszon-Moran, D.; Kit, B.K.; Flegal, K.M. Trends in obesity prevalence among children and adolescents in the United States, 1988–1994 Through 2013–2014. *JAMA* **2016**, *315*, 2292–2299. [CrossRef]

3. Institute of Medicine. *Accelerating Progress in Obesity Prevention: Solving the Weight of the Nation*; The National Academies Press: Washington, DC, USA, 2012; Available online: http://www.nationalacademies.org/hmd/Reports/2012/Accelerating-Progress-in-Obesity-Prevention.aspx (accessed on 1 June 2019).

4. Division of Nutrition, Physical Activity, and Obesity, National Center for Chronic Disease Prevention and Health Promotion. Childhood Obesity Research Demonstration (CORD) 1.0. Available online: https://www.cdc.gov/obesity/strategies/healthcare/cord1.html (accessed on 1 June 2019).

5. Kubicek, K.; Liu, D.; Beaudin, C.; Supan, J.; Weiss, G.; Lu, Y.; Kipke, M.D. A profile of nonurgent emergency department use in an urban pediatric hospital. *Pediatr. Emerg. Care* **2012**, *28*, 977–984. [CrossRef] [PubMed]

6. Chandler, I.; Rosenthal, L.; Carroll-Scott, A.; Peters, S.M.; McCaslin, C.; Ickovics, J.R. Adolescents who visit the emergency department are more likely to make unhealthy dietary choices: An opportunity for behavioral intervention. *J. Health Care Poor Underserv.* **2015**, *26*, 701–711. [CrossRef] [PubMed]

7. Haber, J.J.; Atti, S.; Gerber, L.M.; Waseem, M. Promoting an obesity education program among minority patients in a single urban pediatric Emergency Department (ED). *Int. J. Emerg. Med.* **2015**, *8*, 38. [CrossRef]

8. Prendergast, H.M.; Close, M.; Jones, B.; Furtado, N.; Bunney, E.B.; Mackey, M.; Marquez, D.; Edison, M. On the frontline: Pediatric obesity in the emergency department. *J. Natl. Med. Assoc.* **2011**, *103*, 922–925. [CrossRef]

9. Vaughn, L.M.; Nabors, L.; Pelley, T.J.; Hampton, R.R.; Jacquez, F.; Mahabee-Gittens, E.M. Obesity screening in the pediatric emergency department. *Pediatr. Emerg. Care* **2012**, *28*, 548–552. [CrossRef]

10. Brown, C.L.; Halvorson, E.E.; Cohen, G.M.; Lazorick, S.; Skelton, J.A. Addressing childhood obesity: opportunities for prevention. *Pediatr. Clin. North Am.* **2015**, *62*, 1241–1261. [CrossRef]

11. Gori, D.; Guaraldi, F.; Cinocca, S.; Moser, G.; Rucci, P.; Fantini, M.P. Effectiveness of educational and lifestyle interventions to prevent paediatric obesity: Systematic review and meta-analyses of randomized and non-randomized controlled trials. *Obes. Sci. Pract.* **2017**, *3*, 235–248. [CrossRef]

12. National Cancer Institute, Division of Cancer Control and Population Sciences. Register of Validated Short Dietary Assessment Instruments. Available online: https://epi.grants.cancer.gov/diet/shortreg/ (accessed on 1 June 2019).

13. National Collaborative on Childhood Obesity Research. Available online: http://www.nccor.org/nccor-tools/measures/ (accessed on 1 June 2019).

14. Bel-Serrat, S.; Julian-Almarcegui, C.; Gonzalez-Gross, M.; Mouratidou, T.; Bornhorst, C.; Grammatikaki, E.; Kersting, M.; Cuenca-Garcia, M.; Gottrand, F.; Molnar, D.; et al. Correlates of dietary energy misreporting among European adolescents: The healthy lifestyle in Europe by nutrition in adolescence (HELENA) study. *Br. J. Nutr.* **2016**, *115*, 1439–1452. [CrossRef]

15. Arheiam, A.; Albadri, S.; Laverty, L.; Harris, R. Reasons for low adherence to diet-diaries issued to pediatric dental patients: A collective case study. *Patient Prefer. Adher.* **2018**, *12*, 1401–1411. [CrossRef] [PubMed]

16. Tuorila, H.; Huotilainen, A.; Lähteenmäki, L.; Ollila, S.; Tuomi-Nurmi, S.; Urala, N. Comparison of affective rating scales and their relationship to variables reflecting food consumption. *Food Qual. Prefer.* **2008**, *19*, 51–61. [CrossRef]

17. Lanfer, A.; Knof, K.; Barba, G.; Veidebaum, T.; Papoutsou, S.; de Henauw, S.; Soos, T.; Moreno, L.A.; Ahrens, W.; Lissner, L. Taste preferences in association with dietary habits and weight status in European children: Results from the IDEFICS study. *Int. J. Obes. (Lond.)* **2012**, *36*, 27–34. [CrossRef]

18. Sharafi, M.; Perrachio, H.; Scarmo, S.; Huedo-Medina, T.B.; Mayne, S.T.; Cartmel, B.; Duffy, V.B. Preschool-adapted liking survey (PALS): A brief and valid method to assess dietary quality of preschoolers. *Child. Obes.* **2015**, *11*, 530–540. [CrossRef] [PubMed]

19. Duffy, V.B.; Lanier, S.A.; Hutchins, H.L.; Pescatello, L.S.; Johnson, M.K.; Bartoshuk, L.M. Food preference questionnaire as a screening tool for assessing dietary risk of cardiovascular disease within health risk appraisals. *J. Am. Diet Assoc.* **2007**, *107*, 237–245. [CrossRef] [PubMed]

20. Pallister, T.; Sharafi, M.; Lachance, G.; Pirastu, N.; Mohney, R.P.; MacGregor, A.; Feskens, E.J.; Duffy, V.; Spector, T.D.; Menni, C. Food preference patterns in a UK twin cohort. *Twin Res. Hum. Genet.* **2015**, *18*, 793–805. [CrossRef] [PubMed]

21. Sharafi, M.; Duffy, V.B.; Miller, R.J.; Winchester, S.B.; Sullivan, M.C. Dietary behaviors of adults born prematurely may explain future risk for cardiovascular disease. *Appetite* **2016**, *99*, 157–167. [CrossRef] [PubMed]

22. Smith, S.; Johnson, S.; Oldman, S.; Duffy, V. Pediatric-adapted liking survey: Feasible and reliable dietary screening in clinical practice. *Caries Res.* **2018**, *53*, 153–159. [CrossRef]

23. Vaidya, A.; Oli, N.; Krettek, A.; Eiben, G. Preference of food-items and physical activity of peri-urban children in Bhaktapur. *J. Nepal Health Res. Counc.* **2017**, *15*, 150–158. [CrossRef]

24. Beckerman, J.P.; Alike, Q.; Lovin, E.; Tamez, M.; Mattei, J. The development and public health implications of food preferences in children. *Front. Nutr.* **2017**, *4*, 66. [CrossRef]

25. Wang, Y.; Beydoun, M.A.; Li, J.; Liu, Y.; Moreno, L.A. Do children and their parents eat a similar diet? Resemblance in child and parental dietary intake: Systematic review and meta-analysis. *J. Epidemiol. Community Health* **2011**, *65*, 177–189. [CrossRef] [PubMed]

26. Lipsky, L.M.; Haynie, D.L.; Liu, A.; Nansel, T.R. Resemblance of diet quality in families of youth with type 1 diabetes participating in a randomized controlled behavioral nutrition intervention trial in Boston, MA (2010–2013): A secondary data analysis. *J. Acad. Nutr. Diet.* **2019**, *119*, 98–105. [CrossRef] [PubMed]

27. Sharafi, M.; Rawal, S.; Fernandez, M.L.; Huedo-Medina, T.B.; Duffy, V.B. Taste phenotype associates with cardiovascular disease risk factors via diet quality in multivariate modeling. *Physiol. Behav.* **2018**, *194*, 103–112. [CrossRef] [PubMed]

28. Nicklas, T.A.; Morales, M.; Linares, A.; Yang, S.J.; Baranowski, T.; De Moor, C.; Berenson, G. Children's meal patterns have changed over a 21-year period: The Bogalusa heart study. *J. Am. Diet. Assoc.* **2004**, *104*, 753–761. [CrossRef] [PubMed]

29. Alzaben, A.S.; MacDonald, K.; Robert, C.; Haqq, A.; Gilmour, S.M.; Yap, J.; Mager, D.R. Diet quality of children post-liver transplantation does not differ from healthy children. *Pediatr. Transpl.* **2017**, *21*. [CrossRef] [PubMed]

30. Wilson, T.A.; Liu, Y.; Adolph, A.L.; Sacher, P.M.; Barlow, S.E.; Pont, S.; Sharma, S.; Byrd-Williams, C.; Hoelscher, D.M.; Butte, N.F. Behavior modification of diet and parent feeding practices in a community—Vs. primary care-centered intervention for childhood obesity. *J. Nutr. Educ. Behav.* **2018**, *51*, 150–161. [CrossRef] [PubMed]

31. Thomson, J.L.; Tussing-Humphreys, L.M.; Goodman, M.H.; Landry, A.S. Diet quality in a nationally representative sample of American children by sociodemographic characteristics. *Am. J. Clin. Nutr.* **2019**, *109*, 127–138. [CrossRef] [PubMed]

32. Craike, M.; Wiesner, G.; Hilland, T.A.; Bengoechea, E.G. Interventions to improve physical activity among socioeconomically disadvantaged groups: An umbrella review. *Int. J. Behav. Nutr. Phys. Act.* **2018**, *15*, 43. [CrossRef]

33. King, A.C.; Powell, K.E.; Members, A.C. 2018 Physical Activity Guidelines Advisory Committee Scientific Report. Available online: https://health.gov/paguidelines/second-edition/report/ (accessed on 18 June 2019).

34. Guenther, P.M.; Kirkpatrick, S.I.; Reedy, J.; Krebs-Smith, S.M.; Buckman, D.W.; Dodd, K.W.; Casavale, K.O.; Carroll, R.J. The healthy eating index-2010 is a valid and reliable measure of diet quality according to the 2010 dietary guidelines for Americans. *J. Nutr.* **2014**, *144*, 399–407. [CrossRef]

35. Rabinowitz, A.N.; Martin, J. Community food security in Connecticut: An evaluation and ranking of 169 towns; Zwick Center Outreach Report. 2012. Available online: https://ideas.repec.org/p/ags/ucozfr/154264.html (accessed on 18 June 2019).

36. U.S. Department of Health and Human Services; U.S. Department of Agriculture. *2015–2020 Dietary Guidelines for Americans*, 8th ed.; U.S. Department of Health and Human Services: Washington, DC, USA; U.S. Department of Agriculture: Washington, DC, USA, 2015. Available online: http://health.gov/dietaryguidelines/2015/guidelines/ (accessed on 1 June 2019).

37. Centers for Disease Control and Prevention. Healthy Weight. BMI Percentile Calculator for Child and Teen. Available online: https://www.cdc.gov/healthyweight/bmi/calculator.html (accessed on 14 July 2019).

38. Centers for Disease Control and Prevention. About Child & Teen BMI. Available online: https://www.cdc.gov/healthyweight/assessing/bmi/childrens_bmi/about_childrens_bmi.html# interpreted%20the%20same%20way (accessed on 14 July 2019).

39. Collins, M.E. Body figure perceptions and preferences among preadolescent children. *Int. J. Eat. Disord.* **1991**, *10*, 199–208. [CrossRef]

40. Marshall, S.; Burrows, T.; Collins, C.E. Systematic review of diet quality indices and their associations with health-related outcomes in children and adolescents. *J. Hum. Nutr. Diet.* **2014**, *27*, 577–598. [CrossRef] [PubMed]

41. Hebestreit, A.; Intemann, T.; Siani, A.; De Henauw, S.; Eiben, G.; Kourides, Y.A.; Kovacs, E.; Moreno, L.A.; Veidebaum, T.; Krogh, V.; et al. Dietary patterns of European children and their parents in association with family food environment: results from the I. family study. *Nutrients* **2017**, *9*, 126. [CrossRef] [PubMed]

42. Yee, A.Z.; Lwin, M.O.; Ho, S.S. The influence of parental practices on child promotive and preventive food consumption behaviors: A systematic review and meta-analysis. *Int. J. Behav. Nutr. Phys. Act.* **2017**, *14*, 47. [CrossRef] [PubMed]

43. Bogl, L.H.; Silventoinen, K.; Hebestreit, A.; Intemann, T.; Williams, G.; Michels, N.; Molnar, D.; Page, A.S.; Pala, V.; Papoutsou, S.; et al. Familial resemblance in dietary intakes of children, adolescents, and parents: Does dietary quality play a role? *Nutrients* **2017**, *9*, 892. [CrossRef] [PubMed]

44. Mennella, J.A.; Bobowski, N.K.; Reed, D.R. The development of sweet taste: From biology to hedonics. *Rev. Endocr. Metab. Disord.* **2016**, *17*, 171–178. [CrossRef]

45. Wang, J.; Shang, L.; Light, K.; O'Loughlin, J.; Paradis, G.; Gray-Donald, K. Associations between added sugar (solid vs. liquid) intakes, diet quality, and adiposity indicators in Canadian children. *Appl. Physiol. Nutr. Metab.* **2015**, *40*, 835–841. [CrossRef] [PubMed]

46. Verloigne, M.; Van Lippevelde, W.; Bere, E.; Manios, Y.; Kovacs, E.; Grillenberger, M.; Maes, L.; Brug, J.; De Bourdeaudhuij, I. Individual and family environmental correlates of television and computer time in 10- to 12-year-old European children: The ENERGY-project. *BMC Public Health* **2015**, *15*, 912. [CrossRef]

47. Yao, C.A.; Rhodes, R.E. Parental correlates in child and adolescent physical activity: A meta-analysis. *Int. J. Behav. Nutr. Phys. Act.* **2015**, *12*, 10. [CrossRef]

48. Rhodes, R.E.; Lim, C. Promoting parent and child physical activity together: Elicitation of potential intervention targets and preferences. *Health Educ. Behav.* **2018**, *45*, 112–123. [CrossRef]

49. Bolton, K.A.; Jacka, F.; Allender, S.; Kremer, P.; Gibbs, L.; Waters, E.; de Silva, A. The association between self-reported diet quality and health-related quality of life in rural and urban Australian adolescents. *Aust. J. Rural Health* **2016**, *24*, 317–325. [CrossRef]

50. Hiza, H.A.; Casavale, K.O.; Guenther, P.M.; Davis, C.A. Diet quality of Americans differs by age, sex, race/ethnicity, income, and education level. *J. Acad. Nutr. Diet.* **2013**, *113*, 297–306. [CrossRef]

51. Golley, R.K.; Hendrie, G.A.; McNaughton, S.A. Scores on the dietary guideline index for children and adolescents are associated with nutrient intake and socio-economic position but not adiposity. *J. Nutr.* **2011**, *141*, 1340–1347. [CrossRef] [PubMed]

52. Andreyeva, T.; Tripp, A.S.; Schwartz, M.B. Dietary quality of Americans by Supplemental Nutrition Assistance Program participation status: A systematic review. *Am. J. Prev. Med.* **2015**, *49*, 594–604. [CrossRef]

53. Robson, S.M.; Couch, S.C.; Peugh, J.L.; Glanz, K.; Zhou, C.; Sallis, J.F.; Saelens, B.E. Parent diet quality and energy intake are related to child diet quality and energy intake. *J. Acad. Nutr. Diet.* **2016**, *116*, 984–990. [CrossRef] [PubMed]

54. Shang, L.; O'Loughlin, J.; Tremblay, A.; Gray-Donald, K. The association between food patterns and adiposity among Canadian children at risk of overweight. *Appl. Physiol. Nutr. Metab.* **2014**, *39*, 195–201. [CrossRef] [PubMed]

55. Cagiran Yilmaz, F.; Cagiran, D.; Ozcelik, A.O. Adolescent obesity and its association with diet quality and cardiovascular risk factors. *Ecol. Food Nutr.* **2019**, *58*, 207–218. [CrossRef] [PubMed]

56. Archero, F.; Ricotti, R.; Solito, A.; Carrera, D.; Civello, F.; Di Bella, R.; Bellone, S.; Prodam, F. Adherence to the Mediterranean diet among school children and adolescents living in northern Italy and unhealthy food behaviors associated to overweight. *Nutrients* **2018**, *10*. [CrossRef] [PubMed]

57.   Mellendick, K.; Shanahan, L.; Wideman, L.; Calkins, S.; Keane, S.; Lovelady, C. Diets rich in fruits and vegetables are associated with lower cardiovascular disease risk in adolescents. *Nutrients* **2018**, *10*. [CrossRef] [PubMed]

58.   Murakami, K. Associations between nutritional quality of meals and snacks assessed by the Food Standards Agency nutrient profiling system and overall diet quality and adiposity measures in British children and adolescents. *Nutrition* **2018**, *49*, 57–65. [CrossRef] [PubMed]

59.   Xu, F.; Cohen, S.A.; Greaney, M.L.; Greene, G.W. The association between US adolescents' Weight status, weight perception, weight satisfaction, and their physical activity and dietary behaviors. *Int. J. Environ. Res. Public Health* **2018**, *15*. [CrossRef] [PubMed]

60.   Lee, J.; Kubik, M.Y.; Fulkerson, J.A. Diet quality and fruit, vegetable, and sugar-sweetened beverage consumption by household food insecurity among 8- to 12-year-old children during summer months. *J. Acad. Nutr. Diet.* **2019**. [CrossRef] [PubMed]

61.   Hunt, E.T.; Brazendale, K.; Dunn, C.; Boutte, A.K.; Liu, J.; Hardin, J.; Beets, M.W.; Weaver, R.G. Income, race and its association with obesogenic behaviors of U.S. children and adolescents, NHANES 2003–2006. *J. Community Health* **2019**, *44*, 507–518. [CrossRef] [PubMed]

62.   Ambrosini, G.L.; Emmett, P.M.; Northstone, K.; Howe, L.D.; Tilling, K.; Jebb, S.A. Identification of a dietary pattern prospectively associated with increased adiposity during childhood and adolescence. *Int. J. Obes. (Lond.)* **2012**, *36*, 1299–1305. [CrossRef] [PubMed]

63.   Elmesmari, R.; Martin, A.; Reilly, J.J.; Paton, J.Y. Comparison of accelerometer measured levels of physical activity and sedentary time between obese and non-obese children and adolescents: A systematic review. *BMC Pediatr.* **2018**, *18*, 106. [CrossRef] [PubMed]

64.   Vanhelst, J.; Beghin, L.; Duhamel, A.; De Henauw, S.; Ruiz, J.R.; Kafatos, A.; Androutsos, O.; Widhalm, K.; Mauro, B.; Sjostrom, M.; et al. Do adolescents accurately evaluate their diet quality? The HELENA study. *Clin. Nutr.* **2017**, *36*, 1669–1673. [CrossRef] [PubMed]

65.   Leung, C.W.; DiMatteo, S.G.; Gosliner, W.A.; Ritchie, L.D. Sugar-sweetened beverage and water intake in relation to diet quality in U.S. children. *Am. J. Prev. Med.* **2018**, *54*, 394–402. [CrossRef] [PubMed]

66.   De Miguel-Etayo, P.; Moreno, L.A.; Santabarbara, J.; Martin-Matillas, M.; Azcona-San Julian, M.C.; Marti Del Moral, A.; Campoy, C.; Marcos, A.; Garagorri, J.M.; Group, E.S. Diet quality index as a predictor of treatment efficacy in overweight and obese adolescents: The EVASYON study. *Clin. Nutr.* **2019**, *38*, 782–790. [CrossRef] [PubMed]

67.   Arsenault, B.J.; Lamarche, B.; Despres, J.P. Targeting overconsumption of sugar-sweetened beverages vs. overall poor diet quality for cardiometabolic diseases risk prevention: place your bets! *Nutrients* **2017**, *9*. [CrossRef] [PubMed]

68.   Tovar, A.; Chui, K.; Hyatt, R.R.; Kuder, J.; Kraak, V.I.; Choumenkovitch, S.F.; Hastings, A.; Bloom, J.; Economos, C.D. Healthy-lifestyle behaviors associated with overweight and obesity in US rural children. *BMC Pediatr.* **2012**, *12*, 102. [CrossRef]

69.   Sugiyama, T.; Horino, M.; Inoue, K.; Kobayashi, Y.; Shapiro, M.F.; McCarthy, W.J. Trends of child's weight perception by children, parents, and healthcare professionals during the time of terminology change in childhood obesity in the United States, 2005–2014. *Child. Obes.* **2016**, *12*, 463–473. [CrossRef] [PubMed]

70.   Sisson, S.B.; Shay, C.M.; Broyles, S.T.; Leyva, M. Television-viewing time and dietary quality among U.S. children and adults. *Am. J. Prev. Med.* **2012**, *43*, 196–200. [CrossRef] [PubMed]

71.   Strasburger, V.C.; Jordan, A.B.; Donnerstein, E. Health effects of media on children and adolescents. *Pediatrics* **2010**, *125*, 756–767. [CrossRef] [PubMed]

72.   Bauer, K.W.; Nelson, M.C.; Boutelle, K.N.; Neumark-Sztainer, D. Parental influences on adolescents' physical activity and sedentary behavior: Longitudinal findings from Project EAT-II. *Int. J. Behav. Nutr. Phys. Act.* **2008**, *5*, 12. [CrossRef] [PubMed]

73.   Labonte, M.E.; Kirkpatrick, S.I.; Bell, R.C.; Boucher, B.A.; Csizmadi, I.; Koushik, A.; L'Abbe, M.R.; Massarelli, I.; Robson, P.J.; Rondeau, I.; et al. Dietary assessment is a critical element of health research—Perspective from the partnership for advancing nutritional and dietary assessment in Canada. *Appl. Physiol. Nutr. Metab.* **2016**, *41*, 1096–1099. [CrossRef] [PubMed]

74.   Garnier, S.; Vallee, K.; Lemoine-Morel, S.; Joffroy, S.; Drapeau, V.; Tremblay, A.; Auneau, G.; Mauriege, P. Food group preferences and energy balance in moderately obese postmenopausal women subjected to brisk walking program. *Appl. Physiol. Nutr. Metab.* **2015**, *40*, 741–748. [CrossRef] [PubMed]

75.   Beheshti, R.; Jones-Smith, J.C.; Igusa, T. Taking dietary habits into account: A computational method for modeling food choices that goes beyond price. *PLoS ONE* **2017**, *12*, e0178348. [CrossRef] [PubMed]

76.   Lee, Y.H.; Shelley, M.; Liu, C.T.; Chang, Y.C. Assessing the association of food preferences and self-reported psychological well-being among middle-aged and older adults in contemporary china-results from the china health and nutrition survey. *Int. J. Environ. Res. Public Health* **2018**, *15*. [CrossRef]

77.   Fletcher, S.; Wright, C.; Jones, A.; Parkinson, K.; Adamson, A. Tracking of toddler fruit and vegetable preferences to intake and adiposity later in childhood. *Matern. Child Nutr.* **2017**, *13*. [CrossRef] [PubMed]

78.   Ramsay, S.A.; Rudley, M.; Tonnemaker, L.E.; Price, W.J. A comparison of college students' reported fruit and vegetable liking and intake from childhood to adulthood. *J. Am. Coll. Nutr.* **2017**, *36*, 28–37. [CrossRef]

79.   Park, H.; Shin, Y.; Kwon, O.; Kim, Y. Association of sensory liking for fat with dietary intake and metabolic syndrome in korean adults. *Nutrients* **2018**, *10*. [CrossRef]

80.   Charlot, K.; Malgoyre, A.; Bourrilhon, C. Proposition for a shortened version of the leeds food preference questionnaire (LFPQ). *Physiol. Behav.* **2019**, *199*, 244–251. [CrossRef] [PubMed]

81.   Potter, C.; Griggs, R.L.; Ferriday, D.; Rogers, P.J.; Brunstrom, J.M. Individual variability in preference for energy-dense foods fails to predict child BMI percentile. *Physiol. Behav.* **2017**, *176*, 3–8. [CrossRef] [PubMed]

82.   Low, J.Y.Q.; Lacy, K.E.; McBride, R.L.; Keast, R.S.J. The associations between oral complex carbohydrate sensitivity, BMI, liking, and consumption of complex carbohydrate based foods. *J. Food Sci.* **2018**, *83*, 2227–2236. [CrossRef] [PubMed]

83.   Ledikwe, J.H.; Ello-Martin, J.; Pelkman, C.L.; Birch, L.L.; Mannino, M.L.; Rolls, B.J. A reliable, valid questionnaire indicates that preference for dietary fat declines when following a reduced-fat diet. *Appetite* **2007**, *49*, 74–83. [CrossRef]

84.   Lowenstein, L.M.; Perrin, E.M.; Berry, D.; Vu, M.B.; Pullen Davis, L.; Cai, J.; Tzeng, J.P.; Ammerman, A.S. Childhood obesity prevention: Fathers' reflections with healthcare providers. *Child. Obes.* **2013**, *9*, 137–143. [CrossRef] [PubMed]

85.   Groele, B.; Glabska, D.; Gutkowska, K.; Guzek, D. Mother's fruit preferences and consumption support similar attitudes and behaviors in their children. *Int. J. Environ. Res. Public Health* **2018**, *15*. [CrossRef] [PubMed]

86.   Vollmer, R.L.; Baietto, J. Practices and preferences: Exploring the relationships between food-related parenting practices and child food preferences for high fat and/or sugar foods, fruits, and vegetables. *Appetite* **2017**, *113*, 134–140. [CrossRef] [PubMed]

87.   Nekitsing, C.; Hetherington, M.M.; Blundell-Birtill, P. Developing healthy food preferences in preschool children through taste exposure, sensory learning, and nutrition education. *Curr. Obes. Rep.* **2018**, *7*, 60–67. [CrossRef]

88.   Marty, L.; Miguet, M.; Bournez, M.; Nicklaus, S.; Chambaron, S.; Monnery-Patris, S. Do hedonic- versus nutrition-based attitudes toward food predict food choices? A cross-sectional study of 6- to 11-year-olds. *Int. J. Behav. Nutr. Phys. Act.* **2017**, *14*, 162. [CrossRef]

89.   Jalkanen, H.; Lindi, V.; Schwab, U.; Kiiskinen, S.; Venalainen, T.; Karhunen, L.; Lakka, T.A.; Eloranta, A.M. Eating behaviour is associated with eating frequency and food consumption in 6-8 year-old children: The physical activity and nutrition in children (PANIC) study. *Appetite* **2017**, *114*, 28–37. [CrossRef]

90.   Duffy, V.B.; Smith, S. Leveraging Technology to Deliver Tailored SNAP-Ed Messages. Available online: https://snaped.fns.usda.gov/success-stories/leveraging-technology-deliver-tailored-snap-ed-messages (accessed on 14 July 2019).

91.   Sadeghirad, B.; Duhaney, T.; Motaghipisheh, S.; Campbell, N.R.; Johnston, B.C. Influence of unhealthy food and beverage marketing on children's dietary intake and preference: A systematic review and meta-analysis of randomized trials. *Obes. Rev.* **2016**, *17*, 945–959. [CrossRef] [PubMed]

92.   De Wild, V.W.T.; de Graaf, C.; Jager, G. Use of different vegetable products to increase preschool-aged children's preference for and intake of a target vegetable: A randomized controlled trial. *J. Acad. Nutr. Diet.* **2017**, *117*, 859–866. [CrossRef] [PubMed]

93.   Magarey, A.; Mauch, C.; Mallan, K.; Perry, R.; Elovaris, R.; Meedeniya, J.; Byrne, R.; Daniels, L. Child dietary and eating behavior outcomes up to 3.5 years after an early feeding intervention: The NOURISH RCT. *Obesity (Silver Spring)* **2016**, *24*, 1537–1545. [CrossRef] [PubMed]

94.   Cunningham-Sabo, L.; Lohse, B. Cooking with Kids positively affects fourth graders' vegetable preferences and attitudes and self-efficacy for food and cooking. *Child. Obes.* **2013**, *9*, 549–556. [CrossRef] [PubMed]

95. Wall, D.E.; Least, C.; Gromis, J.; Lohse, B. Nutrition education intervention improves vegetable-related attitude, self-efficacy, preference, and knowledge of fourth-grade students. *J. Sch. Health* **2012**, *82*, 37–43. [CrossRef] [PubMed]

96. Ebneter, D.S.; Latner, J.D.; Nigg, C.R. Is less always more? The effects of low-fat labeling and caloric information on food intake, calorie estimates, taste preference, and health attributions. *Appetite* **2013**, *68*, 92–97. [CrossRef]

97. Carbonneau, E.; Bradette-Laplante, M.; Lamarche, B.; Provencher, V.; Begin, C.; Robitaille, J.; Desroches, S.; Vohl, M.C.; Corneau, L.; Lemieux, S. Development and validation of the food liking questionnaire in a French-Canadian population. *Nutrients* **2017**, *9*, 1337. [CrossRef]

98. Scarmo, S.; Henebery, K.; Peracchio, H.; Cartmel, B.; Lin, H.; Ermakov, I.V.; Gellermann, W.; Bernstein, P.S.; Duffy, V.B.; Mayne, S.T. Skin carotenoid status measured by resonance Raman spectroscopy as a biomarker of fruit and vegetable intake in preschool children. *Eur. J. Clin. Nutr.* **2012**, *66*, 555–560. [CrossRef]

99. Freitas, A.; Albuquerque, G.; Silva, C.; Oliveira, A. Appetite-related eating behaviours: An overview of assessment methods, determinants and effects on children's weight. *Ann. Nutr. Metab.* **2018**, *73*, 19–29. [CrossRef]

100. Fernandez-Alvira, J.M.; Bammann, K.; Eiben, G.; Hebestreit, A.; Kourides, Y.A.; Kovacs, E.; Michels, N.; Pala, V.; Reisch, L.; Russo, P.; et al. Prospective associations between dietary patterns and body composition changes in European children: The IDEFICS study. *Public Health Nutr.* **2017**, *20*, 3257–3265. [CrossRef]

101. Weber, D.R.; Moore, R.H.; Leonard, M.B.; Zemel, B.S. Fat and lean BMI reference curves in children and adolescents and their utility in identifying excess adiposity compared with BMI and percentage body fat. *Am. J. Clin. Nutr.* **2013**, *98*, 49–56. [CrossRef] [PubMed]

102. Oldman, S. Improving Diet & Physical Activity Behaviors through Tailored Mhealth Messages: Application to Childhood Obesity Prevention in a Pediatric Emergency Department. Master's Thesis, Health Promotion Sciences, University of Connecticut, Mansfield, CT, USA, 2018.

103. U.S. Department of Agriculture. SNAP-Ed Connection. Available online: https://snaped.fns.usda.gov/ (accessed on 14 July 2019).

6

Prevalence and Correlates of Preschool Overweight and Obesity Amidst the Nutrition Transition: Findings from a National Cross-Sectional Study in Lebanon

Lara Nasreddine [1,2], Nahla Hwalla [1,2], Angie Saliba [1], Christelle Akl [1] and Farah Naja [1,2,*]

[1]   Department of Nutrition and Food Science, Faculty of Agricultural and Food Sciences, American University of Beirut, P.O. Box 11-0236, Riad El Solh, Beirut, Lebanon; ln10@aub.edu.lb (L.N.); nahla@aub.edu.lb (N.H.); aes10@mail.aub.edu (A.S.); cristell@gmail.com (C.A.)

[2]   Nutrition, Obesity and Related Diseases (NORD), Office of Strategic Health Initiatives, American University of Beirut, P.O. Box 11-0236, Riad El Solh, Beirut, Lebanon

*   Correspondence: fn14@aub.edu.lb

Abstract: There is increasing evidence linking early life adiposity to disease risk later in life. This study aims at determining the prevalence and correlates of overweight and obesity among preschoolers in Lebanon. A national cross-sectional survey was conducted amongst 2–5 years old children ($n = 525$). Socio-demographic, lifestyle, dietary, and anthropometric data were obtained. The prevalence of overweight and obesity was estimated at 6.5% and 2.7%, respectively. Based on stepwise logistic regression for the prediction of overweight and obesity (combined), the variance accounted for by the first block (socioeconomic, parental characteristics) was 11.9%, with higher father's education (OR = 5.31, 95% CI: 1.04–27.26) and the presence of household helper (OR = 2.19, 95% CI: 1.05–4.56) being significant predictors. The second block of variables (eating habits) significantly improved the prediction of overweight/obesity to reach 21%, with eating in front of the television (OR = 1.07, 95% CI: 1.02–1.13) and satiety responsiveness (OR = 0.83, 95% CI: 0.70–0.99) being significantly associated with overweight/obesity. In the third block, fat intake remained a significant predictor of overweight/obesity (OR = 2.31, 95% CI: 1.13–4.75). This study identified specific risk factors for preschool overweight/obesity in Lebanon and characterized children from high socioeconomic backgrounds as important target groups for preventive interventions. These findings may be of significance to other middle-income countries in similar stages of nutrition transition.

Keywords: obesity; preschoolers; prevalence; correlates; diet; socioeconomic status; Lebanon

1. Introduction

Childhood obesity is increasingly recognized as a serious public health concern, with available evidence suggesting a dramatic increase in its worldwide prevalence over the past few decades [1,2]. This increase is documented as early as the preschool years. De Onis et al. [2] showed that the global prevalence of preschool overweight and obesity has escalated from 4.2% in 1990 to 6.7% in 2010, with a projected increase to 9.1% in 2020 [2]. The highest prevalence rates of preschool overweight and obesity in 2010 were reported for the regions of Northern Africa and Western Asia, with an estimate of 17% and 14.7%, respectively [2]. The prevalence of preschool overweight and obesity in these regions, which largely represent the Middle East and North Africa (MENA) region, is projected to rise to over 25% by 2020 [2].

Excess body weight usually results from a complex interaction of genetic, environmental, behavioral and social factors, which may, in concert, modulate the child's propensity for becoming overweight [3]. Increased food intake, frequent consumption of high-calorie sweetened beverages and television viewing have been frequently reported as key determinants of the risk of pediatric overweight and obesity [3,4]. Socioeconomic status (SES) has also been identified as an important modulator of the risk of childhood obesity, although discrepancies have been reported in the direction of the relationship between SES and pediatric obesity [5]. In high-income countries, the risk of childhood obesity has been shown to be the highest in lower socioeconomic groups [5], while the opposite was reported for low-income countries [5,6]. Less is known about the relationship between SES and childhood obesity in middle-income countries, particularly those undergoing the nutrition transition [5,6].

Pediatric obesity is associated with adverse physical and psychological effects that may appear in childhood and track into the adult years [7–9]. Short-term health consequences of pediatric obesity include metabolic abnormalities such as high blood pressure, dyslipidemia, impaired glucose homeostasis, and metabolic syndrome [7]. In the long term, pediatric obesity tends to persist into adulthood, increasing the risk for obesity-associated morbidities such as cardiovascular disease, type 2 diabetes and some types of cancer [8,9]. Psychologically, obese children commonly suffer from negative body image and low self-esteem [7], that often progress into anxiety and depression in adulthood [8]. Consequently, the early prevention of overweight and obesity is increasingly recognized as a vital strategy to decrease the burden of associated short- and long-term morbidity [10]. The preschool years are identified as an important stage for preventive interventions, as eating patterns established in young childhood tend to track into later life [11].

The development of effective intervention programs aiming at the prevention of pediatric obesity should be based on rigorous investigations of its determinants and associated factors [10]. Most of the studies investigating obesity correlates in preschoolers have been conducted in high-income countries [12] and, as such, findings may not be applicable to low and middle-income countries, where the highest increases in preschool obesity are projected to take place. Among the latter, the Middle East and North Africa (MENA) region has been largely under-represented [12]. In Lebanon, an upper-middle income country of the Eastern Mediterranean basin that is currently undergoing the nutrition transition [13], available evidence documents an increase in obesity prevalence amongst 6–18 years old children and adolescents [14]. However, data on the prevalence and correlates of preschool obesity are lacking. Based on a nationally representative survey, the present study aims at (1) determining the prevalence of overweight and obesity among 2–5 years old preschool children in Lebanon and (2) investigating the association of preschool overweight and obesity with socioeconomic factors, parental characteristics, dietary intakes and eating behavior. Gaining greater insight into factors that are associated with preschool overweight and obesity should orient further studies investigating early life obesity and assist policy makers in setting forth successful culture-specific obesity prevention strategies in the region. The present study undertaken in Lebanon, and particularly the identification of factors that modulate the risk of under-five overweight, may be viewed as a case-study for other middle-income countries in similar stages of the nutrition transition. The study responds to the United Nation's call for a worldwide commitment to address preschool overweight and reverse its rising trends, as included in the General Assembly's resolution proclaiming the UN Decade of Action on Nutrition (2016–2025) [15].

2. Materials and Methods

2.1. Study Population

The data for this study was drawn from the national survey, "Early Life Nutrition and Health in Lebanon", conducted on a representative sample of Lebanese children (0–5 years) and their mothers. The survey was undertaken between September 2011 and August 2012. A stratified cluster sampling strategy was followed, whereby the strata were the six Lebanese governorates and the clusters were selected further at the level of districts. Within each district, households were selected following a probability proportional to size approach, whereby a higher number of participating households were drawn from more populous districts. The selection of the households was carried out using systematic sampling. Housing units constituted the primary sampling units in the different districts of Lebanon. To participate in the study, the household ought to include a mother and a child below five years of age. The child had to be Lebanese, born at term (of gestational age at birth ≥37 weeks), not suffering from any chronic illness, inborn errors of metabolism or physical malformations that may interfere with his/her feeding patterns and body composition, and not reported as being ill during the past 24 h (i.e., on the day that would be recalled for food intake). Of the 1194 eligible households that were contacted, 1029 participated in the survey (response rate 86%). The main reasons for refusal were time constraint, child being sick, lack of husband's consent or disinterest in the study. In face to face interviews with participating mothers, trained nutritionists collected data, using age-specific multi-component questionnaires covering information on demographic, socioeconomic, eating habits and dietary intakes. Anthropometric measurements were obtained from both mother and child. Dietary intake was assessed using the United States Department of Agriculture (USDA) multiple pass 24-h recall (24-HR) [16]. Interviews were held in the household setting and lasted for approximately one hour. Quality control measures including pre-testing of the study instruments, equipment and data collection procedure in addition to training and field monitoring, were applied. All questionnaires were designed by a panel of experts including scientists in the fields of epidemiology and nutrition and were tested on a convenience sample of 100 households to check for clarity and cultural sensitivity.

2.2. Ethical Considerations

The design and conduct of the survey were performed according to the guidelines laid down in the Declaration of Helsinki, and all procedures involving human subjects were approved by the Institutional Review Board of the American University of Beirut. A written informed consent was obtained from all mothers prior to participation.

2.3. Data Collection

For the purpose of this study, data of children aged between 2 and 5 years were used ($n = 531$). The availability of this sample size allowed the estimation of a 10% prevalence of overweight and obesity at a 95% confidence interval and a precision of ±2.5% [17]. Survey data used in this study included demographic, socioeconomic, and parental characteristics, eating habits, anthropometric measurements, as well as dietary intakes. Demographic characteristics consisted of the following: sex of the child, age of the child and the mother (in years), mother's marital status (married, not married) and number of children in the family; socioeconomic indicators included father's and mother's education levels (primary or less, intermediate, high school, and above) and household's monthly income, which are the most commonly utilized indicators of socioeconomic status [18], in addition to mother's employment (working, not working), presence of paid household helper, and household crowding index. Moreover, given that the formal age at which children enroll in the preprimary level of schools is three years in Lebanon [19], information on the type of school the child attends (private vs. public) was also obtained as one of the socioeconomic indicators. In fact, in Lebanon, there exist strong social inequalities among those attending private and public schools, with the private schools enrolling the highest proportion of students from a high SES, and the public schools enrolling those from a low SES [19,20]. The assessment of the child's eating habits included weekly frequency of breakfast consumption, eating in front of the television (TV), eating out, and eating the same meal with the family. In addition, early life feeding practices were assessed by the mother's retrospective recall of breastfeeding duration, age of introduction of formula and of solid food. The child satiety responsiveness and food responsiveness were evaluated using questions derived from the Child Eating Behaviour Questionnaire (CEBQ) [21].

2.4. Anthropometric Assessment

Information on birth weight of the child was obtained from the mother. Anthropometric measurements were performed, including weight and height of both mothers and children. Participants were weighed to the nearest 0.1 kg in light indoor clothing and with bare feet or stockings, using a standard clinical balance (Seca, model 770, Hamburg, Germany). Measurements of the weight were taken twice and repeated a third time if the first two measurements differed by more than 0.3 kg. Using a portable stadiometer (Seca, model 213, Hamburg, Germany) height was measured without shoes. Measurements of the height were taken twice and repeated a third time if the first two measurements differ by more than 0.5 cm. The average values of weight and height were used for the calculation of BMI, which is computed as the ratio of weight (kilograms) to the square of height (meters). Weight and height were not collected from women who were pregnant at the time of the interview ($n = 42$), due to the limitations of BMI use during pregnancy.

Overweight and obesity among mothers were assessed using the World Health Organization (WHO) criteria for body mass index (BMI) [22]. For children, the prevalence of overweight and obesity was assessed using the WHO-2006 criteria based on sex and age specific BMI z-scores, which were calculated using the WHO AnthroPlus software (WHO 2009, Department of Nutrition for Health and Development, Switzerland, Geneva) [23,24]. Accordingly, the following cutoffs were adopted: $+1 < $ BMI-for-age z-score $\leq +2$ (at risk of overweight), $+2 < $ BMI-for-age z-score $\leq +3$ (overweight), and BMI-for-age z-score $> +3$ (obesity). In addition, and in order to allow for comparability with other studies, the prevalence of overweight and obesity was assessed using two other definitions, including the Center for Disease Control and Prevention-2000 (CDC-2000) and International Obesity Task Force (IOTF):

1. According to the CDC 2000 reference [25,26] cut-off values were defined based on sex and age specific BMI percentiles: 85th to <95th percentile (overweight) and ≥95th percentile (obesity).
2. According to the IOTF standard [27], overweight and obesity were based on centiles passing at age 18 years through BMI 25 kg/m^2 and 30 kg/m^2, respectively.

2.5. Dietary Intake of Children

Dietary intake of children was assessed by a single multiple pass 24 HR. Even though various methods have been developed for the assessment of dietary consumption, including dietary recalls, food frequency questionnaires (FFQs) and food records [28], the choice of the 24 HR approach in this study may be explained by (1) the lack of validated culture-specific FFQs targeting under-five children in Lebanon and the MENA region; and (2) the practical difficulties of using food records in the context of national surveys, given the burden that this method may impose on participants and given its literacy requirements [28]. In addition, acknowledging the practical challenges of administering repeated multiple 24 HRs in the context of a national survey and the impact that this approach may have on response rate [29], we have opted to use a single 24 HR, with mothers serving as the main proxy. In case another caretaker shared the responsibility of feeding the child, the mother directly consulted with him/her for additional information pertinent to the dietary interview. The 24-HRs were carried using the multiple pass food recall five-step approach, developed by the USDA [16]. This approach has consistently showed attenuation in the 24-HRs' limitations [30]. The steps followed included (1) quick food list recall; (2) forgotten food list probe; (3) time and occasion at which foods were consumed; (4) detailed overall cycle; and (5) a final probe review of the foods consumed. While collecting the dietary data, specific reference was made to solicit information about food that were consumed at daycare or school. The Nutritionist Pro software (version 5.1.0, 2014, First Data Bank, Nutritionist Pro, Axxya Systems, San Bruno, CA, USA) was used for the analysis of the dietary intake data and to estimate energy and macronutrients' intakes. For composite and mixed dishes, standardized recipes were added to the Nutritionist Pro software using single food items. Within the Nutritionist Pro, the USDA database was selected for analysis (SR 24, published September 2011). Food composition of specific Lebanese foods (not included in the Nutritionist Pro software database) was obtained from food composition tables for use in the Middle East [31].

2.6. Data Analysis

Frequencies and percentages, as well as means and standard deviations (SD), were used to describe categorical and continuous variables, respectively. Crowding index was calculated as the total number of co-residents per household divided by the total number of rooms, excluding the kitchen and bathrooms. Bivariate logistic regression was used to examine the sociodemographic, eating habits and dietary intake correlates of overweight and obesity in the study population. In this regression, the dependent variable was 'overweight/obesity', as defined by the WHO-2006 (BMI-for-age z-score > +2) [23]. In order to examine the independent effect of each group of variables (sociodemographic and parental characteristics, eating habits and dietary intake) in predicting overweight and obesity, a stepwise logistic regression was conducted. Block 1 consisted of sociodemographic and parental characteristics, block 2 included eating habits variables and block 3 was comprised of dietary intake data. Variables chosen to be included in the multivariate modeling were either significant in the bi-variate analysis and/or were important according to the literature. Data analysis was carried out using Statistical Package for Social Sciences 22.0 (SPSS for Windows, 2013, SPSS Inc., Chicago, IL, USA). A p-value less than 0.05 was considered statistically significant.

3. Results

Out of the 531 survey participants, six children had incomplete sociodemographic and dietary data and, hence, were excluded from the remaining analyses and results. Among children participating in this study (n = 525), prevalence rates of overweight and obesity using the four definitions are presented in Table 1. According to the WHO-2006 criteria, prevalence estimates of overweight and obesity were 6.5% and 2.7%, respectively. Higher estimates were obtained using IOTF and CDC-2000 reference cutoffs, with the latter presenting the highest estimates (overweight 16.1% and obesity 10.6%). Although the WHO-2006 presented lowest estimates of overweight and obesity compared to other references, it also had the lowest prevalence of normal weight (64.6%) since, according to this reference, a proportion of normal weight are grouped under a distinct category called 'at risk of overweight', with a prevalence of 26.3%. This particular category does not exist within the other references. No significant difference in overweight or obesity rates were observed between boys and girls (Table 1).

Table 1. Overweight/obesity prevalence among 2–5 years old Lebanese preschoolers, according to WHO-2006, IOTF and CDC-2000 criteria.

Weight Status	Total (n = 525)	Boys (n = 281)	Girls (n = 244)
	n (%)		
WHO-2006 reference [a]			
Normal weight [b]	339 (64.6)	177 (63.0)	162 (66.4)
At risk of overweight	138 (26.3)	78 (27.8)	60 (24.6)
Overweight [c]	34 (6.5)	18 (6.4)	16 (6.6)
Obese	14 (2.7)	8 (2.8)	6 (2.5)
Overweight and obese	48 (9.1)	26 (9.3)	22 (9.0)
IOTF reference [d]			
Normal weight [b]	433 (82.8)	235 (84.2)	198 (81.1)
Overweight [c]	70 (13.4)	36 (12.9)	34 (13.9)
Obese	20 (3.8)	8 (2.9)	12 (4.9)
Overweight and obese	90 (17.2)	44 (15.8)	46 (18.8)
CDC-2000 reference [e]			
Normal weight [b]	383 (73.1)	207 (74.2)	176 (72.1)
Overweight [c]	84 (16.1)	41 (14.7)	43 (17.6)
Obese	56 (10.6)	31 (11.1)	25 (10.2)
Overweight and obese	140 (26.8)	72 (25.8)	68 (27.9)

No significant differences between genders were observed. [a] World Health Organization-2006 reference [23]; [b] The normal weight category included thinness, with only one child identified as thin based on the WHO 2006 criteria [23], 18 based on IOTF criteria [32], and 16 based on CDC [25,26]; [c] "Overweight" category does not include "Obese"; [d] International Obesity Task Force reference [27]; [e] Center for Disease Control and Prevention-2000 reference [25,26].

Table 2 presents descriptive statistics for the sociodemographic, socioeconomic, and parental characteristics, eating habits, and dietary intake of study participants, in addition to the univariate associations of these correlates with overweight (including obesity) (BMI-for-age z-score > +2). The mean age of preschoolers was of 3.3 ± 0.87 years, with 53.5% boys and 46.5% girls. Most parents had intermediate level education (62.8% of fathers and 61.5% of mothers). The majority of mothers did not work (85.1%) and most of the households did not have a household helper (84.1%). Average maternal BMI was estimated at 26.71 ± 5.18 kg/m² (Table 2), with the prevalence of overweight and obesity being estimated at 58.4% among mothers (34.3% overweight and 24.1% obese) (data not shown). When looking at early life feeding practices, almost half of the participating preschoolers were breastfed for less than six months (47.8%), 16.8% for 6–11 months (data not shown) and 35.4% for more than 12 months. The average breastfeeding duration was estimated at 8.9 ± 8.7 months, while the average age of formula milk introduction and of solid food introduction were estimated at 1.3 ± 1.7 and 5.8 ± 2.49 months, respectively. In the study sample, the average weekly frequency of eating breakfast was of 6.7 ± 1.6, while the mean frequencies of "eating in front of the TV" and of "eating the same meal as the family" were estimated at 4.8 ± 6 and 10.7 ± 6.2, respectively. As for dietary intake variables, energy and macronutrient consumption were categorized as above or below the respective median values. These median values corresponded to 1509 kcal/day for energy, 39.3% for "energy consumption from fat", 48.6% for "energy consumption from CHO", and 13.15% for energy consumption from protein. As shown in Table 2, lower odds of overweight/obesity were found in families with number of children ≥3, attending a public school, a crowding index ≥1, longer duration of breastfeeding (≥12 months), eating the same meal with the family at home and a higher satiety responsiveness. The odds of overweight/obesity increased significantly with father's education level, mother's education level, presence of paid helper at home, income higher than 1,500,000 Lebanese lira (LL), mother's BMI, higher frequency of eating while watching TV, eating out, and a greater food responsiveness. Among dietary intake variables, energy consumption from fat was associated with a higher odd of overweight/obesity (Table 2).

Table 2. Association of demographic, socioeconomic, eating habits and dietary intakes with preschoolers' weight status, Lebanon (n = 525) [a].

Variables	Total [b] (n = 525)	Normal Weight (Including at Risk of Overweight) (n = 477)	Overweight (Not Including Obese) (n = 34)	Obese (n = 14)	Univariate Analysis [d]
		Children Adiposity Status [c]			
	Demographic, socioeconomic and parental characteristics n (%)				OR [95% CI]
Gender					
Boys	281 (53.5)	255 (53.5)	18 (52.9)	8 (57.1)	1 [ref]
Girls	244 (46.5)	222 (46.5)	16 (47.1)	6 (42.9)	0.97 [0.53–1.76]
Child's Age (years)					
mean ± SD	3.32 + 0.87	3.32 + 0.88	3.33 + 0.78	3.53 + 0.57	1.08 [0.77–1.53]
Mother's Age (years)					
mean ± SD	32.78 + 5.97	32.68 + 5.92	33.11 + 6.49	35.21 + 6.27	1.02 [0.98–1.08]
Mother's marital status					
Married	514 (97.9)	468 (98.1)	33 (97.1)	13 (92.9)	1 [ref]
Unmarried (divorced or widowed)	11 (2.1)	9 (1.9)	1 (2.9)	1 (7.1)	2.26 [0.47–10.77]
Number of children in the family					
≤2 children	272 (51.8)	236 (49.5)	26 (76.5)	10 (71.4)	1 [ref]
≥3 children	253 (48.2)	241 (50.5)	8 (23.5)	4 (28.6)	**0.32 [0.16–0.64]**
Type of school attended [e]					
Private	310 (74.5)	274 (72.9)	25 (89.3)	11 (91.7)	1 [ref]
Public	106 (25.5)	102 (27.1)	3 (10.7)	1 (8.3)	**0.29 [0.10–0.86]**

Table 2. *Cont.*

Variables		Children Adiposity Status [c]			
	Total [b] (*n* = 525)	Normal Weight (Including at Risk of Overweight) (*n* = 477)	Overweight (Not Including Obese) (*n* = 34)	Obese (*n* = 14)	Univariate Analysis [d]
	Demographic, socioeconomic and parental characteristics *n* (%)				OR [95% CI]
Father's education					
Primary or less	116 (22.1)	114 (24.3)	2 (6.1)	0 (0.0)	1 [ref]
Intermediate	324 (62.8)	290 (61.8)	26 (78.8)	8 (57.1)	**6.68** [1.57–28.27]
High school and above	76 (14.7)	65 (13.9)	5 (15.2)	6 (42.9)	**9.64** [2.07–44.86]
Mother's education					
Primary or less	101 (19.2)	98 (20.5)	2 (5.9)	1 (7.1)	1 [ref]
Intermediate	323 (61.5)	292 (61.2)	23 (67.6)	8 (57.1)	**3.46** [1.03–11.59]
High school and above	101 (19.2)	87 (18.2)	9 (26.5)	5 (35.7)	**5.25** [1.46–18.90]
Mother's employment					
Working	78 (14.9)	68 (14.3)	5 (14.7)	5 (35.7)	1 [ref]
Not Working	447 (85.1)	409 (85.7)	29 (85.3)	9 (64.3)	0.63 [0.30–1.32]
Presence of paid helper					
No	439 (84.1)	406 (85.7)	25 (73.5)	8 (57.1)	1 [ref]
Yes	83 (15.9)	68 (14.3)	9 (26.5)	6 (42.9)	**2.71** [1.40–5.26]
Crowding index					
<1 person/room	60 (11.5)	50 (10.5)	6 (17.6)	4 (28.6)	1 [ref]
≥1 person/room	464 (88.5)	426 (89.5)	28 (82.4)	10 (71.4)	**0.45** [0.21–0.96]
Monthly income					
Low (<1,000,000 LL)	172 (39.3)	161 (40.6)	10 (33.3)	1 (9.1)	1 [ref]
Medium (1,000,000–1,500,000 LL)	108 (24.7)	100 (25.2)	8 (26.7)	0 (0.0)	1.17 [0.45–3.01]
High (>1,500,000 LL)	158 (36.1)	136 (34.3)	12 (40.0)	10 (90.9)	**2.36** [1.10–5.05]
Mother's BMI (Kg/m^2) *	26.71 ± 5.18	26.59 ± 5.17	27.99 ± 5.63	27.51 ± 4.40	**1.05** [1.00–1.10]
	Breastfeeding history and eating habits				OR [95% CI]
Breastfeeding duration					
<12 months	339 (64.6)	300 (62.9)	26 (76.5)	13 (92.9)	**1 [ref]**
≥12 months	186 (35.4)	177 (37.1)	8 (23.5)	1 (7.1)	**0.39 [0.18–0.82]**
Breastfeeding duration (in months)	8.94 ± 8.73	9.11 ± 8.92	8.10 ± 6.84	4.92 ± 3.85	1 [ref] 0.97 [0.94–1.01]
Age of formula/cow's milk's introduction (months)	1.34 ± 1.71	1.34 ± 1.70	1.66 ± 2.07	0.70 ± 0.89	1 [ref] 0.99 [0.78–1.27]
Age of solid food's introduction (months)	5.80 ± 2.49	5.75 ± 2.51	6.48 ± 2.57	5.89 ± 1.47	1 [ref] 1.07 [0.98–1.18]
Child's birth weight (kg)	3.19 ± 0.55	3.18 ± 0.56	3.30 ± 0.52	3.32 ± 0.49	1.00 [1.00–1.01]
Eating breakfast (weekly frequency)	6.74 ± 1.64	6.75 ± 1.68	6.88 ± 0.53	6.21 ± 2.00	0.97 [0.81–1.16]
Eating in front of the TV (weekly frequency)	4.81 ± 6.00	4.61 ± 5.59	6.67 ± 9.87	7.14 ± 6.58	**1.04 [1.01–1.09]**
Eating out (weekly frequency)	0.40 ± 0.87	0.38 ± 0.78	0.70 ± 1.65	0.57 ± 0.82	**1.27 [1.01–1.62]**
Eating the same meal as the family at home (weekly frequency)	10.74 ± 6.24	10.92 ± 6.29	9.55 ± 5.55	7.60 ± 5.54	**0.94 [0.89–0.99]**
Satiety responsiveness	8.56 ± 2.15	8.63 ± 2.15	7.94 ± 2.02	7.71 ± 2.05	**0.84 [0.73–0.97]**
Food responsiveness	3.87 ± 1.39	3.82 ± 1.37	3.97 ± 1.50	5.14 ± 1.46	**1.28 [1.03–1.58]**

Table 2. *Cont.*

Variables	Total [b] (*n* = 525)	Normal Weight (Including at Risk of Overweight) (*n* = 477)	Overweight (Not Including Obese) (*n* = 34)	Obese (*n* = 14)	Univariate Analysis [d]
		Children Adiposity Status [c]			
		Dietary intake (per day) [f] *n* (%)			OR [95% CI]
Total energy (Kcal)					
Below the median [f]	258 (50.1)	234 (50.1)	18 (52.9)	61 (42.9)	1 [ref]
Above the median [f]	257 (49.9)	233 (49.9)	16 (47.1)	8 (57.1)	1.00 [0.55–1.81]
Energy consumption from fat (%)					
Below the median [f]	259 (50.3)	243 (52.0)	11 (32.4)	5 (35.7)	1 [ref]
Above the median [f]	256 (49.7)	224 (48.0)	23 (67.6)	9 (64.3)	**2.17 [1.15–4.06]**
Energy consumption from CHO (%)					
Below the median [f]	257 (49.9)	227 (48.6)	22 (64.7)	8 (57.1)	1 [ref]
Above the median [f]	258 (50.1)	240 (51.4)	12 (35.3)	6 (42.9)	0.56 [0.30–1.04]
Energy consumption from protein (%)					
Below the median [f]	260 (50.5)	240 (51.4)	11 (32.4)	9 (64.3)	1 [ref]
Above the median [f]	255 (49.5)	227 (48.6)	23 (67.6)	5 (35.7)	1.48 [0.81–2.70]

OR: odds ratio for overweight/obesity vs. normal weight; CI: confidence interval; TV: television; CHO: carbohydrates. [a] In this table, continuous and categorical variables are presented as mean ± SD and *n* (%), respectively; [b] Lack of corresponding sum of frequencies with total sample size is due to missing data; [c] Children adiposity status based on the WHO 2006 BMI-for-age z-score cut-offs [23]; Normal weight (including at risk of overweight): −2 ≤ z-score ≤ +2; Overweight (not including obese): +2 < z-score ≤ +3; Obese: z-score > +3; [d] Crude logistic regression was conducted with the outcome variable being "overweight" and "obese"combined; [e] The sum of frequencies does not correspond to the total sample size given that preschoolers below the age of three years do not go to school. [f] Median for "total energy" corresponds to 1509 kcal; median for "energy consumption from fat" corresponds to 39.3%; median for "energy consumption from CHO" corresponds to 48.6%; median for "energy consumption from protein" corresponds to 13.15%; * The number of mothers included in this variable is 483, after exclusion of pregnant women (*n* = 42). Bolded numbers are significant at $p < 0.05$.

The results of the stepwise logistic regression examining the independent effects of socioeconomic and parental characteristics, eating habits, as well as dietary intakes on the odds of overweight/obesity are presented in Table 3. The variance accounted for by the first block (socioeconomic and parental characteristics) was 11.9%. Within this block, father's education, mother's BMI, presence of a paid helper, and crowding index made significant contributions ($p < 0.05$) to the prediction of overweight/obesity among study participants. The second block of variables was related to early life feeding and eating habits, including breastfeeding duration, eating while watching TV, eating out, eating the same meal with the family at home, satiety responsiveness, and food responsiveness. After controlling for the socioeconomic and parental characteristics, these variables significantly improved the prediction of overweight/obesity to reach 21% ($p < 0.01$). Eating in front of the TV was associated with an 8% increase in the odds of overweight/obesity (OR: 1.08, 95% CI: 1.02–1.1), while a higher score of satiety responsiveness was associated with lower odds of overweight/obesity in the study population (OR: 0.8, 95% CI: 0.68–0.99). As for the third block (dietary intakes), energy consumption from fat remained a significant predictor of preschool overweight/obesity, after adjusting for other variables (OR: 2.31, 95% CI: 1.13–4.75). (Table 3).

Given the association between preschool overweight/obesity and fat intake, additional analyses were conducted to assess the major food contributors to fat and energy intakes in the study sample. The results showed that, besides milk and dairy products which appeared as the largest contributor to fat intake (24.4%), the main sources of fat were fast food and salty snacks (21.6%), followed by beef, poultry, and eggs (12.3%), rice and rice-based dishes (8.7%), and sweet deserts (8.2%). Similarly, the main contributor to daily energy intake was milk and dairy products (17.6%), followed by fast food and salty snacks (16.2%), breads (12.5%), sweets (9.6%), meat, poultry, and eggs (9.04%), rice and rice-based dishes (7.8%), and sweetened beverages (6.1%) (data not shown).

Table 3. Associations of overweight [a] with selected demographic, socioeconomic, parental, and dietary variables among preschoolers ($n = 525$).

Variables	Model 1 [b]	Model 2 [b]	Model 3 [b]
	OR [95% CI]		
Demographic, socioeconomic and parental variables			
Gender			
Boys	1 [ref]	1 [ref]	1 [ref]
Girls	0.97 [0.52–1.83]	1.07 [0.56–2.07]	0.96 [0.49–1.88]
Child's age (years)			
mean ± SD	0.99 [0.68–1.44]	0.91 [0.63–1.33]	0.92 [0.63–1.35]
Father's education [c]			
Primary or less	1 [ref]	1 [ref]	1 [ref]
Intermediate	**5.16 [1.19–22.41]**	**5.81 [1.27–26.51]**	**5.77 [1.24–26.96]**
High school and above	**5.31 [1.04–27.26]**	5.22 [0.96–28.39]	5.02 [1.03–27.91]
Mother's BMI (Kg/m^2)			
mean ± SD	**1.06 [1.01–1.13]**	**1.09 [1.03–1.16]**	**1.08 [1.02–1.15]**
Presence of paid helper			
No	1 [ref]	1 [ref]	1 [ref]
Yes	**2.19 [1.05–4.56]**	**2.34 [1.05–5.21]**	**2.30 [1.02–5.17]**
Crowding index			
<1 person/room	1 [ref]	1 [ref]	1 [ref]
≥1 person/room	**0.42 [0.19–0.97]**	0.47 [0.19–1.15]	**0.41 [0.17–1.02]**
Breastfeeding history and eating habits			
Breastfeeding duration	------------		
<12 months		1 [ref]	1 [ref]
≥12 months		0.62 [0.27–1.42]	0.62 [0.27–1.44]
Eating in front of the TV	------------	**1.07 [1.02–1.13]**	**1.08 [1.02–1.14]**
Eating out	------------	1.23 [0.93–1.63]	1.22 [0.92–1.62]
Eating the same meal as the family at home	------------	0.95 [0.89–1.01]	0.95 [0.89–1.01]
Satiety responsiveness	------------	**0.83 [0.70–0.99]**	**0.8 [0.68–0.99]**
Food responsiveness	------------	1.14 [0.87–1.49]	1.16 [0.88–1.52]
Dietary variables			
Total daily energy (Kcal) [d]	------------	------------	
Low			1 [ref]
High			0.72 [0.35–1.50]
Energy consumption from Fat (%) [d,e]	------------	------------	
Low			1 [ref]
High			**2.31 [1.13–4.75]**
−2 Log Likelihood	274.89	252.82	247.2
Nagelkerke R^2	0.12	0.21	0.23
Nagelkerke R^2 difference	0.12	0.09	0.02

OR: odds ratio; CI: confidence interval. [a] Overweight (including obesity) defined based on the WHO 2006 sex and age specific + 2 BMI z-scores [23]; [b] Model 1: adjusted for gender, age, father's education, presence of paid helper, crowding index and mother's BMI; Model 2 = Model 1 + adjustment for eating behavior variables; Model 3 = Model 2 + adjustment for dietary variables; [c] Low, medium and high education levels refer to primary or less, intermediate or high school and above, respectively; [d] Low and high total energy and energy from fat refer to first and second median, respectively; [e] Fat intake based on percent contribution to daily energy intake. Bolded numbers are significant at $p < 0.05$.

4. Discussion

This paper reports on the national prevalence of overweight and obesity in Lebanese 2–5 years old preschoolers and provides evidence linking specific socioeconomic, dietary, and lifestyle factors to increased risk of overweight and obesity in this age group. In view of the scarcity of data on the determinants of childhood obesity in the MENA, the present study's findings may be viewed as a case-study for other middle-income countries of the region, in similar stages of the nutrition transition.

Using the WHO-2006 BMI criteria, findings of this study show that the prevalence of overweight/obesity combined (BMI-for-age z-score > +2) (9.1%) amongst Lebanese preschoolers exceeds the global prevalence estimate of preschool overweight/obesity for 2010 (6.7%), as well as the estimate reported for developing countries (6.1%) [2]. The prevalence rates of overweight (6.4% in boys and 6.6% in girls) and obesity (2.8% in boys and 2.5% in girls) amongst Lebanese preschoolers are similar to those reported from several European countries, while being lower than those reported from some other MENA countries such as Bahrain and Qatar [33–44]. (Table 4). To allow for a comparison with findings reported from other countries, data were re-analyzed according to the IOTF and CDC criteria. Based on the IOTF criteria, current prevalence estimates of overweight (12.9% in boys and 13.9% in girls) and obesity (2.9% in boys and 4.9% in girls) amongst Lebanese preschoolers are within the range reported from developed countries such as Australia and Canada [33,44–46]. When using the CDC criteria, the prevalence estimates of preschool overweight (14.7% in boys and 17.6% in girls) and obesity (11.1% in boys and 10.2% in girls) in Lebanon are found to be higher than those reported from Iran (overweight: 9.8 and 10.3% respectively; obesity: 4.8 and 4.5% respectively) [47], with the prevalence of obesity being also higher than that reported from the United States of America [48].

Table 4. Prevalence of overweight and obesity among Lebanese preschool children compared to those in selected countries.

Country	Date of Surveys	Criteria Used	Age (Years)	Overweight [b] (%)		Obesity (%)	
				Boys	Girls	Boys	Girls
		WHO-2006 [c]					
Lebanon [a]	2010		2–5	6.4	6.6	2.8	2.5
China (Beijing) [41]	2004		2–5	4.6	2.7	2.9	1.7
Bahrain [39]	2003		2–5	9.8	10.1	7.1	5.9
Jordan [42]	2010		1–5	6.7	7.3	2.5	1.1
Qatar (Doha) [40]	2009–2010		2–5	10.6	15.2	15.5	12.5
The Netherlands [34]	2002–2006		2–5	6	4.1	5	2.9
Romania [35]	2004		2–5	5.7	4.2	2.1	2.2
Spain [43]	2006		2–5	9.6	12.2	8.8	4.4
Italy [36]	2005		2–5	5.9	5.7	4.1	2.6
Cyprus [37,38]	2004		2–5	3.3	4.7	1.8	1.3
England [44]	2002		2–5	9.8	7.5	2.5	2.2
		IOTF [d]					
Lebanon [a]	2010		2–5	12.9	13.9	2.9	4.9
Canada [46]	2004		2–5	13	19	6	6
Australia [45]	2007		2–3	17	14	4	4
		CDC [e]					
Lebanon [a]	2010		2–5	14.7	17.6	11.1	10.2
Iran (Tehran) [47]	2009–2010		3–6	9.8	10.3	4.8	4.5
United States of America [48]	2011–2012		2–5	23.9	21.7	9.5	7.2
Saudi Arabia (Khobar) [49]	2006		2–4	19.6	16.3	20	18.1

[a] Current study; [b] Overweight (not including obesity); [c] WHO-2006: World Health organization 2006 reference [23]; [d] IOTF: International Obesity Task Force [27]; [e] CDC: Center for Disease Control and Prevention-2000 [25,26].

Pediatric obesity and excess body weight often result from a complex interaction between genetic and lifestyle factors [10]. Our finding of a positive significant association between preschool overweight/obesity and maternal BMI corroborates those reported from other studies and underscores the importance of genetic factors in the etiology of body fatness [10,50]. Our study's findings also underscore the importance of socioeconomic and lifestyle factors in modulating the risk of pediatric overweight. To our knowledge, this study is the first from the MENA region to investigate and document a positive association between preschool overweight/obesity and SES as assessed by several indicators, including type of school attended, father's educational level, mother's educational level, presence of a paid helper, crowding index, and monthly income. Socioeconomic and parental characteristics made the highest contributions to the prediction of overweight/obesity among study participants, accounting for 12% of the model variance. Previous studies conducted in other parts of the world suggest that SES affects the risk of developing obesity in children, but available evidence highlights disparities in the relationship between SES and pediatric obesity in industrialized vs. developing countries [51]. While children from low SES groups are at higher risk of obesity in industrialized countries, pediatric obesity appears to be predominantly a problem of the rich in low-income countries [18,51]. Less is, however, known about the relationship between SES and childhood obesity in middle-income countries, particularly those undergoing the nutrition transition [5,6]. The present study showed that, in Lebanon, a middle-income country undergoing the nutrition transition, the odds of preschool overweight/obesity were positively associated with SES. In fact, higher paternal education, which is one of the most commonly adopted SES indicators [18], was associated with a five-fold increase in the odds of preschool overweight/obesity, and a higher crowding index, which reflects a lower SES, was associated with lower odds of overweight/obesity in this age group. These findings are in agreement with those reported from several developing countries [52,53] and highlight the role of upward mobility and SES in modulating the family's economic and cultural resources, all of which may bear ramifications on lifestyle and, therefore, obesity risk in childhood. The observed positive association between SES and preschool overweight/obesity in Lebanon may be explained by the fact that children from affluent families may have higher access to energy-rich diets and electronic games as well as more opportunities for eating out, putting them at a higher risk for positive energy balance and weight gain [5]. Additional analyses conducted in this study have in fact shown significant associations between "eating out", "eating the same meal with the family", and main drivers of SES, such as paternal education (data not shown).

Of interest, the study findings showed that the presence of a paid helper in the household was associated with a two-fold increase in the odds of overweight/obesity in Lebanese preschoolers, even after adjustment for other SES indicators including father's education and crowding index. It is important to note that in the Lebanese context, the responsibility of feeding the child is often shared with the household helper, and this type of child care is becoming increasingly common in the country. Available estimates suggest that, in 2010, Lebanon hosted 117,941 paid sleep-in domestic workers who come from foreign countries, including the Philippines, Sri Lanka, Ethiopia, and Bangladesh, and who live in their employer's house for the duration of their contract [54]. Our findings of a positive association between preschool overweight/obesity and the presence of a household helper echo those reported by a population-based birth cohort of Chinese children, where "informal" non-parental child care at each of 3, 5, or 11 years of age was independently associated with higher BMI-for-age z-scores and with the presence of childhood overweight levels [55]. Our results are also in agreement with findings stemming from Western societies, where several studies [56–58] have reported an association between pediatric obesity and "informal" rather than parental child care [55]. Needless to say that caregivers, including household helpers, may play an important role in influencing the child's dietary practices and eating habits [59]. While parents may play a more active role in supervising the child's eating behavior, household helpers, who are usually hired for housework as well as child care, may not be able to spend much time and effort on enforcing dietary recommendations, limiting the child's consumption of energy-dense favorite foods or restraining TV viewing [55]. In our study, the time spent on TV viewing was not directly assessed, but a positive association was found between preschool overweight/obesity and eating while watching TV. Several studies have shown that eating in front of the TV is positively associated with higher BMI among children, an association that is independent of the overall time spent watching TV or the sedentary behavior that accompanies it [60,61]. Dubois et al. showed that four- to five-year-old children who frequently ate in front of the TV had higher BMI relative to their peers, while no significant associations were found between the child's BMI and the overall time spent watching TV [3]. There are several mechanisms that could link preschool obesity to the act of eating while watching TV. First, children who eat in front of the TV may miss out on the nutritional and psychosocial benefits of family meals [3,61]. In addition, eating in front of the TV is associated with increased exposure to the advertisements of unhealthy foods at meal time hours and with mindless eating that often results in the consumption of larger food portions [62]. Available evidence suggests that children who are given the opportunity to eat while watching TV may become less sensitive to internal cues of satiety [63]. In this study, higher satiety responsiveness was associated with significantly lower odds of overweight/obesity in preschoolers. These findings are in agreement with previously reported inverse association between satiety response and preschoolers' BMI [64,65].

The results of the present study showed that higher dietary fat intake was associated with a two-fold increase in the prevalence of preschool overweight/obesity. Even though the evidence in the literature is inconsistent, several studies have shown that percentage energy intake from fat was greater in obese children compared with their non-obese counterparts, although total energy intake was not different, a finding that is in agreement with the results of the present study [66–68]. Other studies using BMI and or skinfold measures to estimate adiposity have documented a positive association between the percentage of energy intake from fat and body fatness in children before and after controlling for maternal BMI, a finding that is also in agreement with the results of the present study [69,70]. There are a number of mechanisms through which dietary fat may play a role in the development of overweight and obesity. Compared to protein and carbohydrate, fat is more palatable and energy dense, has less ability to regulate hunger and satiety and, hence, is more likely to lead to passive over-consumption [69,71,72]. In addition, and in contrast to protein and carbohydrate, which have comparatively limited storage capacity and are therefore preferentially oxidized when energy intake exceeds expenditure, there is no regulation of fat balance or limit on storage of excess energy from fat, making it more efficiently (about 96%) stored than excess carbohydrate energy (60% ± 80%) [66,73]. Thus, given the poor regulation of fat at both the levels of consumption and oxidation, a chronically high fat diet may compromise the regulation of energy balance and lead to weight gain [71,72]. The study findings may thus call for dietary intervention strategies aiming at reducing fat intake amongst preschoolers in Lebanon [74]. These interventions should, at least partly, focus on the observed main sources of fat in this age group, which included fast food, salty snacks, and sweets.

The strengths of the study include the national design of the survey, the use of a culture and population specific questionnaire in data collection and the measurements of anthropometric characteristics instead of self-reporting. In addition, several indicators were used in this study for the assessment of SES, all of which have converged in documenting a positive association with preschool overweight/obesity in Lebanon. The results of this study should, however, be considered in light of the following limitations. Though every effort was exerted in order to ensure the representativeness of the sample, a comparison of the study sample distribution across governorates with that of the Lebanese population for the same age group showed a few discrepancies. For instance, while South Lebanon constitutes 21.1% of the population, this percentage was only 16.8% in the study population. This difference was compensated by a higher representation of Mount Lebanon (32% in the study sample vs. 28.8% in the population), and Beirut (10.5% in the study sample vs. 7.7% in the population). Such discrepancies resulted from the fact that the research team faced security clearance challenges in South Lebanon, whereby access to this governorate is controlled by tight security measures. In our study, dietary information was based on the collection of one 24-HR, which may not be representative of dietary intakes at the individual level. However, despite its well-known limitations, such as reliance on memory and day-to-day variation, the 24-HR may provide accurate estimates of energy intake at the population level [75]. In the present study, dietary information was collected by the multiple pass 24-HR approach, which was shown to provide accurate estimates of dietary intake in children [76]. In addition, the recalls were taken by research nutritionists who went through extensive training prior to data collection in order to minimize interviewer errors. Similarly, inter-observer measurement error in anthropometric assessment was minimized by extensive training and follow up to maintain quality of measurement among all research nutritionists. It is important to note that physical activity was not assessed in the present study, and as such its association with preschool overweight/obesity was not investigated. However, variability in physical activity tends to be rather limited in this age group and engagement in structured exercise is quite uncommon [77,78]. It is important to note that no information was available regarding whether the participating mothers have recently delivered and/or are currently breastfeeding at the time of the interview. For these two groups of mothers, given that BMI may not be reflective of their usual weight status, their inclusion in the analysis may have attenuated the results found in this study. Similarly, data on access to non-traditional food markets, body image of children, means of transportation and the built environment, which may play an important role in influencing the risk of childhood obesity [79,80] were not collected in this study. Finally, the cross-sectional design of the study allows us to test associations rather than to assess any causal relationships.

5. Conclusions

This study showed that the rates of overweight and obesity amongst Lebanese preschoolers exceed the global prevalence estimate of preschool overweight/obesity, as well as the estimate reported for developing countries [2]. This study has also provided the first evidence from the MENA region on the link between preschool overweight/obesity and higher SES, thus, potentially serving as a case-study for other middle-income countries in similar stages of the nutrition transition. In addition, specific dietary behaviors, including eating while watching TV and consuming a high fat diet, were shown to be associated with increased risk of overweight and obesity in Lebanese preschoolers, which corroborate findings stemming from previous studies on this age group. Taken together, the study's findings highlight the importance of the home environment in modulating the young child's lifestyle and dietary habits and hence obesity risk early in life. In this context, the results of the study call for education interventions aiming at raising parental awareness on preschool overweight in Lebanon, a country where early life "chubbiness" may not be perceived as a health threat but is rather culturally believed to be a sign of good health and an inherent component of the child's "cuteness".

Recognizing that the development of early life obesity prevention strategies should rely on evidence-based public health approaches, the results of this paper could represent a stepping stone for the formulation of effective interventions and policies aiming at curbing the epidemic of pediatric obesity in Lebanon. Family-focused interventions and behavioral strategies, coupled with school-based interventions and policies, are needed to instill healthy lifestyle and dietary habits early in life [6].

Acknowledgments: Funding for this study was provided by the Lebanese National Council for Scientific Research (Beirut, Lebanon) through its support of the Associated Research Unit (ARU) on 'Nutrition and Non-communicable Diseases in Lebanon' and by the University Research Board (American University of Beirut, Lebanon). The authors are indebted to every subject who took the time to participate in the study. The authors would also like to acknowledge the services of Nada Adra for her help in statistical analyses, Joana Abou-Rizk for her help in dietary analyses and Jennifer Ayoub for editing the manuscript.

Author Contributions: L.N., as the principal investigator, was responsible for the conceptualization of the study objectives and methodology and contributed to the write-up of the manuscript. N.H. critically reviewed the manuscript and provided valuable input for data interpretation. A.S. was involved in data collection and analysis in partial fulfilment of her MSc Degree. C.A. was responsible for the statistical evaluation of the data; F.N. contributed to data analysis and write-up of the manuscript and played a central role in integrating the dietary and anthropometric results. All authors participated in the drafting of the manuscript and have approved the final version of the manuscript.

References

1. Wang, Y.; Lobstein, T. Worldwide trends in childhood overweight and obesity. *Int. J. Pediatr. Obes.* **2006**, *1*, 11–25. [CrossRef] [PubMed]
2. De Onis, M.; Blössner, M.; Borghi, E. Global prevalence and trends of overweight and obesity among preschool children. *Am. J. Clin. Nutr.* **2010**, *92*, 1257–1264. [CrossRef] [PubMed]
3. Dubois, L.; Farmer, A.; Girard, M.; Peterson, K. Social factors and television use during meals and snacks is associated with higher BMI among pre-school children. *Public Health Nutr.* **2008**, *11*, 1267–1279. [CrossRef] [PubMed]
4. Gupta, N.; Goel, K.; Shah, P.; Misra, A. Childhood obesity in developing countries: Epidemiology, determinants, and prevention. *Endocr. Rev.* **2012**, *33*, 48–70. [CrossRef] [PubMed]
5. Mirmiran, P.; Sherafat Kazemzadeh, R.; Jalali Farahani, S.; Azizi, F. Childhood obesity in the Middle East: A review. *East. Mediterr. Health J.* **2010**, *16*, 1009–1017. [PubMed]
6. World Health Organization. Report of the Commission on Ending Childhood Obesity. 2016. Available online: http://www.who.int/end-childhood-obesity/final-report/en/ (accessed on 10 July 2016).
7. Mirza, N.M.; Yanovski, J.A. Prevalence and consequences of pediatric obesity. In *Handbook of Obesity: Epidemiology, Etiology, and Physiopathology*; Taylor & Francis Ltd.: Boca Raton, FL, USA, 2014; pp. 55–74.
8. Kelsey, M.M.; Zaepfel, A.; Bjornstad, P.; Nadeau, K.J. Age-related consequences of childhood obesity. *Gerontology* **2014**, *60*, 222–228. [CrossRef] [PubMed]
9. Park, M.H.; Falconer, C.; Viner, R.M.; Kinra, S. The impact of childhood obesity on morbidity and mortality in adulthood: A systematic review. *Obes. Rev.* **2012**, *13*, 985–1000. [CrossRef] [PubMed]
10. Jouret, B.; Ahluwalia, N.; Cristini, C.; Dupuy, M.; Nègre-Pages, L.; Grandjean, H.; Tauber, M. Factors associated with overweight in preschool-age children in southwestern France. *Am. J. Clin. Nutr.* **2007**, *85*, 1643–1649. [PubMed]
11. World Health Organization. Global Strategy on Diet, Physical Activity and Health. 2004, Resolution WHA55.23. WHO, Geneva. A57/59. 17 April 2004. Available online: http://www.who.int/dietphysicalactivity/strategy/eb11344/en/ (accessed on 10 July 2016).
12. Monasta, L.; Batty, G.; Cattaneo, A.; Lutje, V.; Ronfani, L.; Van Lenthe, F.; Brug, J. Early-life determinants of overweight and obesity: A review of systematic reviews. *Obes. Rev.* **2010**, *11*, 695–708. [CrossRef] [PubMed]
13. World Health Organization. Technical Paper. Regional Strategy on Nutrition 2010–2019. 2010. Fifty-Seventh Session. Agenda Item 4 (b). Available online: http://applications.emro.who.int/docs/EM_RC57_54_en.pdf (accessed on 10 July 2016).
14. Nasreddine, L.; Naja, F.; Chamieh, M.C.; Adra, N.; Sibai, A.-M.; Hwalla, N. Trends in overweight and obesity in Lebanon: Evidence from two national cross-sectional surveys (1997 and 2009). *BMC Public Health* **2012**, *12*, 798. [CrossRef] [PubMed]
15. World Health Organization. Nutrition—General Assembly Proclaims the Decade of Action on Nutrition. Available online: http://www.who.int/nutrition/GA_decade_action/en/ (accessed on 10 July 2016).
16. Moshfegh, A.J.; Borrud, L.; Perloff, B.; LaComb, R. Improved method for the 24-hour dietary recall for use in national surveys. *FASEB J.* **1999**, *13*, A603.
17. Naing, L.; Than, W.; Rusli, B. Practical issues in calculating the sample size for prevalence studies. *Arch. Orofac. Sci.* **2006**, *1*, 9–14.
18. Dinsa, G.; Goryakin, Y.; Fumagalli, E.; Suhrcke, M. Obesity and socioeconomic status in developing countries: A systematic review. *Obes. Rev.* **2012**, *13*, 1067–1079. [CrossRef] [PubMed]
19. Banque Bemo. *Education in Lebanon Growth Drivers, Structure, Primary and Secondary Cycles, Tertiary Cycle, Challenges and Recommendations*; BEMO Industry Report; Banque Bemo: Beirut, Lebanon, 2014.
20. Yaacoub, N.; Badre, L. *Education in Lebanon*; Statistics in Focus (SIF), Central Administration of Statistics: Beirut, Lebanon, 2012.
21. Wardle, J.; Guthrie, C.A.; Sanderson, S.; Rapoport, L. Development of the children's eating behaviour questionnaire. *J. Child Psychol. Psychiatry* **2001**, *42*, 963–970. [CrossRef] [PubMed]
22. National Institutes of Health. Clinical guidelines on the identification, evaluation, and treatment of overweight and obesity in adults: The evidence report. *Obes. Res.* **1998**, *6*, 51–209.

23. WHO Multicentre Growth Reference Study Group. *Who Child Growth Standards: Length/Height-for-Age, Weight-for-Age, Weight-for-Length, Weight-for-Height and Body Mass Index-for-Age: Methods and Development*; World Health Organization: Geneva, Switzerland, 2006; Available online: http://www.who.int/childgrowth/standards/Growth_standard.pdf (accessed on 8 July 2016).

24. World Health Organization. *Who Anthro Plus for Personal Computers Manual: Software for Assessing Growth of the World's Children and Adolescents*; World Health Organization: Geneva, Switzerland, 2009; Available online: http://www.who.int/growthref/tools/who_anthroplus_manual.pdf (accessed on 8 July 2016).

25. Kuczmarski, R.J.; Ogden, C.L.; Grummer-Strawn, L.M.; Flegal, K.M.; Guo, S.S.; Wei, R.; Mei, Z.; Curtin, L.R.; Roche, A.F.; Johnson, C.L. CDC growth charts: United states. *Adv. Data* **2000**, *314*, 1–27.

26. Kuczmarski, R.J.; Ogden, C.L.; Guo, S.S.; Grummer-Strawn, L.M.; Flegal, K.M.; Mei, Z.; Wei, R.; Curtin, L.R.; Roche, A.F.; Johnson, C.L. 2000 CDC growth charts for the united states: Methods and development. *Vital Health Stat.* **2002**, *11*, 1–190.

27. Cole, T.J.; Bellizzi, M.C.; Flegal, K.M.; Dietz, W.H. Establishing a standard definition for child overweight and obesity worldwide: International survey. *BMJ* **2000**, *320*, 1240. [CrossRef] [PubMed]

28. Willett, W. *Nutritional Epidemiology*, 2nd ed.; Oxford University Press: New York, NY, USA, 1998.

29. Shim, J.-S.; Oh, K.; Kim, H.C. Dietary assessment methods in epidemiologic studies. *Epidemiol. Health* **2014**, *36*, e2014009. [CrossRef] [PubMed]

30. Moshfegh, A.; Rhodes, D.; Baer, D.; Murayi, T.; Clemens, J.; Rumpler, W. The U.S. Department of agriculture automated multiple-pass method reduces bias in the collection of energy intakes. *Am. J. Clin. Nutr.* **2008**, *88*, 324–332. [PubMed]

31. Pellet, P.; Shadarevian, S. *Food Composition Tables for Use in the Middle East*; American University of Beirut: Beirut, Lebanon, 2013.

32. Cole, T.J.; Flegal, K.M.; Nicholls, D.; Jackson, A.A. Body mass index cut offs to define thinness in children and adolescents: International survey. *BMJ* **2007**, *335*, 194. [CrossRef] [PubMed]

33. Cattaneo, A.; Monasta, L.; Stamatakis, E.; Lioret, S.; Castetbon, K.; Frenken, F.; Manios, Y.; Moschonis, G.; Savva, S.; Zaborskis, A. Overweight and obesity in infants and pre-school children in the European Union: A review of existing data. *Obes. Rev.* **2010**, *11*, 389–398. [CrossRef] [PubMed]

34. Frenken, F. *Health Interview Survey 1981–2006*; Statistics Netherlands: Herleen, The Netherlands, 2007.

35. Nanu, M. *Nutritional Status of Children under 5 Years Old. National Nutritional Surveillance Programme 1993–2002*; Alfred Rusescu Institute for Mother and Child Care: Bucharest, Romania, 2003.

36. Onyango, A.W.; de Onis, M.; Caroli, M.; Shah, U.; Sguassero, Y.; Redondo, N.; Carroli, B. Field-testing the who child growth standards in four countries. *J. Nutr.* **2007**, *137*, 149–152. [PubMed]

37. Savva, S.; Tornaritis, M.; Chadjigeorgiou, C.; Kourides, Y.; Savva, M.; Panagi, A.; Chrictodoulou, E.; Kafatos, A. Prevalence and socio-demographic associations of undernutrition and obesity among preschool children in Cyprus. *Eur. J. Clin. Nutr.* **2005**, *59*, 1259–1265. [CrossRef] [PubMed]

38. Savva, S.; Tornaritis, M.; Chadjigeorgiou, C.; Kourides, Y.; Epiphaniou-Savva, M.; Panagi, A.; Chrictodoulou, E.; Kafatos, A. *Research and Education Institute of Child Health (REICH) Crosssectional Study, May–June 2004*; Research and Education Institute of Child Health (REICH): Nicosia, Cyprus, 2005.

39. Al-Raees, G.Y.; Al-Amer, M.A.; Musaiger, A.O.; D'Souza, R. Prevalence of overweight and obesity among children aged 2–5 years in Bahrain: A comparison between two reference standards. *Int. J. Pediatr. Obes.* **2009**, *4*, 414–416. [CrossRef] [PubMed]

40. Rady, M.; Al-Muslemani, M.; Salama, R. Determinants of overweight and obesity among Qatari children (2–5 years) in Doha, Qatar-2010. *Can. J. Clin. Nutr.* **2013**, *1*, 16–26. [CrossRef]

41. Shan, X.-Y.; Xi, B.; Cheng, H.; Hou, D.-Q.; Wang, Y.; Mi, J. Prevalence and behavioral risk factors of overweight and obesity among children aged 2–18 in Beijing, china. *Int. J. Pediatr. Obes.* **2010**, *5*, 383–389. [CrossRef] [PubMed]

42. Jordan Ministry of Health. National Micronutrient Survey Jordan 2010. 2011. Available online: http://www.gainhealth.org/wp-content/uploads/2014/05/56.-Jordan-Micronutrient-Survey-Report.pdf (accessed on 15 July 2016).

43. Instituto Nacional de Estadística; Ministerio de Sanidad y Consumo. *Encuesta Nacional de Salud 2006—Estilos de Vida y Prácticas Preventivas*; INE: Madrid, Spain, 2008.

44. Stamatakis, E. Anthropometric measurements, overweight, and obesity. In *Health Survey for England 2002—The Health for Children and Young People*; Sproston, K., Primatesta, P., Eds.; Highline Medical Services Organization: London, UK, 2003; Volume 1.

45. Commonwealth Scientific Industrial Research Organisation (CSIRO); Preventative Health National Research Flagship; The University of South Australia. 2007 Australian National Children's Nutrition and Physical Activity Survey—Main Findings. 2008. Available online: https://www.health.gov.au/internet/main/publishing.nsf/Content/8F4516D5FAC0700ACA257BF0001E0109/\protect\T1\textdollarFile/childrens-nut-phys-survey.pdf (accessed on 16 July 2016).

46. Shields, M. Measured Obesity: Overweight Canadian Children and Adolescents. Statistics Canada, 2005. Nutrition: Findings from the Canadian Community Health Survey; Issue No. 1 2005. Available online: http://www.statcan.gc.ca/pub/82-620-m/2005001/pdf/4193660-eng.pd (accessed on 16 July 2016).

47. Gaeini, A.; Kashef, M.; Samadi, A.; Fallahi, A. Prevalence of underweight, overweight and obesity in preschool children of Tehran, Iran. *J. Res. Med. Sci.* **2011**, *16*, 821–827. [PubMed]

48. Ogden, C.L.; Carroll, M.D.; Kit, B.K.; Flegal, K.M. Prevalence of childhood and adult obesity in the United States, 2011–2012. *J. Am. Med. Assoc.* **2014**, *311*, 806–814. [CrossRef] [PubMed]

49. Al Dossary, S.; Sarkis, P.; Hassan, A.; Ezz El Regal, M.; Fouda, A. Obesity in Saudi children: A dangerous reality. *East. Mediterr. Health J.* **2010**, *16*, 1003–1008. [PubMed]

50. Hui, L.; Nelson, E.; Yu, L.; Li, A.; Fok, T. Risk factors for childhood overweight in 6-to 7-y-old Hong Kong children. *Int. J. Obes.* **2003**, *27*, 1411–1418. [CrossRef] [PubMed]

51. Wang, Y.; Lim, H. The global childhood obesity epidemic and the association between socio-economic status and childhood obesity. *Int. Rev. Psychiatry* **2012**, *24*, 176–188. [CrossRef] [PubMed]

52. Nasreddine, L.; Mehio-Sibai, A.; Mrayati, M.; Adra, N.; Hwalla, N. Adolescent obesity in Syria: Prevalence and associated factors. *Child Care Health Dev.* **2010**, *36*, 404–413. [CrossRef] [PubMed]

53. Mushtaq, M.U.; Gull, S.; Shahid, U.; Shafique, M.M.; Abdullah, H.M.; Shad, M.A.; Siddiqui, A.M. Family-based factors associated with overweight and obesity among Pakistani primary school children. *BMC Pediatr.* **2011**, *11*, 114. [CrossRef] [PubMed]

54. Fakih, A.; Marrouch, W. Determinants of Domestic Workers' Employment: Evidence from Lebanese Household Survey Data. 2012. Available online: http://ftp.iza.org/dp6822.pdf (accessed on 18 July 2016).

55. Lin, S.L.; Leung, G.M.; Hui, L.L.; Lam, T.H.; Schooling, C.M. Is informal child care associated with childhood obesity? Evidence from Hong Kong's "children of 1997" birth cohort. *Int. J. Epidemiol.* **2011**, *40*, 1238–1246. [CrossRef] [PubMed]

56. Benjamin, S.E.; Rifas-Shiman, S.L.; Taveras, E.M.; Haines, J.; Finkelstein, J.; Kleinman, K.; Gillman, M.W. Early child care and adiposity at ages 1 and 3 years. *Pediatrics* **2009**, *124*, 555–562. [CrossRef] [PubMed]

57. Pearce, A.; Li, L.; Abbas, J.; Ferguson, B.; Graham, H.; Law, C. Is childcare associated with the risk of overweight and obesity in the early years? Findings from the UK millennium cohort study. *Int. J. Obes.* **2010**, *34*, 1160–1168. [CrossRef] [PubMed]

58. Schooling, C.M.; Yau, C.; Cowling, B.J.; Lam, T.H.; Leung, G.M. Socio-economic disparities of childhood body mass index in a newly developed population: Evidence from Hong Kong's 'children of 1997' birth cohort. *Arch. Disease Child.* **2010**, *95*, 437–443. [CrossRef] [PubMed]

59. Story, M.; Kaphingst, K.M.; French, S. The role of child care settings in obesity prevention. *Future Child.* **2006**, *16*, 143–168. [CrossRef] [PubMed]

60. Utter, J.; Neumark-Sztainer, D.; Jeffery, R.; Story, M. Couch potatoes or French fries: Are sedentary behaviors associated with body mass index, physical activity, and dietary behaviors among adolescents? *J. Am. Diet. Assoc.* **2003**, *103*, 1298–1305. [CrossRef]

61. Vik, F.N.; Bjørnarå, H.B.; Øverby, N.C.; Lien, N.; Androutsos, O.; Maes, L.; Jan, N.; Kovacs, E.; Moreno, L.A.; Dössegger, A. Associations between eating meals, watching TV while eating meals and weight status among children, ages 10–12 years in eight European countries: The energy cross-sectional study. *Int. J. Behav. Nutr. Phys. Act.* **2013**, *10*, 58. [CrossRef] [PubMed]

62. Chandon, P.; Wansink, B. Does food marketing need to make us fat? A review and solutions. *Nutr. Rev.* **2012**, *70*, 571–593. [CrossRef] [PubMed]

63. Francis, L.A.; Birch, L.L. Does eating during television viewing affect preschool children's intake? *J. Am. Diet. Assoc.* **2006**, *106*, 598–600. [CrossRef] [PubMed]

64. Jansen, P.W.; Roza, S.J.; Jaddoe, V.; Mackenbach, J.D.; Raat, H.; Hofman, A.; Verhulst, F.C.; Tiemeier, H. Children's eating behavior, feeding practices of parents and weight problems in early childhood: Results from the population-based Generation R Study. *Int. J. Behav. Nutr. Phys. Act.* **2012**, *9*, 130. [CrossRef] [PubMed]

65. Santos, J.L.; Ho-Urriola, J.A.; González, A.; Smalley, S.V.; Domínguez-Vásquez, P.; Cataldo, R.; Obregón, A.M.; Amador, P.; Weisstaub, G.; Hodgson, M.I. Association between eating behavior scores and obesity in Chilean children. *Nutr. J.* **2011**, *10*, 108. [CrossRef] [PubMed]

66. Gazzaniga, J.M.; Burns, T.L. Relationship between diet composition and body fatness, with adjustment for resting energy expenditure and physical activity, in preadolescent children. *Am. J. Clin. Nutr.* **1993**, *58*, 21–28. [PubMed]

67. Maffeis, C.; Talamini, G.; Tato, L. Influence of diet, physical activity and parents' obesity on children's adiposity: A four-year longitudinal study. *Int. J. Obes. Relat. Metab. Disord.* **1998**, *22*, 758–764. [CrossRef] [PubMed]

68. United States Department of Agriculture (USDA). Is Intake of Dietary Fat Associated with Adiposity in Children? Available online: http://www.nel.gov/evidence.cfm?evidence_summary_id=250348 (accessed on 20 July 2016).

69. Magarey, A.; Daniels, L.; Boulton, T.; Cockington, R. Does fat intake predict adiposity in healthy children and adolescents aged 2–15 years? A longitudinal analysis. *Eur. J. Clin. Nutr.* **2001**, *55*, 471–481. [CrossRef] [PubMed]

70. Skinner, J.; Bounds, W.; Carruth, B.; Morris, M.; Ziegler, P. Predictors of children's body mass index: A longitudinal study of diet and growth in children aged 2–8 years. *Int. J. Obes. Relat. Metab. Disord.* **2004**, *28*, 476–482. [CrossRef] [PubMed]

71. World Health Organization. *Obesity. Preventing and Managing the Global Epidemic*; Report of a WHO Consultation on Obesity; World Health Organisation: Geneva, Switzerland, 1998; Available online: http://www.who.int/nutrition/publications/obesity/WHO_TRS_894/en/ (accessed on 20 July 2016).

72. Little, T.J.; Horowitz, M.; Feinle-Bisset, C. Modulation by high-fat diets of gastrointestinal function and hormones associated with the regulation of energy intake: Implications for the pathophysiology of obesity. *Am. J. Clin. Nutr.* **2007**, *86*, 531–541. [PubMed]

73. Horton, T.J.; Drougas, H.; Brachey, A.; Reed, G.W.; Peters, J.C.; Hill, J. Fat and carbohydrate overfeeding in humans: Different effects on energy storage. *Am. J. Clin. Nutr.* **1995**, *62*, 19–29. [PubMed]

74. Campbell, K.; Hesketh, K. Strategies which aim to positively impact on weight, physical activity, diet and sedentary behaviours in children from zero to five years. A systematic review of the literature. *Obes. Rev.* **2007**, *8*, 327–338. [CrossRef] [PubMed]

75. Livingstone, M.; Robson, P. Measurement of dietary intake in children. *Proc. Nutr. Soc.* **2000**, *59*, 279–293. [CrossRef] [PubMed]

76. Burrows, T.L.; Martin, R.J.; Collins, C.E. A systematic review of the validity of dietary assessment methods in children when compared with the method of doubly labeled water. *J. Am. Diet. Assoc.* **2010**, *110*, 1501–1510. [CrossRef] [PubMed]

77. Penpraze, V.; Reilly, J.J.; MacLean, C.M.; Montgomery, C.; Kelly, L.A.; Paton, J.Y.; Aitchison, T.; Grant, S. Monitoring of physical activity in young children: How much is enough? *Pediatr. Exerc. Sci.* **2006**, *18*, 483. [CrossRef]

78. Corder, K.; Ekelund, U.; Steele, R.M.; Wareham, N.J.; Brage, S. Assessment of physical activity in youth. *J. Appl. Physiol.* **2008**, *105*, 977–987. [CrossRef] [PubMed]

79. Griffiths, L.J.; Parsons, T.J.; Hill, A.J. Self-esteem and quality of life in obese children and adolescents: A systematic review. *Int. J. Pediatr. Obes.* **2010**, *5*, 282–304. [CrossRef] [PubMed]

80. Booth, K.M.; Pinkston, M.M.; Poston, W.S.C. Obesity and the built environment. *J. Am. Diet. Assoc.* **2005**, *105*, 110–117. [CrossRef] [PubMed]

7

Use of Vitamin and Mineral Supplements Among Adolescents Living in Germany—Results from EsKiMo II

Hanna Perlitz *, Gert B.M. Mensink, Clarissa Lage Barbosa, Almut Richter, Anna-Kristin Brettschneider, Franziska Lehmann, Eleni Patelakis, Melanie Frank, Karoline Heide and Marjolein Haftenberger

Department of Epidemiology and Health Monitoring, Robert Koch Institute, 12101 Berlin, Germany; MensinkG@rki.de (G.B.M.M.); Lage-BarbosaC@rki.de (C.L.B.); RichterA@rki.de (A.R.); BrettschneiderA@rki.de (A.-K.B.); LehmannF@rki.de (F.L.); PatelakisE@rki.de (E.P.); Frank.Melanie@icloud.com (M.F.); Karoline.Heide@t-online.de (K.H.); HaftenbergerM@rki.de (M.H.)
* Correspondence: PerlitzH@rki.de

Abstract: Dietary supplements may contribute to nutrient intake; however, actual data on dietary supplement use among adolescents living in Germany are rare. The aim of this analysis was to describe the current use of dietary supplements, its determinants, and reasons of use. Changes in supplement use over time were evaluated by comparing the results with those from EsKiMo I (2006). Data from the Eating Study as a KiGGS Module EsKiMo II (2015–2017) were used to analyze supplement intake according to sociodemographic, health characteristics, and physical exercise behavior of 12–17-year-olds (n = 1356). Supplement use during the past four weeks was assessed by a standardized computer assisted personal interview. Multivariable logistic regression was used to identify the association between supplement use and its determinants. Between 2015–2017, 16.4% (95%-CI: 13.0–19.7%) of the adolescents used dietary supplements, and its use decreased with lower levels of physical exercise and overweight. Most supplement users used only one supplement, often containing both vitamins and minerals. The most frequently supplemented nutrients were vitamin C and magnesium. The main reported reason to use supplements was 'to improve health'. Prevalence of supplement use was slightly lower in 2015-2017 than in 2006 (18.5%; 95%-CI: 15.8–21.2%). The results underline the importance of including nutrient intake through dietary supplements in nutrition surveys.

Keywords: vitamin; mineral; dietary supplements; adolescents; EsKiMo

1. Introduction

An optimal nutrient supply during the growth period of adolescence is important [1]. The majority of the population living in Germany has an adequate supply of almost all vitamins and minerals. Generally, with a balanced diet the requirements for essential nutrients will be met. However, for some nutrients, like in particular folate, iodine, and vitamin D, the nutrient status is suboptimal for large population groups in Germany. Accordingly, vitamin or mineral supplements are only recommended in Germany for medically diagnosed deficiencies or for vulnerable groups, such as infants, pregnant women, and the elderly. For adolescents, there are no recommendations for the preventive use of dietary supplements [2].

Nevertheless, sales for dietary supplements have increased in Germany and other western countries over the last decades [3,4]. The demand for supplements constituted a sale of 1.4 billion Euro in Germany in 2018 [4]. In light of the mostly adequate nutrient supply and the risks associated with an excessive intake of vitamins and nutrients, this trend should be observed critically [5].

Many studies described an increase in the use of dietary supplements, such as the National Health and Nutrition Examination Survey (NHANES) between 1971–2000 among adults [6]. The proportion of German adults who used dietary supplements during a period of seven days increased by six percent (12.3% to 18.1%) between 1997–1999 and 2008–2011 [7]. Up-to-date and representative information on supplement use among children and adolescents living in Germany is lacking. There are some studies on supplement use, but these are mainly regional and/or older studies and include different age groups. Among children and adolescents (2–18 years) who participated in the regional Dortmund Nutritional and Anthropometric Longitudinally Designed Study (DONALD) between 1986–2003, 7.5% reported the use of dietary supplements in a three-day-weighted dietary record [8]. 9.2% of children (9–12 years) from two German birth cohort studies (GINIplus and LISAplus) used dietary supplements (2005–2009) [9]. In the first representative German Eating Study as a KiGGS Module (EsKiMo) from 2006, one fifth of the adolescents (12–17 years) had used dietary supplements in the previous four weeks [10]. Current data about dietary supplement use and its determinants may help to estimate the risk of oversupply of micronutrients in specific groups. EsKiMo II, conducted from 2015 to 2017 by the Robert Koch Institute (RKI), provides recent data on the use of dietary supplements. The present analysis aims to quantify the use of vitamin and mineral supplements in association with some determinants, and to evaluate the reasons for dietary supplement use among adolescents living in Germany. A major advantage of the current analysis is the possibility to describe the change in the prevalence of dietary supplement use between 2006 and 2015–2017 by comparing results from EsKiMo I and EsKiMo II.

2. Methods

2.1. Study Design and Study Population

EsKiMo II was conducted from June 2015 until September 2017 as part of the second wave of the German Health Interview and Examination Survey for Children and Adolescents (KiGGS Wave 2). The aim of the cross-sectional EsKiMo II was to assess the dietary behavior of children and adolescents and to identify changes in food consumption in the last decade by comparison with the previous study EsKiMo I, conducted in 2006. The EsKiMo II study protocol was consented with the Federal Commissioners for Data Protection and approved by the Hannover Medical School ethics committee in June 2015 (Number 2275–2015). Written informed consent was obtained from all parents or legal guardians and participants aged 14 years and older prior to the study interviews and examinations. Details on the methodology of EsKiMo II can be found elsewhere [11–13].

Altogether, 2644 children and adolescents aged 6–17 years who took part in KiGGS Wave 2 participated in EsKiMo II (participation rate 59.4%). The current analysis is limited to 1356 adolescents aged 12–17 years, as supplement use for this age group was assessed in the same way as in EsKiMo I, which allows describing changes in supplement use between 2006 and 2015–2017. Data of 1272 adolescents who participated in EsKiMo I was included for trend analysis of vitamin and mineral supplement use over time.

2.2. Assessment of Supplement Use

Dietary supplement use was assessed using a standardized computer assisted interview within the Dietary Interview Software for Health Examination Studies DISHES [14] by trained nutritionists during home visits. The use of dietary supplements was ascertained by the following question: "Have you taken dietary supplements (like vitamins or minerals) in form of tablets, drops etc. in the last four weeks?" In case of a positive response, types (name and brand), frequencies of use, dosage form, and amounts of the supplement and reasons for using were asked. Dietary supplements were selected from a database, which was integrated in the software. This supplement database is an update from previous dietary surveys conducted in Germany by the RKI and the Max Rubner Institute. Supplements which were not included in the database were recorded as a free text with the name, brand, and dosage form.

If available, a photo of the supplement packaging was taken. Afterwards, nutrient composition of all recorded supplements was checked with the information from the package, from the internet and/or from the manufacturer, and, if necessary, updated or added in the database. Reasons for supplement use were asked by predefined categories ('to improve health', 'based on a doctor's recommendation', 'increase of physical and mental performance', 'read/heard about beneficial information', 'compensation of low fruit/vegetables consumption', 'based on a pharmacist's recommendation'), with the possibility of free texts for other reasons (more than one answer was possible).

The current analysis is limited to dietary supplements containing vitamins or minerals and considers both freely available and medically prescribed dietary supplements. Supplements containing neither vitamins nor minerals or containing vitamins or minerals in homeopathic doses were assigned to the category 'other dietary supplements' and excluded from this analysis. Protein and dietetic products were assigned to foods and not considered in this analysis. Vitamin and mineral supplements were categorized as: vitamins, minerals, and combined preparations containing both vitamin/s and mineral/s.

2.3. Assessment of Other Variables

EsKiMo II participants were visited about three to six months after participation in KiGGS Wave 2. Sociodemographic, lifestyle, and health characteristics were assessed within KiGGS Wave 2 by self-administered questionnaires completed by the parents and by the adolescents aged 11 years old and older themselves [15]. Socio-economic status (SES) was based on information about education level, occupational status, and net household income of the parents and categorized into low, medium, and high SES [16]. Attended school types were categorized as lower secondary school, upper secondary school, and other school types. Participants were defined as having a migration background, when they or at least one parent were not born in Germany or did not have the German nationality. Three categories for residence region were constructed according to federal states: north (Schleswig-Holstein, Hamburg, Lower Saxony, Bremen, Berlin, Brandenburg, Mecklenburg-Western Pomerania), middle (North Rhine-Westphalia, Hesse, Saxony, Saxony-Anhalt, Thuringia), and south (Rhineland-Palatinate, Baden-Wuerttemberg, Bavaria, Saarland). Community size was categorized as: <5000 inhabitants, 5000 to 20,000 inhabitants, 20,000 to under 100,000 inhabitants, and >100,000 inhabitants. During the personal interviews in EsKiMo II, questions about the body height and weight of the adolescents were asked. Based on this self-reported information, body mass index (BMI) (body weight in kg/body size in m^2) was calculated and assigned into age- and sex-specific BMI categories according to Kromeyer-Hauschild (underweight, normal weight, overweight) [17,18]. Furthermore, subjective health status was rated by adolescents of 11 years and older themselves in four categories, ranging from excellent to poor. Physical exercise as a specific and more intensive type of physical activity includes all kinds of sports, but without physical education at school. Questions about the usual duration (hours/minutes per week) of physical exercise were asked and replies were categorized into 'low' (less than one hour /week), 'medium' (1–3 h/week) and 'high' (more than 3 h/week).

2.4. Statistical Analysis

Prevalence of supplement use is presented according to sociodemographic and other characteristics. In addition, multivariate logistic regression was conducted to analyze the independent associations of these sociodemographic and other characteristics with supplement use. The associations were adjusted for all other variables. For supplement users, the type, number, and frequency as well as the reasons for vitamin or mineral supplement use are described. Finally, changes in the prevalence of dietary supplement use between 2006 and 2015–2017 are examined. All analyses were performed with SAS Version 9.4 (SAS Institute, Cary, NC, USA). The criterion for statistical significance was set at p-value< 0.05. A weighting factor was applied to correct for deviations from the population structure according to age (in years), sex, region (as of 31.12.2015), nationality (as of 31.12.2014), and education level of the parents (Mikrozensus 2013), as well as to consider differences in participation´s probability according to seasonality, SES of the family, and school type. In order to take the clustered design into account (with a stronger correlation of the participants within a community compared to a totally random group), the SAS survey procedures were applied. Data of 1267 adolescents from EsKiMo I are included for trend analysis. Study procedures and instruments of EsKiMo I are generally the same as for EsKiMo II and are described elsewhere [19]. Prior analyses of EsKiMo I were calculated using a weighting factor to correct for the disproportional higher number of participants from the Eastern part of Germany as well as deviations in age, sex, and nationality from the general population [10]. For the present analysis, these prevalence estimates were recalculated with a weighting factor constructed as described above and correcting deviations from the population structure of 2004. For comparison of prevalence estimates from EsKiMo I and EsKiMo II taking into account demographic changes over time, the EsKiMo I prevalence estimates were standardized to the sex- and age-structure of the population underlying the EsKiMo II data.

3. Results

In total, 16.4% of the adolescents (girls: 18.8%, boys: 14.0%) aged 12 to 17 years had used vitamin or mineral supplements in the previous four weeks (Table 1). The proportion of supplement use was similar across age groups, SES, type of school, migration background, region of residence, and community size (Table 1). Additionally, there was no association between self-assessed health status and dietary supplement use (data not shown).

The multivariable logistic regression showed that sex, weight status, and physical exercise were independent determinants of dietary supplement use. Boys use dietary supplements less frequently than girls (OR: 0.60 (0.38–0.94) and adolescents with overweight use dietary supplements less frequently compared to adolescents with normal weight (OR: 0.41 (0.21–0.79) (Table 1). The use of dietary supplements was lower for adolescents with low levels of physical exercise (OR: 0.56 (0.33–0.95) compared to those with a high level of physical exercise (Table 1).

Table 1. Associations between vitamin and/or mineral supplement use among adolescents (12–17 years) and determinants (sociodemographic characteristics, weight status, and physical exercise) in EsKiMo II (2015–2017), $n = 1356$.

Vitamin and/or Mineral Supplement Use	Prevalence [1]	Multivariate Logistic Regression Analysis [1]
	$n = 1356$ % (95% CI)	$n = 1223$ adjusted OR (95% CI) [2]
Total	16.4 (13.0–19.7)	-
Sex		
Girls	18.8 (14.5–23.2)	Ref.
Boys	14.0 (9.9–18.1)	0.60 (0.38–0.94) *
Age group		
12–13 years	14.4 (10.3–18.4)	0.76 (0.46–1.26)
14–15 years	19.4 (13.2–25.5)	1.30 (0.77–2.20)
16–17 years	15.2 (10.4–20.0)	Ref.
Socio-economic status (SES) [3]		
Low	12.3 (5.4–19.2)	0.63 (0.26–1.53)
Medium	15.3 (11.7–19.0)	0.66 (0.42–1.05)
High	22.3 (16.2–28.3)	Ref
Type of school [4]		
Lower secondary school	14.5 (10.9–18.1)	0.84 (0.53–1.32)
Upper secondary school	19.2 (14.4–24.0)	Ref.
Other school types	13.4 (4.8–22.0)	1.02 (0.40–2.59)
Migration background [5]		
Yes	15.4 (6.9–23.9)	0.89 (0.48–1.67)
No	16.5 (13.2–19.9)	Ref.

Table 1. *Cont.*

Vitamin and/or Mineral Supplement Use	Prevalence [1]	Multivariate Logistic Regression Analysis [1]
Region of residence		
North	13.8 (8.5–19.0)	0.74 (0.40–1.39)
Middle	16.7 (11.7–21.6)	1.11 (0.62–1.96)
South	17.7 (11.2–24.3)	Ref.
Community size		
<5000 inhabitants	15.0 (8.5–21.5)	Ref.
5000–<20,000 inhabitants	19.9 (11.6–28.2)	1.04 (0.52–2.09)
20000–<100,000 inhabitants	16.9 (10.9–22.9)	0.83 (0.39–1.74)
≥100,000 inhabitants	13.4 (8.2–18.6)	0.76 (0.36–1.63)
Weight status		
Underweight	20.7 (11.2–30.1)	1.33 (0.73–2.41)
Normal weight	17.0 (13.1–21.0)	Ref
Overweight	9.3 (3.9–14.7)	0.41 (0.21–0.79) *
Physical Exercise		
<1 h/week	11.5 (7.2–15.9)	0.56 (0.33–0.95) *
1–3 h/week	14.8 (10.9–18.8)	0.73 (0.47–1.12)
>3 h/week	19.9 (15.0–24.9)	Ref.

[1] weighted for the German population of 2015; [2] adjusted for all other variables; [3] Socio-economic status: n (missing) = 19; [4] Type of school n (missing) = 62, including participants who already finished school; [5] migration background n (missing) = 9; n = number of subjects; OR = odds ratio; CI = confidence interval; * OR is statistical significantly different from the reference with p-value < 0.05.

Among the dietary supplement users, 36.9% utilize vitamin supplements, 40.8% mineral supplements, and 46.4% a combination of both vitamins and minerals (Table 2), with no differences regarding sex (data not shown). During the previous four weeks, the majority of the users had consumed only one kind of dietary supplement (72.7%), and about a quarter (27.3%) had consumed more than one (Table 2). Around 28% of the vitamin and mineral supplements were used daily (6–7 times a week) (data not shown). The most commonly used vitamin supplements contained vitamin C (43.9%), followed by vitamin D (41.1%) and vitamin B12 (30.4%). The reported mineral supplements most often contained magnesium (45.9%), zinc (28.1%), and iron (24.1%; Table 2).

Table 2. Frequency [1] of the number and type of dietary supplements used among adolescents (12–17 years) in EsKiMo II (2015–2017), $n = 1356$.

	Total	Supplement User
	$n = 1356$ % (95% CI)	$n = 234$ % (95% CI)
Type of supplement [2]		
Vitamin/s	6.0 (4.3–7.7)	36.9 (29.4–44.5)
Mineral/s	6.7 (4.5–8.8)	40.8 (31.9–49.8)
Combination of vitamin/s and mineral/s	7.6 (5.5–9.7)	46.4 (38.8–54.1)
Number of supplements		
1 supplement	11.9 (9.3–14.4)	72.7 (64.8–80.6)
>1 supplement	4.5 (2.8–6.2)	27.3 (19.4–35.2)
Vitamins [1]		
Vitamin A	1.2 (0.6–1.9)	7.5 (3.7–11.9)
Thiamin	4.2 (2.7–5.7)	25.6 (17.3–34.0)
Riboflavin	4.0 (2.5–5.5)	24.2 (16.0–32.4)
Niacin	3.6 (2.1–5.1)	22.3 (14.3–30.3)
Pantothenic acid	3.3 (2.0–4.6)	20.5 (13.7–27.7)
Vitamin B6	4.2 (2.8–5.5)	25.7 (18.1–33.3)
Biotin	3.6 (2.3–5.0)	22.2 (15.7–28.6)
Folate	4.1 (2.6–5.6)	25.2 (17.6–32.8)
Vitamin B12	5.0 (3.3–6.7)	30.4 (22.1–38.7)

Table 2. *Cont.*

	Total	Supplement User
Vitamin C	7.2 (5.4–9.0)	43.9 (35.8–52.1)
Vitamin D	6.7 (4.6–8.8)	41.1 (32.6–49.5)
Vitamin E	3.6 (2.3–5.0)	22.3 (15.1–29.6)
Vitamin K	0.9 (0.3–1.6)	5.7 (2.3–9.2)
Minerals [1]		
Calcium	3.2 (1.6–4.9)	19.8 (11.9–27.7)
Copper	1.5 (0.5–2.5)	8.9 (3.1–14.6)
Fluoride	0.4 (0.0–0.9)	2.3 (0.0–5.4)
Iron	3.9 (2.2–5.7)	24.1 (15.1–33.0)
Iodine	1.4 (0.4–2.4)	8.5 (2.7–14.4)
Potassium	0.3 (0.1–0.5)	1.9 (0.5–3.4)
Magnesium	7.5 (5.1–9.9)	45.9 (36.9–54.9)
Manganese	1.3 (0.4–2.2)	17.5 (2.6–13.0)
Molybdenum	1.3 (0.4–2.3)	8.2 (2.6–14.0)
Sodium	0.1 (0.0–0.2)	0.7 (0.0–1.5)
Phosphorus	0.4 (0.0–0.9)	2.7 (0.2–5.2)
Selenium	1.9 (0.8–2.9)	11.5 (5.6–17.4)
Zinc	4.6 (2.9–6.3)	28.1 (19.1–36.4)

[1] weighted for the German population of 2015; [2] due to multiple supplement use and multiple active components the sum of the prevalences by type of supplements or active components may deviate from the prevalence of total supplement use as displayed in Table 1; CI = confidence interval.

The most common reason for using vitamin and mineral supplements during the last four weeks was 'to improve health' (59.3%). One fifth of the participants (20.7%) reported to use supplements 'based on a doctor's recommendation', followed by 17.7% of the adolescents who reported an 'increase of physical and mental performance' as motivation. Further, less frequently reported reasons for using supplements were 'read/heard about beneficial information' (7.2%), 'compensation for low fruit/vegetables consumption' (7.2%), 'based on a pharmacist's recommendation' (3.6%). Among other reasons assessed as free text, the most often answer was 'based on KiGGS examination results' (2%) (Figure 1).

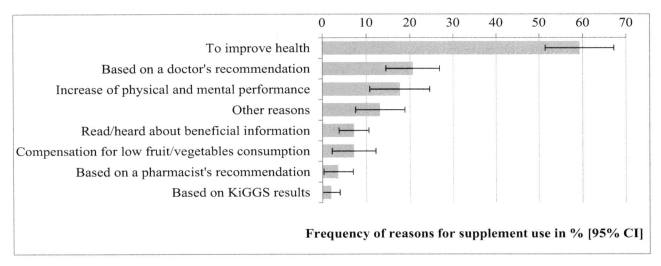

Figure 1. Prevalence and 95%-confidence intervals (CI) of reasons for dietary supplement use among adolescents (12–17 years) in EsKiMo II (2015–2017), *n* = 228 (weighted for the German population of 2015).

The prevalence of dietary supplement use in the previous four weeks decreased slightly, but not statistically significantly, from 18.5% to 16.4% between Eskimo I (2006) and Eskimo II (2015–2017) (Table 3).

Table 3. Trend analysis of dietary supplement use among adolescents (12–17 years) between EsKiMo I (2006) and EsKiMo II (2015–2017).

	EsKiMo I	EsKiMo I	EsKiMo II
	$n = 1267$ % (95% CI) Weighted for 2004	$n = 1267$ % (95% CI) Weighted for 2015	$n = 1356$ % (95% CI) Weigthed for 2015
Total	18.5 (15.8–21.2)	18.5 (15.8–21.2)	16.4 (13.0–19.7)
Girls	19.3 (15.3–23.4)	19.4 (15.3–23.5)	18.8 (14.5–23.2)
Boys	17.7 (14.3–21.1)	17.7 (14.3–21.1)	14.0 (9.9–18.1)
Type of supplement [1]			
Vitamin/s	6.2 (4.7–7.8)	6.2 (4.7–7.8)	6.0 (4.3–7.7)
Mineral/s	9.9 (7.6–12.2)	9.9 (7.6–12.3)	6.7 (4.5–8.8)
Combination of vitamin/s and mineral/s	6.1 (4.4–7.8)	6.1 (4.4–7.8)	7.6 (5.5–9.7)
Number of supplements			
1 supplement	13.6 (11.1–16.1)	13.7 (11.2–16.2)	11.9 (9.3–14.4)
>1 supplement	4.9 (3.2–6.5)	4.9 (3.2–6.5)	4.5 (2.8–6.2)

[1] due to multiple dietary supplement use and multiple active components, the sum of the prevalences by type of dietary supplements or active components may deviate from the prevalence of total dietary supplement use; CI = confidence interval.

4. Discussion

To our knowledge, no nationwide overview of recent dietary supplement use among adolescents has been presented for Germany since EsKiMo I in 2006. Our analysis show that 16.4% of the adolescents aged 12 to 17 years had used vitamin or mineral supplements in the last four weeks.

In EsKiMo II, supplement use is associated with sex, weight status, and physical exercise. Dietary supplement use was similar across age groups, SES, type of school, migration background, region of residence, community size, and subjective health status.

Comparison of our study results with other studies is difficult due to differences in methods of data collection, definitions of dietary supplements, timeframes, and age groups. In most western countries, the use of dietary supplements among children and adolescents is higher than in Germany [20–23], which is also confirmed for adults [24]. A third of the participants aged 9–18 years of the American dietary survey NHANES (2011–2014) reported dietary supplement use during the last month [20]. In an Australian study (2014–2015), 20.1% of the adolescents (10–17 years old) had used dietary supplements during the past two weeks [21].

Previous studies including children and adolescents showed inconsistent findings considering sex differences in dietary supplement use. Many studies observed no significant differences in dietary supplement use by sex [21,22,25]. Parents probably determine the supplement use for their children, which may largely explain the absence of sex differences. The German DONALD study showed a higher prevalence of dietary supplement use among boys [26]. A Polish study observed that supplement use was more common among girls [23]. Other studies observed higher supplement use among children and adolescents with underweight, which is similar to our observations [25,27,28]. Previous findings regarding the effect of physical exercise on dietary supplement use are heterogeneous and only partly comparable due to differences in data assessment and definition of physical exercise. In EsKiMo II, adolescents who reported less than one hour of physical exercise per week used less frequently dietary supplements. This finding is consistent with the results from EsKiMo I and NHANES, although different definitions for physical exercise were applied [10,27].

Previous studies were also inconsistent with regard to the effect of age on dietary supplement use. NHANES and a Korean study found a higher prevalence of dietary supplement use for younger age groups [20,22]. However, unlike our study, these studies also included children under the age of 12 years.

Other studies observed a higher prevalence of supplement use for older age groups (15–18 years; 16–18 years) [8,23]. In EsKiMo II, dietary supplement use is similar regarding SES. Previous studies consistently showed that a higher prevalence of dietary supplement use was associated with higher SES, higher education of the parents or higher household income [21,22,25,26,29]. For EsKiMo I, supplement use significantly differed by school type [10], whereas such differences were not significant for EsKiMo II, but the categories are not exactly the same. EsKiMo II did not observe differences in supplement use by migration status. The definition of migration status is very different between studies and countries, making it difficult to compare results. Although a Polish study with a small sample size observed a higher supplement use among adolescents living in bigger cities [23], dietary supplement use among adolescents was similar through different community sizes in EsKiMo II. This is similar to the results of the German Health Interview and Examination Survey (DEGS1; 2008–2011), which also observed no statistically significant differences in supplement use according to the community size and region of residence among German adults [7].

In EsKiMo II, the most frequently dietary supplements used were a combination of vitamins and minerals. Vitamin C and magnesium were the most supplemented micronutrients, similarly to results of an Australian study [21]. Other studies showed related results: in NHANES and DONALD, the most frequently dietary supplement used was also vitamin C, but the most frequent mineral supplemented was calcium and not magnesium [26,30]. A German consumer survey with adults observed similar results to EsKiMo II, with even higher prevalences for vitamin C (53%) and magnesium (59%) [31]. Vitamin C and magnesium are also the most commonly supplemented micronutrients by adults [24,31–33]. However, there are no recommendations and no need for adolescents to supplement vitamin C and magnesium [2,34].

Reasons for dietary supplements use can be diverse. Within EsKiMo II, the most commonly reported reason for vitamin or mineral supplements use was 'to improve health' (59.3%), which was also identified as the most frequent motive in previous studies (CRN Consumer survey: 58%; NHANES 2011–2014: 38.0%) [30,35]. The German NEMONIT study, for example, indicated 'prevention of nutrient deficiencies (or covering increased nutrient requirements)' (62.4%) and 'achievement or improvement of general well-being' (34.7%) as the most common motives for dietary supplement use among German adults [36]. For the participants of EsKiMo II, the recommendations of a physician were reported as the second most important reason for dietary supplements use, but this only applies to one in five adolescents (20.7%). 2% of the supplement users indicated using dietary supplements as a consequence of the personal evaluation they received after taking part on KiGGS Wave 2, from which the EsKiMo II study sample was drawn.

The prevalence of dietary supplement intake decreased slightly, but not significantly, between EsKiMo I (2006) and EsKiMo II (2015–2017). Data from the longitudinal DONALD-study among children and adolescents aged 2–18 in Germany were used to describe a time trend in dietary supplement use from 1986–2003. Supplement use peaked between 1994 and 1996 [26]. One study among adolescents in the US showed similar prevalences between 2003–2004 and 2013–2014 [37]. While former studies for adults reported an increase in dietary supplement intake [6,38], more recent results showed a stagnation in its intake and a declining trend for some particular dietary supplements [39,40]. The observed stagnation may seem surprising, considering the many lifestyle changes detected in the last decades. However, in Germany, the supply of most vitamins and minerals through natural sources meets the recommended level and this situation has not changed substantially during the last ten years.

Currently, there are no recommendations for the use of vitamin and mineral supplements among adolescents in Germany. The German Nutrition Society recommends a balanced diet to meet the requirements for essential nutrients. The use of dietary supplements is only recommended for individuals with certain medically diagnosed diseases [1]. Nevertheless, a deficit for some vitamins, such as vitamin D, folic acid, and iodine has been reported among adolescents [41]. In addition, there is a certain risk of overconsumption, in particular when more than one dose of supplements or several different supplements containing the same nutrients are consumed every day in combination with fortified foods. For the latter, the consumer is often unaware of the specific fortifications. The growing market for both product groups, including a less controllable sale and distribution over the internet, may increase the risk of side effects. Therefore, in Germany, the Federal Institute for Risk Assessment defined a recommendation for maximum levels of the amount of vitamins and minerals contained in dietary supplements [5]. Furthermore, within the observed time period, results of large randomized controlled trials could not confirm the expected additional benefits of a regular supplement intake, e.g. for vitamin D. This may have counteracted marketing and promoting activities, therefore slowing down further increases in supplement intake.

Among the strengths of our study are the representative study population and the assessment through standardized personal interviews, which took place mainly at the participant's home. Data collection of vitamin and mineral supplements was carried out using a comprehensive supplement database. For more detailed information, pictures of the dietary supplement packages were taken. The nutrient composition of all dietary supplements reported was checked. The cross-sectional design of the study can represent a limitation for certain research questions, since no direct causalities can be derived from the observed correlations. In addition, selection bias is possible due to the previous participation of the adolescents in KiGGS Wave 2. To minimize the effect of selective participation, population weights were applied to correct deviations from the German population. A further limitation could be the use of self-reported body height and weight to estimate weight status. Self-reported body weight and height of a subgroup of participants who had also taken part in physical examinations of KiGGS Wave 2 were individually compared with the measured data from KiGGS Wave 2. This comparison showed only small differences and a high correlation between the measured and self-reported data.

5. Conclusions

Almost one fifth of adolescents reported to use dietary supplements within the last four weeks; most of them took one dietary supplement. Vitamin C and magnesium were the most commonly supplemented nutrients, although predominantly no nutrient deficiency exists for these nutrients. Nevertheless, critical nutrients, such as vitamin B12 and vitamin D, were also taken frequently [34,41]. Boys, adolescents with lower physical exercise levels and with overweight were less likely to use dietary supplements. The considerable use of dietary supplements among adolescents underlines the importance of considering dietary supplements intake into account for assessing nutrient intake in nutrition surveys. Furthermore, possible oversupply should be monitored and information on the risk and benefits of specific dietary supplements should be provided to the population.

Author Contributions: G.B.M.M. conceptualized and managed the EsKiMo studies. A.R. had major contributions to the design of the studies and the conduct of EsKiMo I. H.P. and M.H. performed analyses, drafted the initial manuscript, and interpreted the data. A.-K.B., M.F., K.H., C.L.B., F.L., E.P., A.R. and G.B.M.M. reviewed and revised the manuscript. All authors were involved in the conduction and data aggregation and read and approved the final manuscript.

Acknowledgments: We would like to thank all study participants and their families, and our colleagues from the Robert Koch Institute who supported the conduction of EsKiMo II. We are especially grateful to Janet Frotscher for her support on the verification of the supplement composition data.

References

1. Deutsche Gesellschaft für Ernährung; Österreichische Gesellschaft für Ernährung; Schweizerische Gesellschaft für Ernährungsforschung. *Referenzwerte für die Nährstoffzufuhr*; Deutsche Gesellschaft für Ernährung (DGE), Österreichische Gesellschaft für Ernährung (ÖGE), Schweizerische Gesellschaft für Ernährung (SGE): Bonn, Germany, 2015; Volume 2.

2. Bechthold, A.; Albrecht, V.; Leschik-Bonnet, E.; Heseker, H. Beurteilung der Vitaminversorgung in Deutschland. Teil 1: Daten zur Vitaminzufuhr. *Ernährungs Umschau* **2012**, *6*, 324–336.

3. Statista, Retail Sales of Vitamins & Nutritional Supplements in the United States from 2000 to 2017 (in billion U.S. dollars). 2017. Available online: http://www.statista.com/statistics/235801/retail-sales-of-vitamins-and-nutritional-supplements-in-the-us/ (accessed on 16 November 2017).

4. Bund für Lebensmittelrecht und Lebensmittelkunde e. V. (BLL) Markt für Nahrungsergänzungsmittel in Deutschland 2018. Available online: https://www.bll.de/de/verband/organisation/arbeitskreise/arbeitskreis-nahrungsergaenzungsmittel-ak-nem/20181029-zahlen-nahrungsergaenzungsmittel-markt-2018 (accessed on 4 May 2019).

5. Weißenborn, A.; Bakhiya, N.; DeMuth, I.; Ehlers, A.; Ewald, M.; Niemann, B.; Richter, K.; Trefflich, I.; Ziegenhagen, R.; Hirsch-Ernst, K.I.; et al. Höchstmengen für Vitamine und Mineralstoffe in Nahrungsergänzungsmitteln. *J. Consum. Prot. Food Saf.* **2018**, *13*, 25–39. [CrossRef]

6. Briefel, R.R.; Johnson, C.L. Secular trends in dietary intake in the United States. *Annu. Nutr.* **2004**, *24*, 401–431. [CrossRef] [PubMed]

7. Knopf, H. Selbstmedikation mit Vitaminen, Mineralstoffen und Nahrungsergänzungsmitteln in Deutschland. *Bundesgesundheitsblatt Gesundheitsforschung Gesundheitsschutz* **2017**, *60*, 268–276. [CrossRef]

8. Sichert-Hellert, W.; Wenz, G.; Kersting, M. Vitamin Intakes from Supplements and Fortified Food in German Children and Adolescents: Results from the DONALD Study. *J. Nutr.* **2006**, *136*, 1329–1333. [CrossRef]

9. Sausenthaler, S.; Standl, M.; Buyken, A.; Rzehak, P.; Koletzko, S.; Bauer, C.P.; Schaaf, B.; Von Berg, A.; Berdel, D.; Borte, M.; et al. Regional and socio-economic differences in food, nutrient and supplement intake in school-age children in Germany: results from the GINIplus and the LISAplus studies. *Public Health Nutr.* **2011**, *14*, 1724–1735. [CrossRef]

10. Six, J.; Richter, A.; Rabenberg, M.; Hintzpeter, B.; Vohmann, C.; Ståhl, A.; Heseker, H.; Mensink, G.B.M. Supplementenkonsum bei Jugendlichen in Deutschland. *Bundesgesundheitsblatt Gesundheitsforschung Gesundheitsschutz* **2008**, *51*, 1202–1209. [CrossRef]

11. Lage Barbosa, C.; Brettschneider, A.-K.; Haftenberger, M.; Lehmann, F.; Frank, M.; Heide, K.; Patelakis, E.; Perlitz, H.; Krause, L.; Houben, R.; et al. Comprehensive assessment of food and nutrient intake of children and adolescents in Germany: EsKiMo II—The eating study as a KiGGS module. *BMC Nutr.* **2017**, *3*, 75. [CrossRef]

12. Mensink, G.B.M.; Haftenberger, M.; Brettschneider, A.-K.; Barbosa, C.L.; Perlitz, H.; Patelakis, E.; Heide, K.; Frank, M.; Lehmann, F.; Krause, L.; et al. EsKiMo II—The Eating study as a KiGGS Module in KiGGS Wave 2. *J. Health Monitoring* **2017**, *2*, 38–46.

13. Brettschneider, A.-K.; Barbosa, C.L.; Haftenberger, M.; Heide, K.; Frank, M.; Patelakis, E.; Perlitz, H.; Lehmann, F.; Richter, A.; Mensink, G.B.M. The nutrition survey EsKiMo II—Design, execution and public health policy relevance. *Ernährungs Umschau* **2018**, *65*, 80–88.

14. Mensink, G.B.M.; Haftenberger, M.; Thamm, M. Validity of DISHES 98, a computerised dietary history interview: energy and macronutrient intake. *Eur. J. Clin. Nutr.* **2001**, *55*, 409–417. [CrossRef]

15. Mauz, E.; Gößwald, A.; Kamtsiuris, P.; Hoffmann, R.; Lange, M.; von Schenck, U.; Allen, J.; Butschalowsky, H.; Frank, L.; Hölling, H.; et al. New data for action. Data collection for KiGGS Wave 2 has been completed. *J. Health Monitoring* **2017**, *2*, 2–27.

16. Lampert, T.; Hoebel, J.; Kuntz, B.; Müters, S.; Kroll, L.E. Socioeconomic status and subjective social status measurement in KiGGS Wave 2. *J. Health Monitoring* **2018**, *3*, 108–125.

17. Kromeyer-Hauschild, K.; Wabitsch, M.; Kunze, D.; Geller, F.; Geiß, H.C.; Hesse, V.; Von Hippel, A.; Jaeger, U.; Johnsen, D.; Korte, W.; et al. Perzentile für den Body-mass-Index für das Kindes- und Jugendalter unter Heranziehung verschiedener deutscher Stichproben. *Monatsschrift Kinderheilkd* **2001**, *149*, 807–818. [CrossRef]

18. Kromeyer-Hauschild, K.; Moss, A.; Wabitsch, M. Body Mass index reference values for German children, adolescents and adults. Modification of the AGA BMI reference in the age range between 15 and 18 years. *Adipositas* **2015**, *9*, 123–127.

19. Mensink, G.B.M.; Bauch, A.; Vohmann, C.; Stahl, A.; Six, J.; Kohler, S.; Fischer, J.; Heseker, H. EsKiMo—Das Ernährungsmodul im Kinder- und Jugendgesundheitssurvey (KiGGS). *Bundesgesundheitsblatt Gesundheitsforschung Gesundheitsschutz* **2007**, *50*, 902–908. [CrossRef] [PubMed]

20. Jun, S.; Cowan, A.E.; Tooze, J.A.; Gahche, J.J.; Dwyer, J.T.; Eicher-Miller, H.A.; Bhadra, A.; Guenther, P.M.; Potischman, N.; Dodd, K.W.; et al. Dietary Supplement Use among U.S. Children by Family Income, Food Security Level, and Nutrition Assistance Program Participation Status in 2011(-)2014. *Nutrients* **2018**, *10*, 1212. [CrossRef]

21. O'Brien, S.K.; Malacova, E.; Sherriff, J.L.; Black, L.J. The Prevalence and Predictors of Dietary Supplement Use in the Australian Population. *Nutrients* **2017**, *9*, 1154. [CrossRef]

22. Kang, M.; Kim, D.W.; Lee, H.; Lee, Y.J.; Jung, H.J.; Paik, H.Y.; Song, Y.J. The nutrition contribution of dietary supplements on total nutrient intake in children and adolescents. *Eur. J. Clin. Nutr.* **2016**, *70*, 257–261. [CrossRef]

23. Gajda, K.; Zielinska, M.; Ciecierska, A.; Hamulka, J. Determinants of the use of dietary supplements among secondary and high school students. *Rocz. Panstw. Zakl. Hig.* **2016**, *67*, 383–390.

24. Skeie, G.; Braaten, T.; Hjartaker, A.; Lentjes, M.; Amiano, P.; Jakszyn, P.; Pala, V.; Palanca, A.; Niekerk, E.M.; Verhagen, H.; et al. Use of dietary supplements in the European Prospective Investigation into Cancer and Nutrition calibration study. *Eur. J. Clin. Nutr.* **2009**, *63*, S226–S238. [CrossRef]

25. Bailey, R.L.; Gahche, J.J.; Thomas, P.R.; Dwyer, J.T. Why US children use dietary supplements. *Pediatr. Res.* **2013**, *74*, 737–741. [CrossRef] [PubMed]

26. Sichert-Hellert, W.; Kersting, M. Vitamin and Mineral Supplements Use in German Children and Adolescents between 1986 and 2003: Results of the DONALD Study. *Ann. Nutr. Metab.* **2004**, *48*, 414–419. [CrossRef]

27. Shaikh, U.; Byrd, R.S.; Auinger, P. Vitamin and mineral supplement use by children and adolescents in the 1999–2004 National Health and Nutrition Examination Survey: relationship with nutrition, food security, physical activity, and health care access. *Arch. Pediatr. Adolesc. Med.* **2009**, *163*, 150–157. [CrossRef] [PubMed]

28. Picciano, M.; Dwyer, J.T.; Radimer, K.L.; Wilson, D.H.; Fisher, K.D.; Thomas, P.R.; Yetley, E.A.; Moshfegh, A.J.; Levy, P.S.; Nielsen, S.J.; et al. Dietary supplement use among infants, children, and adolescents in the united states, 1999–2002. *Arch. Pediatr. Adolesc. Med.* **2007**, *161*, 978–985. [CrossRef]

29. Dwyer, J.; Nahin, R.L.; Rogers, G.T.; Barnes, P.M.; Jacques, P.M.; Sempos, C.T.; Bailey, R. Prevalence and predictors of children's dietary supplement use: The 2007 National Health Interview Survey. *Am. J. Clin. Nutr.* **2013**, *97*, 1331–1337. [CrossRef] [PubMed]

30. Bailey, R.L.; Gahche, J.J.; Miller, P.E.; Thomas, P.R.; Dwyer, J.T. Why US Adults Use Dietary Supplements. *JAMA Intern. Med.* **2013**, *173*, 355. [CrossRef]

31. Heinemann, M.; Willers, J.; Bitterlich, N.; Hahn, A. Verwendung von Nahrungsergänzungsmitteln mit Vitaminen und Mineralstoffen—Ergebnisse einer deutschlandweiten Verbraucherbefragung. *J. Verbraucherschutz Lebensmittelsicherheit* **2015**, *10*, 131–142. [CrossRef]

32. Pouchieu, C.; Andreeva, V.A.; Péneau, S.; Kesse-Guyot, E.; Lassale, C.; Hercberg, S.; Touvier, M. Sociodemographic, lifestyle and dietary correlates of dietary supplement use in a large sample of French adults: results from the NutriNet-Santé cohort study. *Br. J. Nutr.* **2013**, *110*, 1480–1491. [CrossRef] [PubMed]

33. Bailey, R.L.; Gahche, J.J.; Lentino, C.V.; Dwyer, J.T.; Engel, J.S.; Thomas, P.R.; Betz, J.M.; Sempos, C.T.; Picciano, M.F. Dietary supplement use in the United States, 2003–2006. *J. Nutr.* **2011**, *141*, 261–266. [CrossRef]

34. Lage Barbosa, C.; Brettschneider, A.K.; Haftenberger, M.; Lehmann, F.; Frank, M.; Perlitz, H.; Heide, K.; Patelakis, E.; Mensink, G.B.M. Aktueller Überblick der Ernährungssituation von Kindern und Jugendlichen in Deutschland: Ergebnisse aus EsKiMo II. Available online: https://www.dge.de/fileadmin/public/doc/wk/2019/DGE-Proc-Germ-Nutr-Soc-Vol-25-2019.pdf (accessed on 5 April 2019).

35. Dickinson, A.; Blatman, J.; El-Dash, N.; Franco, J.C. Consumer Usage and Reasons for Using Dietary Supplements: Report of a Series of Surveys. *J. Am. Nutr.* **2014**, *33*, 176–182. [CrossRef] [PubMed]

36. Frey, A.; Hoffmann, I.; Heuer, T. Characterisation of vitamin and mineral supplement users differentiated according to their motives for using supplements: results of the German National Nutrition Monitoring (NEMONIT). *Public Heal. Nutr.* **2017**, *20*, 2173–2182. [CrossRef]

37. Qato, D.M.; Alexander, G.C.; Guadamuz, J.S.; Lindau, S.T. Prevalence of Dietary Supplement Use in US Children and Adolescents, 2003–2014. *JAMA Pediatr.* **2018**, *172*, 780. [CrossRef]

38. Kim, H.J.; Giovannucci, E.; Rosner, B.; Willett, W.C.; Cho, E. Longitudinal and secular trends in dietary supplement use: Nurses' Health Study and Health Professionals Follow-Up Study, 1986–2006. *J. Acad. Nutr. Diet.* **2014**, *114*, 436–443. [CrossRef]

39. Kantor, E.D.; Rehm, C.D.; Du, M.; White, E.; Giovannucci, E.L. Trends in Dietary Supplement Use among US Adults From 1999–2012. *JAMA* **2016**, *316*, 1464–1474. [CrossRef]

40. Marques-Vidal, P.; Vollenweider, P.; Waeber, G. Trends in vitamin, mineral and dietary supplement use in Switzerland. The CoLaus study. *Eur. J. Clin. Nutr.* **2017**, *71*, 122–127. [CrossRef] [PubMed]
41. Mensink, G.B.M.; Heseker, H.; Stahl, A.; Richter, A.; Vohmann, C. Die aktuelle Nährstoffversorgung von Kindern und Jugendlichen in Deutschland. *Ernährungs Umschau* **2007**, *11*, 636–646.

Emotional Eating, Health Behaviours and Obesity in Children

Elli Jalo [1,*], Hanna Konttinen [1,2], Henna Vepsäläinen [1], Jean-Philippe Chaput [3], Gang Hu [4], Carol Maher [5], José Maia [6], Olga L. Sarmiento [7], Martyn Standage [8], Catrine Tudor-Locke [9], Peter T. Katzmarzyk [4] and Mikael Fogelholm [1]

[1]   Department of Food and Nutrition, University of Helsinki, 00014 Helsinki, Finland; hanna.konttinen@helsinki.fi (H.K.); henna.vepsalainen@helsinki.fi (H.V.); mikael.fogelholm@helsinki.fi (M.F.)

[2]   Sociology, University of Helsinki, 00014 Helsinki, Finland

[3]   Children's Hospital of Eastern Ontario Research Institute, Ottawa, ON K1H 8L1, Canada; jpchaput@cheo.on.ca

[4]   Pennington Biomedical Research Center, Baton Rouge, LA 70808, USA; gang.hu@pbrc.edu (G.H.); peter.katzmarzyk@pbrc.edu (P.T.K.)

[5]   Alliance for Research In Exercise Nutrition and Activity (ARENA), School of Health Sciences, University of South Australia, Adelaide, SA 5001, Australia; carol.maher@unisa.edu.au

[6]   CIFI2D, Faculdade de Desporto, University of Porto, 4200-450 Porto, Portugal; jmaia@fade.up.pt

[7]   School of Medicine, Universidad de los Andes, Bogotá 11001000, Colombia; osarmien@uniandes.edu.co

[8]   Department for Health, University of Bath, Bath BA2 7AY, UK; m.standage@bath.ac.uk

[9]   Department of Kinesiology, School of Public Health and Health Sciences, University of Massachusetts Amherst, MA 01003, USA; ctudorlocke@umass.edu

*   Correspondence: elli.jalo@helsinki.fi

Abstract: Eating in response to negative emotions (emotional eating, EE) may predispose an individual to obesity. Yet, it is not well known how EE in children is associated with body mass index (BMI) and health behaviours (i.e., diet, physical activity, sleep, and TV-viewing). In the present study, we examined these associations in a cross-sectional sample of 5426 (54% girls) 9–11-year-old children from 12 countries and five continents. EE, food consumption, and TV-viewing were measured using self-administered questionnaires, and physical activity and nocturnal sleep duration were measured with accelerometers. BMI was calculated using measured weights and heights. EE factor scores were computed using confirmatory factor analysis, and dietary patterns were identified using principal components analysis. The associations of EE with health behaviours and BMI z-scores were analyzed using multilevel models including age, gender, and household income as covariates. EE was positively and consistently (across 12 study sites) associated with an unhealthy dietary pattern (β = 0.29, SE = 0.02, p < 0.0001), suggesting that the association is not restricted to Western countries. Positive associations between EE and physical activity and TV viewing were not consistent across sites. Results tended to be similar in boys and girls. EE was unrelated to BMI in this sample, but prospective studies are needed to determine whether higher EE in children predicts the development of undesirable dietary patterns and obesity over time.

Keywords: eating behaviour; psychological eating style; negative emotions; Emotion-Induced Eating Scale; health behaviour; BMI

1. Introduction

Childhood obesity rates are high in both developed and developing countries [1]. It is likely that the most important contributors are the increased availability of energy-dense foods and a reduced need for physical activity—the current obesogenic environment. Many individual characteristics could be relevant for explaining the differential susceptibility to the development of obesity among individuals in the same environment. One example is emotional eating (EE), which refers to a tendency to eat more in response to negative emotions [2,3]. According to the EE theory (also called the psychosomatic theory), individuals with EE use eating to reduce the intensity of negative emotions [2]. This is considered a poor coping strategy, and such difficulties in emotion regulation may be one possible mechanism underlying EE [4]. Foods consumed in response to negative emotions are usually high in sugar and/or fat [3]. These palatable foods provide hedonic pleasure and instant reward, which may distract from the experience of negative emotions [3]. Because an expected normal physiological reaction to negative emotions is a suppressed appetite [3,5], EE may interfere with physiological regulation. It may therefore represent a risk factor for becoming overweight and obese. Several studies have indeed suggested this might be the case in adults, since EE has been found to correlate positively with body mass index (BMI) [6–9] and to predict weight gain [10,11].

However, in children, empirical evidence regarding the association between EE and obesity is far from conclusive. Cross-sectional studies conducted with children (mean age between 7 and 13 years) have reported a positive association [12–18], no association [19,20], or even an inverse association [21–23] between EE and BMI/being overweight. It is possible that some of these inconsistencies are related to the use of different approaches to measure EE in previous work. Even though it has been shown that there is a good agreement between self-reported and parent-reported EE [13], the majority of the studies reporting positive associations with BMI/being overweight have employed parent-reported EE [12,14–18]. In contrast, self-reported EE has been employed in studies reporting an inverse association with BMI/being overweight [21–23]. Regardless, broader measures of emotion dysregulation have also been associated with obesity in children. For example, emotion-driven impulsiveness was associated with increased BMI z-scores in a large sample of 12–18-year-old children [24]. In longitudinal studies, parent-reported EE at the age of 5 to 6 years predicted higher BMI in 7–8-year-old children [25], but parent-reported EE at the age of 6 years was not associated with changes in BMI standard deviation scores in children aged 6 to 8 years [26].

Health behaviours, such as adhering to a healthy diet and getting adequate physical activity and sleep, are potentially important in prevention of childhood obesity [27–29]. As in adults, EE has been associated with a higher consumption of salty and sweet energy-dense foods and soft drinks in 12–15-year-old children [30] and a higher consumption of sweets and soft drinks in 12-year-old girls [31]. In contrast, in children aged between 5 and 12 years, no association between EE and the consumption of snacks [20,32], sweet foods [32], or fatty foods [32] has been reported. Even though these contradictory findings may be due to methodological issues (e.g., crude measure for snacking, and parent- vs. self-reported food consumption data), it is currently unclear whether EE is associated with diet in children under the age of 12 years. The clustering of health behaviours in children [33,34] raises the question of whether EE is also related to physical activity, sedentary behaviour (such as TV viewing), and/or sleep duration. Given that these behaviours do not occur in isolation, it is important to study them simultaneously.

The aim of this study was to examine the associations between self-reported EE, health behaviours (i.e., dietary patterns, physical activity, sleep duration, and TV viewing), and BMI in 9–11-year-old children. Because of inconsistent evidence and the limited number of previous studies, the analyses were exploratory, and we did not have specific hypotheses regarding the directions of these associations. Previous studies on EE in children have been mainly conducted in Western countries (in Europe and North America). In this work, we used a large sample from 12 countries and five continents, which gave us a unique opportunity to examine whether EE is consistently linked to behaviours that predispose individuals to obesity across countries representing diversity in terms of development, culture, socioeconomic status, and ethnic backgrounds.

2. Materials and Methods

2.1. Study Setting and Participants

The present study is a secondary analysis of the International Study of Childhood Obesity, Lifestyle and the Environment (ISCOLE), which aimed to determine the relationships between lifestyle behaviours and obesity in children. The details of the ISCOLE protocol have been reported previously [35]. The cross-sectional sample consisted of 9–11-year-old children from study sites located in urban and semi-urban areas in 12 different countries from all parts of the world (Australia, Brazil, Canada, China, Colombia, Finland, India, Kenya, Portugal, South Africa, the United Kingdom, and the United States). Rural areas were excluded due to logistical concerns. Each study site identified one or more school districts with a sufficient population to provide a sample of 500 children. The primary sampling unit within sites was schools, and the secondary sampling unit was classes within the schools. Schools were stratified by socio-economic status before sampling in order to maximize variability within sites see [35]. The Institutional Review Board at the Pennington Biomedical Research Center (coordinating center) approved the overarching ISCOLE protocol, and the Institutional/Ethical Review Boards at each participating institution approved the local protocols. Parents or legal guardians provided written informed consent, and children provided their written assent before participation, as required by local ethics boards. Data were collected from September 2011 through December 2013.

In total, 7372 children participated in ISCOLE [36], of which 5426 (74%) were included in the present analytical sample. Children who were missing data on one or several of the following variables were excluded: emotional eating (0.7% were excluded due to lacking data on this variable), dietary patterns (2.3%), accelerometry (moderate to vigorous physical activity (MVPA) and/or sleep, 16.5%), TV viewing (0.6%), BMI (0.4%), and household income (11.1%).

2.2. Emotional Eating

EE was measured via the Emotion-Induced Eating Scale (EIES), which was developed using a sample of over 2000 girls aged 9 to 10 years from the United States by Striegel-Moore et al. [21]. Children completed the EIES as part of a six-page questionnaire. The original EIES consists of seven items pertaining to emotionally-induced eating, as follows: eating in response to feeling sad, worried, mad, bored, or happy (e.g., "I eat more when I'm sad"), eating when not hungry, and using food as a reward. Responses were recorded on a 3-point scale (1 = never or almost never, 2 = sometimes, 3 = usually or always). See Supplementary Materials, Figure S1 for item level frequencies of the original EIES. However, taking a closer look at the wordings of the original EIES items reveals that two items out of the seven do not describe eating in response to emotions ("I eat between meals even if I'm not hungry" and "When I do something well I give myself a food treat"), and one item describes eating in response to a positive affective state ("I eat more when I'm happy"). EE is traditionally defined as "eating induced by negative emotions" [2], and it is also suggested that the desire to eat in response to negative emotions vs. positive emotions are two different constructs [5]. We wanted to adhere to this definition, and therefore used only the four items describing eating in response to negative emotions (sad, mad, worried, and bored) to assess EE in this study.

A confirmatory factor analysis (CFA) using a weighted least squares estimation with robust standard errors and a mean and variance adjusted test statistic (Lavaan package version 0.5.-23.1097 in the R system of statistical computing) was applied to test whether the four items describing eating in response to negative emotions loaded onto a one-factor latent construct. The items were used as ordinal variables in the analysis. The CFA was first conducted for the pooled data and then repeated for each study site and both genders separately. When evaluating the model fit, Comparative Fit Index (CFI) and Tucker–Lewis Index (TLI) values ≥ 0.95, a Root Mean Square Error of the Approximation (RMSEA) value ≤ 0.06, and a Standardized Root Square Mean Residuals (SRMR) value ≤ 0.08 were considered to indicate a good fit between the model and data [37]. Based on these criteria, the model showed an excellent fit for the pooled data (χ^2(df) = 2.660(2), p for χ^2 = 0.264, CFI = 1.000, TLI = 1.000,

RMSEA = 0.007 and SRMR = 0.006, Table 1). The Cronbach's alpha value for the four EE items was 0.60. For comparison, we tested also the original 7-item scale. CFA indicated a poorer fit compared to 4-item model (x^2(df) = 364.68(14), p for x^2 < 0.001, CFI = 0.96, TLI = 0.94, RMSEA = 0.06, and SRMR = 0.04). Furthermore, the Cronbach's alpha value for the 7-item scale (0.65) was not substantially higher than the respective value for the 4-item scale, especially because alpha always increases when more items are added [38]. These results further supported our initial decision to include only the four items measuring eating in response to negative emotions.

In the gender-stratified analysis, standardized factor loadings were highly comparable between boys and girls (Table 1). The test of the measurement invariance also indicated strong invariance, since CFI values changed less than 0.01 [39] when loadings (ΔCFI = 0.001, p for Δx^2 = 0.416), thresholds (ΔCFI < 0.001, p for Δx^2 = 0.874), and residual variances (ΔCFI = 0.001, p for Δx^2 = 0.182) were forced equal across the genders in a stepwise manner. There were some differences in factor loadings between the study sites in the site-stratified analysis, especially regarding the item about eating in response to boredom (factor loadings ranged from 0.31 to 0.87 between the sites). The test of the measurement invariance also indicated that loadings were not equal across the study sites (ΔCFI = 0.03, p for Δx^2 < 0.001). Yet, since partial metric invariance (equality of factor structure and factor loadings) was achieved after releasing an equality constraint only for one factor loading (the "bored" item, ΔCFI=0.008, p for Δx^2 = 0.064), we decided to use the EE factor scores from the pooled data in the present analyses. However, we also repeated all analyses by using the site-specific EE factor scores and found that the results remained highly similar (data not shown). EE factor scores were computed using the Empirical Bayes approach.

Table 1. Confirmatory factor analysis [a] for Emotion-Induced Eating Scale (EIES) negative emotion items.

| | n | x^2 (df) | p-Value | CFI | TLI | RMSEA | SRMR | Standardized Factor Loadings for EIES Items [b] | | | |
								Sad	Worried	Mad	Bored
All	7319	2.66 (2)	0.264	1.00	1.00	0.01	0.01	0.79	0.69	0.62	0.46
Gender											
Boys	3393	0.32 (2)	0.854	1.00	1.00	<0.01	<0.01	0.79	0.70	0.61	0.44
Girls	3926	6.53 (2)	0.038	1.00	0.99	0.02	0.013	0.78	0.69	0.63	0.49
Country (city/cities)											
Australia (Adelaide)	526	0.89 (2)	0.642	1.00	1.01	<0.01	0.01	0.82	0.69	0.65	0.52
Brazil (Sao Paulo)	569	0.26 (2)	0.878	1.00	1.01	<0.01	0.01	0.75	0.70	0.43	0.85
Canada (Ottawa)	566	0.14 (2)	0.932	1.00	1.02	<0.01	0.01	0.94	0.66	0.66	0.41
China (Tianjin)	549	3.27 (2)	0.195	1.00	0.99	0.03	0.03	0.75	0.61	0.83	0.37
Colombia (Bogota)	919	4.20 (2)	0.123	0.99	0.96	0.04	0.03	0.61	0.55	0.53	0.36
Finland (Helsinki, Espoo, Vantaa)	535	1.29 (2)	0.524	1.00	1.01	<0.01	0.02	0.72	0.79	0.58	0.59
India (Bangalore)	620	0.79 (2)	0.675	1.00	1.03	<0.01	0.02	0.62	0.60	0.48	0.44
Kenya (Nairobi)	559	5.11 (2)	0.078	0.99	0.95	0.05	0.03	0.85	0.58	0.47	0.31
Portugal (Porto)	777	3.42 (2)	0.181	1.00	1.00	0.03	0.02	0.74	0.81	0.79	0.87
South Africa (Cape Town)	541	7.31 (2)	0.026	0.98	0.95	0.07	0.04	0.81	0.62	0.62	0.38
United Kingdom (Bath and Somerset)	525	1.08 (2)	0.583	1.00	1.01	<0.01	0.01	0.85	0.69	0.63	0.52
Unites States of America (Baton Rouge)	633	2.02 (2)	0.365	1.00	1.00	<0.01	0.02	0.84	0.76	0.76	0.60

(a) The weighted least squares estimation with robust standard errors and a mean and variance adjusted test statics was used, and items were used as ordinal variables. The model fit was evaluated with several types of fit indices including Chi-Square statistics, the Comparative Fit Index (CFI), the Tucker–Lewis Index (TLI), the Root Mean Square Error of Approximation (RMSEA), the and Standardized Root Mean Square Residual (SRMR). As suggested by Hu and Bentler [37], CFI and TLI values $\geq$0.95, RMSEA values $\leq$0.06, and SRMR values $\leq$0.08 were considered to indicate a good fit for the data. Results are presented for pooled data and separately for each gender and country (city/cities). (b) Sad = "I eat more when I'm sad", worried = "I eat more, when I'm worried", mad = "I eat when I'm mad", bored = "I eat more, when I'm bored".

2.3. Dietary patterns

Dietary patterns were defined using data from a self-administered food frequency questionnaire (FFQ), in which children reported their usual consumption frequency of 23 different food groups, according to seven response categories ranging from "never" to "more than once a day". The FFQ was validated within ISCOLE against 3-day pre-coded food diaries [40]. The identification of the two dietary patterns has been reported in detail elsewhere [41]. In short, principal components analysis

(PCA) with an orthogonal Varimax transformation was carried out using weekly portions of the FFQ food groups as input variables. From the 23 FFQ food groups, fruit juices were excluded from PCA due to low validity of reporting [40]. Two components were identified and named: (1) an unhealthy diet pattern, with high loadings for fast foods, ice cream, fried food, French fries, potato chips, cakes and sugar-sweetened sodas, and (2) a healthy diet pattern, with high loadings for dark-green vegetables, orange vegetables, vegetables in general, and fruits and berries. The naming was based on previous knowledge of associations between health and food items that loaded highly on the two dietary patterns. In total, the two dietary patterns explained 36% of the total variance in reported food consumption. The unhealthy diet pattern was stronger with an eigenvalue of 4.8 (22% of variance explained), and the healthy diet pattern was slightly weaker with an eigenvalue of 3.1 (14% of variance explained). The PCA was also repeated for each site separately, and the resulting site-specific diet patterns were very similar to the patterns that emerged with the pooled data. In the present paper, we used the pattern scores from the pooled data in accordance with the EE factor scores.

2.4. Physical Activity and Sleep

The average daily time spent in MVPA and average nocturnal sleep duration were assessed using the Actigraph GT3X+ accelerometer (Pensacola, FL, USA). The device was worn at the waist on an elastic belt for 24 hours per day (removing only for water-related activities, such as swimming or taking a shower) for at least seven days. The minimal amount of data considered adequate to calculate the average daily MVPA was at least four days with 10 or more hours of daily awake wear time, including at least one weekend day. MVPA was defined as $\geq$574 counts per 15 s [42]. Nocturnal sleep duration was estimated using an algorithm for 24-h accelerometers that was previously validated for the ISCOLE [43]. This algorithm captures the total nocturnal sleep time from sleep onset to the end of sleep and distinguishes it from daytime sleep episodes, and its accuracy was shown to be acceptable when compared to sleep logs [43]. Only nights with valid sleep (total sleep time $\geq$160 min) were used to calculate the mean nocturnal sleep duration of the week and adequate data for calculating the average value was considered at least 3 valid nights, including one weekend night (Friday or Saturday).

2.5. TV Viewing

TV viewing time was determined with a self-administered questionnaire, which was adapted from the U.S. Youth Risk Behaviour Surveillance system [44]. Children were asked how many hours they typically watched TV for weekdays and weekend days separately. The response categories (respective scores) were "I did not watch TV" (0), less than 1 h (0.5), 1 h (1), 2 h (2), 3 h (3), 4 h (4), and 5 or more h (5). The total score was calculated by weighing the responses for weekdays by 5/7 and weekend days by 2/7. The TV viewing questions were shown to have adequate reliability ($r = 0.55$–0.68) and validity ($r = 0.47$) in a sample of 11–15-year-old U.S. children [45].

2.6. BMI

Anthropometric measurements were conducted during the school day by trained study assistants. Height was measured without shoes using a Seca 213 portable stadiometer (Hamburg, Germany) and weight was measured when participants were barefoot, in light indoor clothing, and without any pocket items, using a portable Tanita SC-240 Body Composition Analyzer (Arlington Heights, IL). Two measurements were obtained, and the average was used for analysis. If the first two measurements were more than 0.5 cm or 0.5 kg apart for height and weight, respectively, a third measurement was done, and the closest two measurements were averaged for analysis. BMI was calculated dividing the weight by the height squared (kg/m^2). Age- and gender-specific reference data from the World Health Organization were used to compute the BMI z-scores [46].

2.7. Covariates

Age, gender, and household income were used as covariates. Parents reported the annual household income using eight to ten predefined categories designed for each study site. Country-specific income categories were merged into four levels. It was not possible to achieve exact quartiles, but the aim of the merging was to ensure the distribution of income was as balanced as possible.

2.8. Statistical analyses

The descriptive results were calculated using IBM SPSS Statistics 24 (IBM SPSS, Chicago, IL, USA). An independent samples t-test and a χ^2 test were used to compare the analytical sample with excluded children. Since the sample was clustered at three levels (students nested within schools nested within study sites), the associations between the EE factor scores and dependent variables were assessed using multilevel linear regression models (PROC MIXED of SAS statistical package version 9.4; SAS Institute Inc., Cary; NC, USA). Study sites and schools nested within study sites were both considered to have random effects. The denominator degrees of freedom for statistical tests pertaining to fixed effects were calculated using the Kenward and Roger approximation [47]. The first adjusted models included age, gender, and household income as covariates. In addition to that, second fully adjusted models included other health behaviours and BMI z-scores. Since a few earlier studies found a gender difference in the association between EE and BMI [22,23], we tested the interaction between the EE factor scores and gender in the fully adjusted models. Multilevel linear regression models were repeated for each site separately, and in these analyses, schools were considered as having random effects. Due to the skewness of the EE factor score variable, it was also studied as a categorical variable with five categories. This variable was formed with two steps: first, children who answered "never" for all four EE items were categorized into one group, and second, remaining children were categorized into quarters based on the EE factor scores.

3. Results

3.1. Descriptive Results

The analytical sample of the present study comprised 5426 children (74% of the overall study sample). Children who were excluded because of missing data showed more tendency towards EE than the included children (mean (SD) score 0.09 (0.58) vs. 0.03 (0.56), $p < 0.001$). In addition, as compared with the analytical sample, they had higher scores for the unhealthy diet pattern (0.22 (1.18) vs. −0.07 (0.93), $p < 0.001$), watched more TV (TV viewing score 1.8 (1.3) vs. 1.7 (1.2), $p = 0.001$), and had higher BMI z scores (0.61 (1.28) vs. 0.44 (1.25), $p < 0.001$). Also, more boys were excluded from the analytical sample than girls (28% vs. 25%, $p = 0.002$). Parents of the excluded children belonged more frequently to the lowest income group compared with those in the analytical sample (30% vs. 25%, $p < 0.001$). There were no differences in the scores for the healthy diet pattern, the amount of MVPA, sleep duration, or age between the excluded and included children.

Out of the analytical sample, 32% of the children answered "never or almost never" to all four EE items, and 25% answered "never or almost never" to three items and "sometimes" to one item. Only 18 (0.3%) children answered "usually or always" to all four EE items. Descriptive results stratified by gender and study site including the EE factor scores are presented in Table 2. There were no significant differences in the EE factor scores between boys and girls (data not shown), except in the United Kingdom, where girls showed a higher tendency towards EE compared with boys (mean (SD) score 0.10 (0.55) in girls vs. −0.04 (0.50) in boys, t-test = −2.37, $p = 0.018$).

Table 2. Descriptive results of the analytical sample by gender and country (city/cities).

	Number of Participants (% Girls)	Mean (SD)								Household Classified Lowest Income [e], n (%)	Household Classified Highest Income [e], n (%)
		Emotional Eating Score [a]	Unhealthy Diet Score [b]	Healthy Diet Score [b]	MVPA (min/day) [c]	Sleep (min/day) [c]	TV Viewing [d]	BMI z-Score	Age (years)		
All	5426 (55)	0.03 (0.56)	−0.07 (0.93)	0.00 (0.99)	60 (25)	528 (53)	1.7 (1.2)	0.43 (1.25)	10.4 (0.6)	1376 (25)	1466 (27)
Gender											
Boys	2461 (0)	0.03 (0.56)	0.00 (0.98)	−0.06 (1.00)	70 (26)	524 (52)	1.8 (1.2)	0.53 (1.30)	10.4 (0.6)	596 (24)	696 (28)
Girls	2965 (100)	0.03 (0.56)	−0.14 (0.89)	0.04 (0.99)	52 (21)	532 (53)	1.6 (1.2)	0.36 (1.21)	10.4 (0.6)	780 (26)	770 (26)
Country (city/cities)											
Australia (Adelaide)	407 (54)	0.05 (0.54)	−0.30 (0.73)	0.24 (0.94)	65 (23)	565 (43)	1.7 (1.1)	0.57 (1.13)	10.7 (0.4)	88 (22)	94 (23)
Brazil (Sao Paulo)	378 (50)	0.24 (0.61)	0.09 (0.90)	−0.45 (1.05)	60 (27)	512 (49)	2.2 (1.4)	0.92 (1.43)	10.5 (0.5)	144 (38)	52 (14)
Canada (Ottawa)	481 (59)	−0.10 (0.51)	−0.50 (0.57)	0.49 (0.98)	59 (20)	544 (51)	1.4 (1.2)	0.42 (1.21)	10.5 (0.4)	88 (18)	186 (39)
China (Tianjin)	430 (48)	−0.09 (0.47)	−0.24 (0.96)	0.05 (0.90)	45 (16)	527 (39)	1.2 (1.1)	0.73 (1.54)	9.9 (0.5)	86 (20)	135 (31)
Colombia (Bogota)	810 (51)	−0.02 (0.52)	−0.08 (0.55)	−0.45 (0.74)	68 (25)	525 (49)	2.1 (1.1)	0.20 (1.05)	10.5 (0.6)	279 (34)	185 (23)
Finland (Helsinki, Espoo, Vantaa)	426 (55)	−0.08 (0.52)	−0.57 (0.43)	−0.15 (0.85)	70 (27)	508 (56)	1.4 (0.9)	0.27 (1.04)	10.5 (0.4)	81 (19)	174 (41)
India (Bangalore)	500 (55)	0.06 (0.51)	−0.10 (0.83)	−0.09 (0.89)	48 (21)	516 (44)	1.2 (0.9)	0.22 (1.36)	10.4 (0.5)	121 (24)	188 (38)
Kenya (Nairobi)	434 (54)	0.19 (0.57)	0.11 (1.01)	0.28 (0.99)	73 (32)	515 (52)	1.6 (1.3)	−0.06 (1.20)	10.2 (0.7)	101 (23)	126 (29)
Portugal (Porto)	490 (57)	−0.09 (0.56)	−0.36 (0.63)	0.25 (1.04)	56 (22)	497 (51)	1.5 (1.0)	0.83 (1.13)	10.4 (0.3)	96 (20)	105 (21)
South Africa (Cape Town)	267 (60)	0.35 (0.67)	1.08 (1.25)	0.26 (1.08)	62 (25)	552 (43)	2.0 (1.3)	0.20 (1.27)	10.2 (0.7)	133 (45)	37 (13)
United Kingdom (Bath and Somerset)	355 (57)	0.04 (0.53)	−0.17 (0.73)	0.03 (0.91)	64 (23)	569 (43)	1.7 (1.0)	0.40 (1.08)	10.9 (0.4)	95 (27)	81 (23)
Unites States of America (Baton Rouge)	418 (60)	0.00 (0.59)	0.59 (1.36)	−0.14 (1.14)	50 (19)	533 (55)	2.0 (1.4)	0.71 (1.27)	9.9 (0.6)	64 (15)	103 (25)

(a) Confirmatory factor analysis with weighted least squares estimation with robust standard errors and a mean and variance adjusted test statistic was conducted. Factor scores were computed using the Empirical Bayes approach, and the range of scores was −0.55 to 1.93. (b) Component scores identified with principal components analysis with an orthogonal varimax rotation. (c) The average amount of moderate to vigorous physical activity (MVPA) during the day and the average amount of night-time sleep, measured with accelerometers. (d) TV viewing score obtained from a questionnaire: minimum 0 points, maximum 5 points. (e) Annual household income was reported by parents using site-specific categories, which were merged into four levels.

3.2. Associations between Emotional Eating, Health Behaviours and BMI

The results from the multilevel linear regression models using the EE score as an independent variable are presented in Table 3. In the unadjusted models, EE was positively associated with the unhealthy diet pattern, MVPA, and TV viewing, and inversely associated with the BMI z-score. No associations were observed between the EE and the healthy diet pattern or sleep duration. The associations with the unhealthy diet pattern, MVPA, and TV viewing remained significant after adjusting for covariates (age, gender, and income), other health behaviours, and BMI z-scores. There was an interaction between the EE score and gender only in association with MVPA ($p = 0.02$). The association between EE and MVPA was positive for both genders, but it was stronger in boys ($\beta = 3.31$, SE $= 0.86$, $p = 0.0001$) than in girls ($\beta = 1.28$, SE $= 0.60$, $p = 0.035$, Table 4).

The adjusted multilevel linear regression models were repeated for each site separately (Table 4). The positive association observed between the EE score and the unhealthy diet pattern was consistent across the study sites, but the significant positive association between EE and MVPA was observed only in Colombia and South Africa, and the significant positive association between EE and TV viewing was observed only in Canada and China.

When EE was included in the adjusted multilevel linear regression models as a categorical variable to account for the skewness of the original continuous variable, the results remained highly similar (Table 5). Compared to children with no EE, children in all EE quarters had higher unhealthy diet pattern scores, and this association followed a linear pattern according to the EE score quarters. A linear positive association was also found between the categorical EE variable and MVPA, and there was a significant, but not very strong, interaction with gender ($p = 0.04$). The association was significant for both genders, but it was stronger for boys. The categorical EE variable was also associated with TV viewing, but the association was not linear. Similar to the continuous EE score, the categorical EE variable was not associated with the healthy diet pattern, sleep duration, or BMI z-score.

Table 3. The associations [a] between emotional eating factor scores (as the independent variable) and outcome variables [b]. $n = 5426$.

	Unhealthy Diet Pattern		Healthy Diet Pattern		MVPA		Sleep		TV Viewing		BMI z-Score	
	Beta (SE)	p-Value	Beta (SE)	p-Value	Beta (SE)	p-Value	Beta (SE)	p-Value	Beta (SE)	p-Value	Beta (SE)	p-Value
Unadjusted [c]	0.33 (0.02)	<0.0001	−0.03 (0.02)	0.739	2.95 (0.55)	<0.0001	−0.04 (1.20)	0.977	0.16 (0.03)	<0.0001	−0.09 (0.03)	0.004
1. Adjusted model [d]	0.32 (0.02)	<0.0001	−0.03 (0.02)	0.291	2.65 (0.51)	<0.0001	0.01 (1.19)	0.993	0.15 (0.03)	<0.0001	−0.09 (0.03)	0.004
2. Adjusted model [e]	0.29 (0.02)	<0.0001	−0.04 (0.02)	0.138	2.01 (0.51)	<0.0001	0.65 (1.22)	0.594	0.07 (0.03)	0.010	−0.06 (0.03)	0.055

(a) Analyzed with a multilevel (site, schools nested within sites) linear regression. (b) The unhealthy and healthy diet pattern scores identified using principal components analysis, daily moderate to vigorous physical activity (min, MVPA), nightly sleep duration (min), TV viewing scores, and BMI z-scores. (c) Only using the emotional eating factor score as an independent variable. (d) Adjusted by age, gender, and household income. (e) Adjusted by age, gender, household income, and other outcome variables.

Table 4. The association between emotional eating [a] and outcome variables [b] in gender-stratified [c] and site-stratified [d] analyses.

	N	Unhealthy Diet Pattern		Healthy Diet Pattern		MVPA		Sleep		TV Viewing		BMI z-Score	
		Beta (SE)	p-Value	Beta (SE)	p-Value	Beta (SE)	p-Value	Beta (SE)	p-Value	Beta (SE)	p-Value	Beta (SE)	p-Value
Gender													
Boys	2461	0.29 (0.03)	<0.0001	−0.03 (0.04)	0.346	3.31 (0.86)	0.0001	−0.91 (1.80)	0.613	0.08 (0.04)	0.068	−0.11 (0.05)	0.014
Girls	2965	0.30 (0.03)	<0.0001	−0.03 (0.03)	0.392	1.28 (0.60)	0.035	1.60 (1.67)	0.337	0.05 (0.04)	0.157	−0.03 (0.04)	0.493
Study sites													
Australia (Adelaide)	407	0.35 (0.06)	<0.0001	−0.01 (0.09)	0.911	0.00 (1.95)	0.998	−2.43 (4.01)	0.544	0.09 (0.10)	0.390	0.17 (0.11)	0.117
Brazil (Sao Paulo)	378	0.19 (0.08)	0.014	−0.06 (0.09)	0.546	3.60 (1.92)	0.062	3.95 (4.04)	0.329	0.05 (0.12)	0.674	0.07 (0.12)	0.562
Canada (Ottawa)	481	0.18 (0.05)	0.0001	−0.01 (0.09)	0.903	1.06 (1.63)	0.515	−0.69 (4.08)	0.867	0.27 (0.10)	0.008	−0.09 (0.11)	0.392
China (Tianjin)	378	0.43 (0.10)	<0.0001	−0.04 (0.10)	0.710	−0.75 (1.57)	0.634	0.66 (4.17)	0.874	0.34 (0.10)	0.001	−0.19 (0.16)	0.227
Colombia (Bogota)	810	0.20 (0.04)	<0.0001	0.10 (0.05)	0.045	3.33 (1.51)	0.028	2.97 (3.44)	0.389	0.10 (0.08)	0.186	−0.16 (0.07)	0.021
Finland (Helsinki, Espoo, Vantaa)	426	0.18 (0.04)	<0.0001	0.02 (0.08)	0.809	1.09 (2.25)	0.630	−2.47 (5.15)	0.632	−0.04 (0.09)	0.624	−0.21 (0.10)	0.032
India (Bangalore)	500	0.21 (0.07)	0.004	−0.10 (0.08)	0.197	−0.10 (1.50)	0.945	1.24 (3.98)	0.756	−0.04 (0.08)	0.583	−0.14 (0.12)	0.246
Kenya (Nairobi)	434	0.30 (0.08)	0.0003	−0.09 (0.09)	0.283	2.80 (1.89)	0.139	1.08 (4.71)	0.819	0.01 (0.11)	0.933	0.12 (0.10)	0.243
Portugal (Porto)	490	0.27 (0.05)	<0.0001	0.05 (0.09)	0.587	2.86 (1.56)	0.068	−0.51 (4.37)	0.907	0.13 (0.08)	0.110	−0.11 (0.10)	0.287
South Africa (Cape Town)	267	0.62 (0.11)	<0.0001	−0.21 (0.11)	0.052	5.12 (2.23)	0.022	2.41 (4.46)	0.589	0.09 (0.13)	0.475	0.06 (0.13)	0.633
United Kingdom (Bath and Somerset)	355	0.23 (0.07)	0.0007	0.01 (0.09)	0.913	−1.98 (1.97)	0.317	−4.68 (4.27)	0.273	−0.04 (0.10)	0.684	0.01 (0.11)	0.920
Unites States of America (Baton Rouge)	418	0.47 (0.09)	<0.0001	−0.03 (0.10)	0.788	0.53 (1.44)	0.715	1.78 (4.52)	0.695	−0.03 (0.11)	0.791	−0.06 (0.11)	0.600

(a) Emotional eating factor scores as the independent variable. (b) The unhealthy and healthy diet pattern scores identified using principal components analysis, daily moderate to vigorous physical activity (min, MVPA), nightly sleep duration (min), TV viewing scores, and BMI z-scores. (c) Analyzed with a multilevel (site, schools nested within sites) linear regression, adjusted with age, household income, and other outcome variables. (d) Analyzed with a multilevel (schools) linear regression, adjusted by age, gender, household income, and other outcome variables.

Table 5. The associations [a] between categorized emotional eating factor scores [b] and outcome variables [c].

	n (%)	Unhealthy Diet Pattern		Healthy Diet Pattern		MVPA		Sleep		TV Viewing		BMI z-Score	
		Beta (SE)	p-Value	Beta (SE)	p-Value	Beta (SE)	p-Value	Beta (SE)	p-Value	Beta (SE)	p-Value	Beta (SE)	p-Value
All			<0.0001		0.190		0.0008		0.105		0.002		0.248
No emotional eating	1759 (32)	ref.		ref.		ref.		ref.		ref.		ref.	
1. quarter	943 (17)	0.11 (0.03)	0.0006	−0.05 (0.04)	0.201	−0.15 (0.82)	0.853	4.42 (1.95)	0.023	0.11 (0.05)	0.014	−0.09 (0.05)	0.065
2. quarter	771 (14)	0.14 (0.03)	<0.0001	−0.08 (0.04)	0.044	0.51 (0.86)	0.551	−1.20 (2.05)	0.557	0.08 (0.05)	0.105	−0.01 (0.05)	0.889
3. quarter	1017 (19)	0.27 (0.03)	<0.0001	−0.06 (0.04)	0.145	1.27 (0.79)	0.109	2.28 (1.89)	0.230	0.18 (0.04)	<0.0001	−0.06 (0.05)	0.239
4. quarter	936 (17)	0.43 (0.03)	<0.0001	−0.08 (0.04)	0.050	3.36 (0.84)	<0.0001	1.74 (2.01)	0.387	0.09 (0.05)	0.047	−0.09 (0.05)	0.093
Boys			<0.0001		0.573		0.001		0.833		0.097		0.052
No emotional eating	789 (32)	ref.		ref.		ref.		ref.		ref.		ref.	
1. quarter	432 (18)	0.10 (0.05)	0.060	−0.03 (0.06)	0.656	−0.96 (1.37)	0.486	−0.09 (2.87)	0.974	0.06 (0.07)	0.371	−0.17 (0.07)	0.021
2. quarter	356 (15)	0.15 (0.05)	0.007	−0.08 (0.06)	0.190	1.45 (1.45)	0.316	−2.40 (3.03)	0.427	0.05 (0.07)	0.512	−0.10 (0.08)	0.215
3. quarter	452 (18)	0.29 (0.05)	<0.0001	−0.08 (0.06)	0.182	2.28 (1.35)	0.093	0.74 (2.83)	0.795	0.19 (0.07)	0.006	−0.17 (0.07)	0.020
4. quarter	432 (18)	0.41 (0.05)	<0.0001	−0.07 (0.06)	0.261	5.09 (1.42)	0.0003	−2.14 (2.96)	0.470	0.09 (0.07)	0.224	−0.18 (0.08)	0.020
Girls			<0.0001		0.615		0.046		0.025		0.038		0.737
No emotional eating	970 (33)	ref.		ref.		ref.		ref.		ref.		ref.	
1. quarter	511 (17)	0.12 (0.04)	0.004	−0.06 (0.05)	0.265	−0.08 (0.96)	0.932	8.01 (2.67)	0.003	0.14 (0.06)	0.017	−0.02 (0.07)	0.727
2. quarter	415 (14)	0.15 (0.04)	0.001	−0.06 (0.06)	0.256	−0.34 (1.01)	0.736	−0.46 (2.81)	0.870	0.09 (0.06)	0.149	0.07 (0.07)	0.321
3. quarter	565 (19)	0.25 (0.04)	<0.0001	−0.03 (0.05)	0.610	−0.08 (0.93)	0.932	3.48 (2.58)	0.177	0.16 (0.06)	0.005	0.02 (0.06)	0.727
4. quarter	504 (17)	0.45 (0.04)	<0.0001	−0.07 (0.05)	0.193	2.62 (1.00)	0.009	4.24 (2.77)	0.126	0.07 (0.06)	0.240	−0.03 (0.07)	0.700

(a) Analyzed with multilevel (site, schools nested within sites) linear regression. All models adjusted with age, household income, other outcome variables, and model for all participants adjusted also for gender. (b) The emotional eating factor scores were categorized by first setting the participants with no emotional eating as reference group and then dividing rest of the participants to quarters based on emotional eating factor scores. The emotional eating score in "No emotional eating" -group was −0.552 and minimum and maximum values of emotional eating factor score was −0.26 and −0.06 in 1st quarter, −0.05 and 0.20 in 2nd quarter, 0.21 and 0.65 in 3rd quarter, and 0.66 and 1.93 in 4th quarter. (c) The unhealthy and the healthy diet pattern scores identified using principal components analysis, daily moderate to vigorous physical activity (min, MVPA), nightly sleep duration (min), TV viewing scores, and BMI z-scores.

4. Discussion

In this large, international sample of 9–11-year-old children, we found a positive association between EE and an unhealthy diet pattern. The novel finding of this study was that this positive association appeared to be consistent across the 12 study sites representing very different cultural and environmental settings. This is an important contribution to the current literature which has been almost completely focused on Western countries. We also found that EE was positively associated with both MVPA and TV viewing, yet these patterns were not consistent across all study sites. There were no associations between EE and healthy diet pattern, nocturnal sleep duration, or BMI z-score.

Our findings regarding the positive association between EE and the unhealthy diet pattern and the lack of association between EE and the healthy diet pattern support the earlier findings mainly in adults [3] that EE is especially associated with increased consumption of sweet and high-fat foods, which are generally considered to be highly palatable. Previous studies in 12–15-year-old children have also indicated that EE is associated with higher consumption of energy-dense foods and soft drinks, but it is not associated with the consumption of fruits and vegetables [30,31]. It must be noted that in addition to the palatability and nutrient composition of foods, food choice in response to emotional state might also reflect the availability and accessibility of foods. Many foods included in the unhealthy diet pattern (i.e., fast foods, ice cream, fried food, French fries, potato chips, cakes, and sugar-sweetened sodas) are ready to eat and are easily obtainable, even for 9–11-year-olds. However, one cause of EE may be poor emotion regulation in general [4], and it has been shown that adolescents (mean age 13.6 years) who are having difficulties with adequately regulating their negative emotions consume snacks, especially energy-dense snacks, more frequently [48]. Yet, because our study, as well as most of the earlier research regarding the association between emotional eating and diet, was cross-sectional, we cannot rule out the possibility of a reverse relationship. That might be the case if an unhealthier diet is associated with a decreased mood, or impaired hunger control, making it easier to eat in emotional states.

Interestingly, in 5–12-year-old children, an age group closer to the present sample age range, no association between self-reported EE and food consumption has been reported previously [20,32]. One explanation for these contradictory findings may be differences in how diet was measured. Van Strien and Oosterveld [20] asked one simple question about the weekly frequency of consumption of sweet and/or savoury snacks with four answer options (never/sometimes/often/everyday), which might not have allowed enough variance to detect a possible association. In the study by Michels et al. [32], food consumption was reported by the parents, and it is possible that foods eaten in response to emotions are eaten without the knowledge of the parents. It has also been suggested that in children aged 6 to 18 years, self-reporting of dietary intake is more valid than parental reports [49,50].

As mentioned above, the positive association between EE and the unhealthy diet pattern appeared to be similar in all 12 countries. All beta estimates were positive, but there were some differences in the sizes of the estimates. The significance of these differences was not tested, because comparing each country against all of the remaining countries was outside of the scope of this study. Yet, similar findings across different countries suggest that the association between EE and the unhealthy diet pattern is not restricted to Western countries and their cultural and food environments. A normal physiological reaction to negative emotions is expected to be a suppressed appetite [5]. So, rather than being an innate characteristic, EE is most likely learned [51], and, for example, the home environment [52] and parenting [53] may affect this process. Our results suggest that the association between EE and unhealthy food consumption in children is independent, or at least not fully dependent, on the culture and culturally learned behavioural patterns.

We found a small but significant positive association between EE and the amount of both daily MVPA and TV viewing. However, in contrast to the association with the unhealthy diet pattern, these associations were not consistent between all study sites. The significant positive associations between EE and these outcomes were observed only in two out of 12 sites (Colombia and South Africa for of MVPA and Canada and China for TV viewing). These findings need further clarification and replication in other study samples, because unassessed local factors may influence the observed relationships. For example, children undertake MVPA under a variety of contexts, and given that accelerometry was used to measure MVPA, we have detailed information on the level and pattern of MVPA but not the cultural, social or environmental context under which MVPA was performed.

We hypothesized that EE might be related to MVPA and TV-viewing, because unhealthy behaviours tend to cluster in children [33,34]. The observed positive association between EE and MVPA was in contrast to that hypothesis. To our knowledge, only one study has previously examined the association between EE and physical activity in children, with no association between EE and weekly frequency of doing sports reported [20]. However, in that study, the amount of physical activity was measured with one simple question, whereas in the present study, MVPA was measured objectively using accelerometers. A few earlier studies support our finding regarding a positive association between EE and TV viewing. Ouwens et al. [54] reported a small but significant positive correlation between EE and TV viewing, and in another study, a significant positive correlation was found, but only in girls [20].

As the present study was cross-sectional, future studies are needed to determine the causal relationship and possible mechanisms for the association between EE and both MVPA and TV viewing. One might only speculate that children with high EE could compensate for this behaviour with a higher amount of MVPA. On the other hand, it may be that children with high MVPA eat more overall as well as during emotional situations. There is also a possibility that children with high MVPA have more hobbies, including those involving physical activity in competing environments, which might lead to more stress and subsequently EE. TV viewing is associated with higher intakes of sweet and salty snacks and carbonated beverages [55], and Ouwens et al. [54] found that the association between TV viewing and snacking was stronger in children with high EE. Distraction caused by the television can lead to diminished awareness of hunger and satiety, and eating in front of television can be considered "mindless eating", which has been shown to be closely related to EE in children [56]. It is also possible that there is a third unmeasured variable explaining the association. For example, children with high negative affectivity could watch more TV as well as display more EE.

We did not find an association between EE and BMI z-scores in the fully adjusted model. In line with our findings, other studies have also reported no difference in self-reported [20] and parent-reported [19] EE between normal weight and overweight 7 to 15-year-old children. However, several studies have also found a positive association [12–18]. In children, EE has been measured using self-reported or parent-reported questionnaires, and it has been shown that there is good concordance between these two approaches [13]. However, it seems that the majority of the studies reporting positive associations with BMI/being overweight have used parent-reported EE [12,14–18], and some studies using self-reported EE have even found an inverse association with BMI/being overweight [21–23]. It remains an interesting question for future studies as to whether inconsistent findings could be partially explained by the different reporting methods for EE.

We found a weak but significant negative association between self-reported EE and BMI z-scores in the unadjusted model, but after adjusting for other health behaviours (including MVPA), it was no longer significant. This result is probably due to including MVPA in the model, since EE was positively associated with MVPA in our sample, and MVPA was the strongest significant predictor of a lower BMI [36]. In earlier studies that reported a negative association [21–23], physical activity was not taken into account. Altogether, our results strengthen the existing literature that, in children, EE does not seem to be as clearly associated with obesity as in adults.

It is interesting and somewhat controversial that EE was associated with the unhealthy diet pattern but not with BMI. However, in the ISCOLE sample, the unhealthy diet pattern was not associated with BMI [36]. It should be noted that the diet pattern scores describe dietary quality instead of energy intake per se, which may be more closely related to BMI. Nevertheless, it has been shown that food choices determined by dietary patterns track into adulthood [57]. It might be that EE already leads to the unhealthy diet pattern during childhood, but its consequences, such as excess weight gain, are visible only later in life. To our knowledge, there are no prospective studies examining these associations from childhood to adolescence or adulthood, but in one previous study, parent-reported EE of 5 to 6-year-old children predicted a higher BMI in 7 to 8-year-old children [25]. In adults, EE has also been shown to predict weight gain [10,11].

We did not find any interactions between EE and gender in association with dietary patterns, TV viewing, sleep duration, or BMI z-scores. Yet, the positive association between EE and MVPA was significantly stronger in boys. Further studies are needed to clarify and explain this observed interaction. In our study, there was no difference in reported EE between boys and girls, which is consistent with some previous findings [12,23], but not all, since Snoek et al. [22] found that 11–16-year-old girls reported more EE than boys. In site-specific analyses, we found that in the United Kingdom, higher amounts of EE were reported among girls than boys. The difference between mean EE scores was small (0.10 (0.55) in girls vs. −0.04 (0.50) in boys), and it is possible that the significant difference emerged by chance due to multiple testing (type I error).

A potential limitation of the present study was that EE was self-reported. However, Braet et al. [13] compared children's self-reported EE vs. parent-reported EE and found that the agreement between reporting was good enough to conclude that it is possible to rely on either of the informants, especially for children aged 10 years and older. We measured EE using the EIES, which was developed in a similar age group as our sample. Even though the internal consistency was less than optimal for the four EIES items (Cronbach's alpha value 0.6), the excellent fit of the one-factor CFA model and high factor loadings supported the unidimensionality of the scale. In addition, the percentage of children reporting no EE in our study was 32%. Similar percentages have been reported previously, regardless of the questionnaire or the reporter. In one study using the child-version of the Dutch Eating Behaviour Questionnaire to measure self-reported EE, 45% of the children reported that they never expressed EE [54], and in the other study, approximately 35% of the parents reported that their child never displays EE using the Children's Eating Behavior Questionnaire [18]. As well as EE, diet was also self-reported. It has been suggested that in children aged 6 to 18 years, self-reporting of dietary intake is more valid than parental reporting [49,50]. Furthermore, in that age group, a relatively short (20–60 items) FFQ without requirement for portion size estimation, as used in the present study, has been suggested to be a valid method for measuring self-reported diet [49].

A further limitation was that the excluded children reported more EE, had higher scores on the unhealthy dietary pattern, watched more TV, and had higher BMI z-scores. This finding fits well with the hypothesis that unhealthy behaviours tend to cluster [33,34]. It is possible that this selection effect has attenuated the observed associations, and it may affect the generalizability of the results, although the observed differences between two groups were quite small, albeit statistically significant. Furthermore, it should also be mentioned that children's opportunities to eat in response to negative emotions depend on how often they experience these emotions. Unfortunately, no measures of emotions, mood, or stress were included in the present study, because it was a secondary analysis of existing ISCOLE, and the questionnaire was originally designed to address the main research questions. Finally, the cross-sectional nature of the data does not allow any conclusions about the causality of the observed associations or their direction to be formed. However, a particular strength and novel aspect of this study is that the same EE questionnaire and outcome measures were used in a large and truly international study sample. We were also able to study multiple health behaviours simultaneously, and MVPA, sleep duration, and BMI were measured objectively.

5. Conclusions

In conclusion, we found a significant positive association between EE and an unhealthy diet pattern, which was consistent across the 12 different study sites. As previous studies have been almost completely focused on Western countries, this extends the present knowledge by suggesting that the association between EE and unhealthy diet pattern is not restricted to Western countries and their cultural and food environments. It is possible that EE can already lead to an unhealthy diet pattern during childhood, but its consequences, such as excess weight gain, are visible only later in life. The associations between EE and other health behaviours were either inconsistent between sites or not significant. We observed no association between EE and BMI z-scores. Prospective studies in different cultural contexts are needed to determine whether higher EE in children leads to an undesirable diet and subsequent obesity over time.

Author Contributions: Conceptualization, E.J., H.K., H.V. and M.F.; Formal analysis, E.J. and H.K.; Investigation, E.J., J.-P.C., G.H., C.M., J.M., O.L.S., M.S., C.T.-L., P.T.K. and M.F.; Methodology, E.J., H.K., H.V., J.-P.C., G.H., J.M., O.L.S., C.T.-L., P.T.K. and M.F.; Project administration, P.T.K. and M.F.; Visualization, E.J.; Writing—original draft, E.J.; Writing—review & editing, H.K., H.V., J.-P.C., G.H., C.M., J.M., O.L.S., M.S., C.T.-L., P.T.K. and M.F.

Acknowledgments: We wish to thank the ISCOLE External Advisory Board, ISCOLE participants and their families, and the ISCOLE Research Group.

References

1. Ng, M.; Fleming, T.; Robinson, M.; Thomson, B.; Graetz, N.; Margono, C.; Mullany, E.C.; Biryukov, S.; Abbafati, C.; Abera, S.F.; et al. Global, regional, and national prevalence of overweight and obesity in children and adults during 1980–2013: a systematic analysis for the Global Burden of Disease Study 2013. *Lancet (London, England)* **2014**, *384*, 766–781. [CrossRef]

2. Kaplan, H.I.; Kaplan, H.S. The psychosomatic concept of obesity. *J. Nerv. Ment. Dis.* **1957**, *125*, 181–201. [CrossRef] [PubMed]

3. Macht, M. How emotions affect eating: A five-way model. *Appetite* **2008**, *50*, 1–11. [CrossRef] [PubMed]

4. van Strien, T. Causes of Emotional Eating and Matched Treatment of Obesity. *Curr. Diab. Rep.* **2018**, *18*, 35. [CrossRef] [PubMed]

5. van Strien, T.; Donker, M.H.; Ouwens, M.A. Is desire to eat in response to positive emotions an 'obese' eating style: Is Kummerspeck for some people a misnomer? *Appetite* **2016**, *100*, 225–235. [CrossRef] [PubMed]

6. Keskitalo, K.; Tuorila, H.; Spector, T.D.; Cherkas, L.F.; Knaapila, A.; Kaprio, J.; Silventoinen, K.; Perola, M. The Three-Factor Eating Questionnaire, body mass index, and responses to sweet and salty fatty foods: a twin study of genetic and environmental associations. *Am. J. Clin. Nutr.* **2008**, *88*, 263–271. [CrossRef] [PubMed]

7. van Strien, T.; Herman, C.P.; Verheijden, M.W. Eating style, overeating, and overweight in a representative Dutch sample. Does external eating play a role? *Appetite* **2009**, *52*, 380–387. [CrossRef]

8. Konttinen, H.; Silventoinen, K.; Sarlio-Lähteenkorva, S.; Männistö, S.; Haukkala, A. Emotional eating and physical activity self-efficacy as pathways in the association between depressive symptoms and adiposity indicators. *Am. J. Clin. Nutr.* **2010**, *92*, 1031–1039. [CrossRef]

9. Péneau, S.; Ménard, E.; Méjean, C.; Bellisle, F.; Hercberg, S. Sex and dieting modify the association between emotional eating and weight status. *Am. J. Clin. Nutr.* **2013**, *97*, 1307–1313. [CrossRef]

10. Koenders, P.G.; van Strien, T. Emotional eating, rather than lifestyle behavior, drives weight gain in a prospective study in 1562 employees. *J. Occup. Environ. Med.* **2011**, *53*, 1287–1293. [CrossRef]

11. van Strien, T.; Konttinen, H.; Homberg, J.R.; Engels, R.C.M.E.; Winkens, L.H.H. Emotional eating as a mediator between depression and weight gain. *Appetite* **2016**, *100*, 216–224. [CrossRef] [PubMed]

12. Braet, C.; Van Strien, T. Assessment of emotional, externally induced and restrained eating behaviour in nine to twelve-year-old obese and non-obese children. *Behav. Res. Ther.* **1997**, *35*, 863–873. [CrossRef]

13. Braet, C.; Soetens, B.; Moens, E.; Mels, S.; Goossens, L.; Van Vlierberghe, L. Are two informants better than one? Parent–child agreement on the eating styles of children who are overweight. *Eur. Eat. Disord. Rev.* **2007**, *15*, 410–417. [CrossRef] [PubMed]

14. Viana, V.; Sinde, S.; Saxton, J.C. Children's Eating Behaviour Questionnaire: associations with BMI in Portuguese children. *Br. J. Nutr.* **2008**, *100*, 445–450. [CrossRef] [PubMed]

15. Webber, L.; Hill, C.; Saxton, J.; Van Jaarsveld, C.H.M.; Wardle, J. Eating behaviour and weight in children. *Int. J. Obes.* **2009**, *33*, 21–28. [CrossRef] [PubMed]

16. dos Passos, D.R.; Gigante, D.P.; Maciel, F.V.; Matijasevich, A. Children's eating behaviour: comparison between normal and overweight children from a school in Pelotas, Rio Grande do Sul, Brazil. *Rev. Paul. Pediatr.* **2015**, *33*, 42–49. [PubMed]

17. Sánchez, U.; Weisstaub, G.; Santos, J.L.; Corvalán, C.; Uauy, R. GOCS cohort: children's eating behavior scores and BMI. *Eur. J. Clin. Nutr.* **2016**, *70*, 925–928. [CrossRef]

18. Steinsbekk, S.; Barker, E.D.; Llewellyn, C.; Fildes, A.; Wichstrøm, L. Emotional Feeding and Emotional Eating: Reciprocal Processes and the Influence of Negative Affectivity. *Child Dev.* **2017**. [CrossRef] [PubMed]

19. Caccialanza, R.; Nicholls, D.; Cena, H.; Maccarini, L.; Rezzani, C.; Antonioli, L.; Dieli, S.; Roggi, C. Validation of the Dutch Eating Behaviour Questionnaire parent version (DEBQ-P) in the Italian population: A screening tool to detect differences in eating behaviour among obese, overweight and normal-weight preadolescents. *Eur. J. Clin. Nutr.* **2004**, *58*, 1217–1222. [CrossRef] [PubMed]

20. van Strien, T.; Oosterveld, P. The children's DEBQ for assessment of restrained, emotional, and external eating in 7- to 12-year-old children. *Int. J. Eat. Disord.* **2008**, *41*, 72–81. [CrossRef] [PubMed]

21. Striegel-Moore, R.; Morrison, J.A.; Schreiber, G.; Schumann, B.C.; Crawford, P.B.; Obarzanek, E. Emotion-induced eating and sucrose intake in children: the NHLBI Growth and Health Study. *Int. J. Eat. Disord.* **1999**, *25*, 389–398. [CrossRef]

22. Snoek, H.M.; van Strien, T.; Janssens, J.M.A.M.; Engels, R.C.M.E. Emotional, external, restrained eating and overweight in Dutch adolescents. *Scand. J. Psychol.* **2007**, *48*, 23–32. [CrossRef] [PubMed]

23. Braet, C.; Claus, L.; Goossens, L.; Moens, E.; Van Vlierberghe, L.; Soetens, B. Differences in eating style between overweight and normal-weight youngsters. *J. Health Psychol.* **2008**, *13*, 733–743. [CrossRef] [PubMed]

24. Coumans, J.M.J.; Danner, U.N.; Ahrens, W.; Hebestreit, A.; Intemann, T.; Kourides, Y.A.; Lissner, L.; Michels, N.; Moreno, L.A.; Russo, P.; et al. The association of emotion-driven impulsiveness, cognitive inflexibility and decision-making with weight status in European adolescents. *Int. J. Obes.* **2018**, *42*, 655–661. [CrossRef] [PubMed]

25. Parkinson, K.N.; Drewett, R.F.; Le Couteur, A.S.; Adamson, A.J. Do maternal ratings of appetite in infants predict later Child Eating Behaviour Questionnaire scores and body mass index? *Appetite* **2010**, *54*, 186–190. [CrossRef] [PubMed]

26. Steinsbekk, S.; Wichstrøm, L. Predictors of Change in BMI from the Age of 4 to 8. *J. Pediatr. Psychol.* **2015**, *40*, 1056–1064. [CrossRef] [PubMed]

27. Pate, R.R.; O'Neill, J.R.; Liese, A.D.; Janz, K.F.; Granberg, E.M.; Colabianchi, N.; Harsha, D.W.; Condrasky, M.M.; O'Neil, P.M.; Lau, E.Y.; Taverno Ross, S.E. Factors associated with development of excessive fatness in children and adolescents: a review of prospective studies. *Obes. Rev.* **2013**, *14*, 645–658. [CrossRef]

28. Huang, J.; Qi, S. Childhood obesity and food intake. *World J. Pediatr.* **2015**, *11*, 101–107. [CrossRef]

29. Felső, R.; Lohner, S.; Hollódy, K.; Erhardt, É; Molnár, D. Relationship between sleep duration and childhood obesity: Systematic review including the potential underlying mechanisms. *Nutr. Metab. Cardiovasc. Dis.* **2017**, *27*, 751–761.

30. Nguyen-Michel, S.; Unger, J.B.; Spruijt-Metz, D. Dietary correlates of emotional eating in adolescence. *Appetite* **2007**, *49*, 494–499. [CrossRef]

31. Elfhag, K.; Tholin, S.; Rasmussen, F. Consumption of fruit, vegetables, sweets and soft drinks are associated with psychological dimensions of eating behaviour in parents and their 12-year-old children. *Public Health Nutr.* **2008**, *11*, 914–923. [CrossRef] [PubMed]

32. Michels, N.; Sioen, I.; Braet, C.; Eiben, G.; Hebestreit, A.; Huybrechts, I.; Vanaelst, B.; Vyncke, K.; De Henauw, S. Stress, emotional eating behaviour and dietary patterns in children. *Appetite* **2012**, *59*, 762–769. [CrossRef] [PubMed]

33. Fernández-Alvira, J.M.; De Bourdeaudhuij, I.; Singh, A.S.; Vik, F.N.; Manios, Y.; Kovacs, E.; Jan, N.; Brug, J.; Moreno, L.A. Clustering of energy balance-related behaviors and parental education in European children: the ENERGY-project. *Int. J. Behav. Nutr. Phys. Act.* **2013**, *10*, 5. [CrossRef]

34. Leech, R.M.; McNaughton, S.A.; Timperio, A. The clustering of diet, physical activity and sedentary behavior in children and adolescents: A review. *Int. J. Behav. Nutr. Phys. Act.* **2014**, *11*, 4. [CrossRef] [PubMed]

35. Katzmarzyk, P.T.; Barreira, T.V.; Broyles, S.T.; Champagne, C.M.; Chaput, J.; Fogelholm, M.; Hu, G.; Johnson, W.D.; Kuriyan, R.; Kurpad, A.; et al. The International Study of Childhood Obesity, Lifestyle and the Environment (ISCOLE): design and methods. *BMC Public Health* **2013**, *13*, 900.

36. Katzmarzyk, P.T.; Barreira, T.V.; Broyles, S.T.; Champagne, C.M.; Chaput, J.; Fogelholm, M.; Hu, G.; Johnson, W.D.; Kuriyan, R.; Kurpad, A.; et al. Relationship between lifestyle behaviors and obesity in children ages 9–11: Results from a 12-country study. *Obesity (Silver Spring)* **2015**, *23*, 1696–1702. [CrossRef] [PubMed]

37. Hu, L.; Bentler, P.M. Cutoff criteria for fit indexes in covariance structure analysis: Conventional criteria versus new alternatives. *Struct. Equ. Model. Multidiscip. J.* **1999**, *6*, 1–55. [CrossRef]

38. Tavakol, M.; Dennick, R. Making sense of Cronbach's alpha. *Int. J. Med. Educ.* **2011**, *2*, 53–55. [CrossRef]

39. Cheung, G.W.; Rensvold, R.B. Evaluating Goodness-of-Fit Indexes for Testing Measurement Invariance. *Struct. Equ. Model. Multidiscip. J.* **2002**, *9*, 233–255. [CrossRef]

40. Saloheimo, T.; González, S.A.; Erkkola, M.; Milauskas, D.M.; Meisel, J.D.; Champagne, C.M.; Tudor-Locke, C.; Sarmiento, O.; Katzmarzyk, P.T.; Fogelholm, M. The reliability and validity of a short food frequency questionnaire among 9–11-year olds: A multinational study on three middle-income and high-income countries. *Int. J. Obes. Suppl.* **2015**, *5*, S22–S28. [CrossRef]

41. Mikkilä, V.; Vepsäläinen, H.; Saloheimo, T.; Gonzalez, S.A.; Meisel, J.D.; Hu, G.; Champagne, C.M.; Church, T.S.; Katzmarzyk, P.T.; Kuriyan, R.; et al. An international comparison of dietary patterns in 9–11-year-old children. *Int. J. Obes. Suppl.* **2015**, *5*, S17–S21.

42. Evenson, K.R.; Catellier, D.J.; Gill, K.; Ondrak, K.S.; McMurray, R.G. Calibration of two objective measures of physical activity for children. *J. Sports Sci.* **2008**, *26*, 1557–1565. [CrossRef] [PubMed]

43. Barreira, T.V.; Schuna, J.M.; Mire, E.F.; Katzmarzyk, P.T.; Chaput, J.; Leduc, G.; Tudor-Locke, C. Identifying children's nocturnal sleep using 24-h waist accelerometry. *Med. Sci. Sports Exerc.* **2015**, *47*, 937–943. [CrossRef]

44. US Centers for Disease Control and Prevention: Youth Risk Behavior Surveillance System (YRBSS). 2012. Available online: https://www.cdc.gov/healthyyouth/data/yrbs/index.htm (accessed on 21 June 2017).

45. Schmitz, K.H.; Harnack, L.; Fulton, J.E.; Jacobs, D.R.; Gao, S.; Lytle, L.A.; Coevering, P.V. Reliability and Validity of a Brief Questionnaire to Assess Television Viewing and Computer Use by Middle School Children. *J. Sch. Health* **2004**, *74*, 370–377. [CrossRef] [PubMed]

46. de Onis, M.; Onyango, A.W.; Borghi, E.; Siyam, A.; Nishida, C.; Siekmann, J. Development of a WHO growth reference for school-aged children and adolescents. *Bull. World Health Organ.* **2007**, *85*, 660–667. [CrossRef] [PubMed]

47. Kenward, M.G.; Roger, J.H. Small sample inference for fixed effects from restricted maximum likelihood. *Biometrics* **1997**, *53*, 983–997. [CrossRef] [PubMed]

48. Coumans, J.M.J.; Danner, U.N.; Intemann, T.; De Decker, A.; Hadjigeorgiou, C.; Hunsberger, M.; Moreno, L.A.; Russo, P.; Stomfai, S.; Veidebaum, T.; et al. Emotion-driven impulsiveness and snack food consumption of European adolescents: Results from the I.Family study. *Appetite* **2018**, *123*, 152–159. [CrossRef]

49. Kolodziejczyk, J.K.; Merchant, G.; Norman, G.J. Reliability and Validity of Child/Adolescent Food Frequency Questionnaires That Assess Foods and/or Food Groups. *J. Pediatr. Gastroenterol. Nutr.* **2012**, *55*, 4. [CrossRef]

50. Burrows, T.L.; Truby, H.; Morgan, P.J.; Callister, R.; Davies, P.S.W.; Collins, C.E. A comparison and validation of child versus parent reporting of children's energy intake using food frequency questionnaires versus food records: Who's an accurate reporter? *Clin. Nutr.* **2013**, *32*, 613–618. [CrossRef]

51. Herle, M.; Fildes, A.; Steinsbekk, S.; Rijsdijk, F.; Llewellyn, C.H. Emotional over- and under-eating in early childhood are learned not inherited. *Sci. Rep.* **2017**, *7*, 9092. [CrossRef]

52. Herle, M.; Fildes, A.; Rijsdijk, F.; Steinsbekk, S.; Llewellyn, C. The Home Environment Shapes Emotional Eating. *Child Dev.* **2017**. [CrossRef]

53. Bjørklund, O.; Wichstrøm, L.; Llewellyn, C.H.; Steinsbekk, S. Emotional Over-and Undereating in Children: A Longitudinal Analysis of Child and Contextual Predictors. *Child Dev.* **2018**. [CrossRef] [PubMed]

54. Ouwens, M.A.; Cebolla, A.; van Strien, T. Eating style, television viewing and snacking in pre-adolescent children. *Nutr. Hosp.* **2012**, *27*, 1072–1078. [PubMed]

55. Coon, K.A.; Tucker, K.L. Television and children's consumption patterns. A review of the literature. *Minerva Pediatr.* **2002**, *54*, 423–436. [PubMed]
56. Hart, S.R.; Pierson, S.; Goto, K.; Giampaoli, J. Development and initial validation evidence for a mindful eating questionnaire for children. *Appetite* **2018**, *129*, 178–185. [CrossRef] [PubMed]
57. Mikkilä, V.; Räsänen, L.; Raitakari, O.T.; Pietinen, P.; Viikari, J. Consistent dietary patterns identified from childhood to adulthood: The cardiovascular risk in Young Finns Study. *Br. J. Nutr.* **2005**, *93*, 923–931. [CrossRef] [PubMed]

9

Which Diet-Related Behaviors in Childhood Influence a Healthier Dietary Pattern? From the Ewha Birth and Growth Cohort

Hye Ah Lee [1,*], **Hyo Jeong Hwang** [2], **Se Young Oh** [3], **Eun Ae Park** [4], **Su Jin Cho** [4], **Hae Soon Kim** [4] and **Hyesook Park** [1,*]

[1]   Department of Preventive Medicine, School of Medicine, Ewha Womans University, Seoul 07985, Korea
[2]   Biomaterials Research Institute, Sahmyook University, Seoul 01795, Korea; fullmoon0118@naver.com
[3]   Department of Food & Nutrition, Research Center for Human Ecology, College of Human Ecology, Kyung Hee University, Seoul 02447, Korea; seyoung@khu.ac.kr
[4]   Department of Pediatrics, School of Medicine, Ewha Womans University, Seoul 07985, Korea; pea8639@ewha.ac.kr (E.A.P.); sujin-cho@ewha.ac.kr (S.J.C.); hyesk@ewha.ac.kr (H.S.K.)
*   Correspondence: khyeah@naver.com (H.A.L.); hpark@ewha.ac.kr (H.P.);

Abstract: This study was performed to examine how childhood dietary patterns change over the short term and which changes in diet-related behaviors influence later changes in individual dietary patterns. Using food frequency questionnaire data obtained from children at 7 and 9 years of age from the Ewha Birth and Growth Cohort, we examined dietary patterns by principal component analysis. We calculated the individual changes in dietary pattern scores. Changes in dietary habits such as eating a variety of food over two years were defined as "increased", "stable", or "decreased". The dietary patterns, termed "healthy intake", "animal food intake", and "snack intake", were similar at 7 and 9 years of age. These patterns explained 32.3% and 39.1% of total variation at the ages of 7 and 9 years, respectively. The tracking coefficient of snack intake had the highest coefficient ($\gamma = 0.53$) and that of animal food intake had the lowest ($\gamma = 0.21$). Intra-individual stability in dietary habits ranged from 0.23 to 0.47, based on the sex-adjusted weighted kappa values. Of the various behavioral factors, eating breakfast every day was most common in the "stable" group (83.1%), whereas consuming milk or dairy products every day was the least common (49.0%). Moreover, changes in behavior that improved the consumption of milk or dairy products or encouraged the consumption of vegetables with every meal had favorable effects on changes in healthy dietary pattern scores over two years. However, those with worsened habits, such as less food variety and more than two portions of fried or stir-fried food every week, had unfavorable effects on changes in healthy dietary pattern scores. Our results suggest that diet-related behaviors can change, even over a short period, and these changes can affect changes in dietary pattern.

Keywords: children; dietary pattern; diet-related behavior; longitudinal study

---

1. Introduction

To improve diet, understanding how dietary patterns develop is important in epidemiological studies related to chronic diseases and public health planning [1]. The critical period for the development of certain dietary patterns, during which time the development should be tracked, remains a major issue in nutritional epidemiology. Several studies have suggested that dietary patterns are determined in childhood [2–4]. One large prospective cohort study, the Avon Longitudinal Study of Pregnancy and Childhood (ALSPAC), indicated that the dietary pattern at 7 years old was a determinant of later dietary patterns based on the results of tracking coefficients from diverse statistical approaches [4]. However, previous studies focusing on the stability of dietary patterns yielded mixed results with only moderate [5,6] or slight tracking [1,7].

With regard to the critical period, children learn what, when, and how to eat through direct experience observing others [8]. Thus, it is important to identify critical intervention factors to suggest appropriate strategies for improving dietary behaviors. However, the effectiveness of interventions to modify dietary behaviors remains unclear [9,10]. One recent observational study from the NEXT Generation Health Study among American teens indicated within-individual correlations of 41%–51% in food group intake and meal practices over four years. It was also reported that time-varied frequencies of intake of fruit/vegetables or snacks were associated with time-varied meal practices, such as the frequency of fast food intake [6]. However, this study focused on intakes of specific food groups or eating behaviors.

Childhood dietary patterns could be reflected in underlying food preferences, diet-related behaviors, as well as environmental factors, such as household income and parental education level [8]. Studying dietary patterns is a reasonable approach because the net effect of a single food or nutrient cannot be separated from the total. Several methodologies have been introduced to explore dietary patterns [11,12]. Of these, principal component analysis (PCA) is a multidimensional reduction analysis method to examine the correlations of food intakes, and is commonly used in nutritional epidemiology [13]. Several studies using PCA reported several dietary patterns in children and adolescents as "healthy", "traditional", "Western", and "junk or processed food intakes", among others [5,14,15]. However, Hu suggested that much more research is necessary in diverse populations due to sociocultural differences [12]. In addition, many previous studies did not take into consideration changes in dietary pattern or related behaviors. A better understanding of changes in diet-related behaviors and dietary patterns may provide an opportunity to explore appropriate intervention strategies.

Using data from a Korean cohort study, we evaluated how childhood dietary patterns change in the short term, and which changes in diet-related behavior influence later changes in individual dietary patterns.

2. Methods

2.1. Study Subjects

This study was part of an ongoing Ewha Birth and Growth Cohort study by the Ewha Woman's University Mokdong Hospital, Seoul, Korea. It was established to longitudinally evaluate the growth and health of children, and it commenced in the early life of the subjects. Briefly, mothers ($n = 940$) were enrolled in the study between 2001 and 2006 during prenatal care visits when they were 24–28 weeks pregnant, and a follow-up was done with their children 3, 5, and 7 years later. About 30% of all possible subjects agreed to participate in the study [16]. A detailed description of the cohort composition, including methodology, has been published elsewhere [17]. Through follow-up at 7 or 9 years of age, a diet-related questionnaire survey was performed using a food frequency questionnaire (FFQ) and questions related to dietary habits. Follow-up at 7 years of age began in 2009, but data were collected using FFQs from 2010. A total of 364 and 380 children participated in follow-up at 7 years (follow-up years from 2009 to 2014) and 9 years of age (follow-up years from 2011 to 2015), respectively. Of these, completed FFQs were obtained for 279 and 360 children, respectively. FFQ data for both follow-up times were obtained for 154 children. Approximately 41.9% of cohort subjects were lost to follow-up (they changed their telephone numbers or withdrew) at the time of the 7-year follow-up, and an additional 3.4% were lost to follow-up at 9 years. Written informed consent for participation in the study was obtained from the parents or guardians of all study participants at the time of follow-up. The study protocol was approved by the Institutional Review Board of the Ewha Womans University Hospital.

2.2. Dietary Data and Dietary Pattern Analysis

Individual dietary data for the past year were collected by the parents or guardians and validated by trained interviewers using the FFQ (90 food items). Both the reproducibility (r value = 0.5–0.8) and validity (r value = 0.3–0.6) of the instrument were acceptable, as reported elsewhere [18,19]. We used the same questionnaire at both follow-ups. These food items were placed into nine non-overlapping categories according to the frequency of consumption, ranging from "rarely eaten" to "more than three times per day" during the preceding year, and portion size, namely, small, average, or large. In this study, we used food intake frequencies to construct dietary patterns [20]. Weekly intake from the FFQ was calculated by multiplying the consumption frequency of each food by the following values for each frequency option: never = 0; once a month = 0.23; two-to-three times a month = 0.58; one-to-two times a week = 1.5; three-to-four times a week = 3.5; five-to-six times a week = 5.5; once a day = 7; twice a day = 14; and three times a day = 21. Of the 90 food items, similar items were grouped to form 22 food groups (Table S1). Prior to PCA, data were standardized using means and standard deviations, and the dietary patterns at each time point were analyzed via PCA with varimax rotation. The first three components were appropriate, based on the screen plots and eigenvalues ≥ 1. The factor-loading values by dietary pattern are shown in Table 1. Factors with loading >0.3 were considered the principal contributors to a dietary pattern [5]. Factor scores were used as outcomes, which were defined as dietary pattern scores. To assess changes in the same dietary patterns over time, we calculated the z scores of food group intake from children aged 9 years using the means and standard deviations obtained when they were 7 years of age. These were multiplied by factor-loading values for each dietary pattern (it was obtained using the data for 7 years old), and then summed. This approach has been used in previous studies [5,21].

Table 1. Factor loading scores for the first three components derived from principal component analysis.

	Healthy Intake		Animal Food Intake		Snack Intake	
	7 Years	9 Years	7 Years	9 Years	7 Years	9 Years
Variance	13.83%	15.12%	10.23%	16.20%	8.21%	7.77%
Yellow vegetables	0.840	0.820	0.070	0.108	−0.020	0.050
Green vegetables	0.800	0.795	0.149	0.105	0.045	0.074
White vegetables	0.475	0.417	0.268	0.014	−0.040	0.057
Mushrooms	0.802	0.677	−0.066	0.081	−0.037	0.126
Beans	0.476	0.522	0.181	0.089	0.198	0.091
Potatoes	0.280	0.468	0.071	0.056	0.227	0.277
Fruit	0.271	0.341	0.160	0.038	0.151	0.148
Nuts	0.222	0.418	0.200	0.090	0.044	0.150
Shellfish	0.106	0.019	0.798	0.948	0.073	0.047
White fish	0.092	0.009	0.714	0.938	0.152	0.022
Blue fish	0.144	0.200	0.598	0.909	0.257	0.063
Meat	0.444	0.081	0.587	0.853	0.125	0.239
Eggs	0.276	0.136	0.120	0.400	0.268	−0.007
Rice	0.066	0.089	0.224	−0.037	0.063	0.072
Bread	0.108	0.078	−0.023	0.033	0.712	0.399
Jam	−0.006	0.192	0.023	0.005	0.617	0.396
Soda	0.047	0.226	0.094	0.024	0.394	0.559
Milk	0.235	0.388	0.028	0.065	0.346	0.459
Candy	−0.047	0.048	0.109	0.011	0.339	0.509
Pizza	−0.030	0.042	0.240	0.059	0.322	0.424
Noodles	0.054	0.070	0.175	0.075	0.251	0.433
Seaweed	0.089	0.529	0.138	0.083	0.234	0.127

2.3. Dietary Habits

We collected data regarding dietary habits using the following questions:

DH1. Do you eat more than two servings of milk or dairy products every day?

DH2. Do you eat meat, fish, egg, beans, or tofu with every meal?

DH3. Do you eat vegetables other than kimchi with every meal?

DH4. Do you eat one serving size of fruit or drink one portion of fruit juice every day?

DH5. Do you eat more than two servings of fried or stir-fried food every week?

DH6. Do you eat more than two servings of fatty meat (e.g., bacon, ribs, eel) every week?

DH7. Do you generally add table salt or soy sauce to food?

DH8. Do you eat three regular meals per day?

DH9. Do you eat ice cream, cake, snacks, and soda (e.g., cola, cider) as snacks more than twice a week?

DH10. Do you eat a variety of food every day?

The possible responses were "always", "generally", and "seldom". Questions DH1–4, DH8, and DH10 evaluated healthy dietary habits, and questions DH5–7 and DH9 evaluated unhealthy dietary habits. This mini-dietary assessment tool has been validated in previous studies [22,23]. In addition, the subjects were also asked "Do you eating breakfast every day?" to which they responded either "yes" or "no". Changes in individual behaviors were classified as "increased", "stable", or "decreased". If one subject at 7 years old replied "seldom" to the question "Do you eat over two servings of milk or dairy products every day?" and answered "always" or "generally" to the same question at 9 years old, the behavior was defined as "increased", while the opposite was classified as "decreased". Finally, those who gave the same answer at both follow-ups were defined as "stable".

2.4. Other Variables

We also evaluated data on household income, parental education, parental obesity, time spent watching television (TV), and child body mass index (BMI); previous studies have shown that these were potentially important factors [2,6,15,21]. Monthly household income was grouped as "low" (<3 million South Korean Won (KRW)), "middle" (3.0–4.9 million KRW), or "high" (>5 million KRW). Parental education level was classified into two levels (graduated from high school; some college or higher). Parental obesity was defined as BMI $\geq$ 25 kg/m^2, calculated by dividing weight by height squared. These data were collected by a self-reported questionnaire at follow-up. The daily amount of time spent watching TV was categorized as <1 h, 1–2 h, and >2 h. Child BMI was calculated by measuring height and weight at both follow-ups.

2.5. Statistical Analysis

The associations between dietary pattern scores and socioeconomic factors, parental factors, and dietary habits were analyzed using the t test or analysis of variance (ANOVA). Based on the findings from the univariate analyses, we selected potentially significant factors ($p < 0.2$) for inclusion in the multiple regression analyses. A factor was considered relevant if it was potentially related to any dietary pattern. However, paternal education was not considered, being strongly associated with household income (an indicator of socioeconomic status). In multiple regression analysis, responses to dietary habits were treated as continuous variables (e.g., "always" = 2, "generally" = 1 and "seldom" = 0 for questions related to healthy dietary habits and applied in reverse for questions about unhealthy dietary habits) by considering multicollinearity. Multicollinearity in multiple regression was assessed based on variance inflation factors and it had a value <2 across our results. Correlations between dietary pattern scores at the two time points were estimated using Spearman's correlation, and the changes in dietary pattern scores within an individual were assessed using the paired t test. To determine the changes in dietary habits, we used weighted kappa and proportion of dietary habit changes stratified according to sex. The independent effects of changes in individual behaviors were expressed as "increased", "stable", or "decreased" over time in terms of changes in dietary patterns after taking sex, household income, and other parameters, into consideration. The change in watching TV was excluded due to data on this variable being missing for a large proportion of the subjects (13.6%). In all analyses, $p < 0.05$ (two-tailed test) was taken to indicate statistical significance. All statistical analyses were conducted using SAS 9.3 (SAS Institute, Cary, NC, USA).

3. Results

With regard to the characteristics of the study subjects, about half were boys (49.46%) with an average BMI of 15.95 kg/m^2 (95% confidence interval: 15.71–16.20 kg/m^2). Most of the children ate breakfast daily (84.84%). Of all of the children, 41.73% watched television for more than 2 h per day. In terms of household income (an indicator of socioeconomic status), 20.59%, 41.54%, and 37.87% of children were in the low, middle, and high groups, respectively. Table 1 shows dietary patterns derived from PCA at each time point. The first three components accounted for 32.27% (PC1: 13.83%, PC2: 10.23%, and PC3: 8.21% at 7 years old) and 39.10% (PC1: 15.12%, PC2: 16.20%, and PC3: 7.77% at 9 years old) of total variation. The three components were referred to as "healthy intake", "animal food intake", and "snack intake". Healthy intake was positively associated with vegetable and bean items. Animal food intake showed weighted loading factors in meat and fish items. Finally, snack intake showed positive loading factors in candy, soda, and bread items. The patterns were similar at the older age, but some food types had more weighted loading factors. Healthy intake at 9 years of age showed more weighted loading factors in fruit, milk, nut, and seaweed food groups than at the younger age.

The results of univariate association are presented in Table S2. Higher household income status tended to show higher mean health intake pattern scores at 7 years of age. In addition, healthy intake was significantly associated with eating breakfast every day and all of the related healthy dietary habits. Animal food intake was associated with sex, eating fatty meat, and generally adding table salt or soy sauce to food. Subjects that spent a longer time watching TV had higher mean snack pattern scores. Snack intake also showed a significant association with eating milk or dairy products; eating fruit or drinking fruit juice every day; eating fried or stir-fried food; generally adding table salt or soy sauce to food; and eating ice cream, cake, snacks, and soda (e.g., cola, cider) as snacks.

In multiple regression analysis, eating breakfast every day and eating a variety of food every day showed independent effects on the healthy pattern with positive coefficients ($\beta = 0.24$, $\beta = 0.19$, respectively). With regard to animal food intake, female gender showed higher pattern scores, while unusual behaviors with regard to fatty meat and generally adding table salt or soy sauce to food showed lower pattern scores. Pattern scores in snack intake were also positively associated with watching TV ($\beta = 0.15$) and negatively associated with eating vegetables other than kimchi ($\beta = -0.23$). Moreover, several factors showed independent effects at both follow-up times. Eating a variety of food was consistently associated with healthy intake at both follow-up times. Eating vegetables other than kimchi with every meal was also negatively associated with snack intake. Otherwise, there were no significant associations with animal food intake (Table 2).

Table 3 shows the results regarding changes in dietary pattern scores and tracking coefficients of dietary patterns. The tracking coefficient of snack intake showed the highest coefficient (0.53, $p < 0.0001$) and animal food intake showed the lowest coefficient (0.21, $p < 0.01$). The mean dietary pattern scores from the earlier time point showed increasing tendencies across dietary patterns, and this score was highest for animal food intake ($\Delta = 0.20$, $p < 0.001$).

Figure 1 shows the intra-individual stability of dietary habits over two years by sex. The weighted kappa values of eating breakfast every day, watching TV, eating three regular meals a day, and eating ice cream, cake, snacks, and soda were markedly higher in girls than in boys, while those of eating a variety of food every day and eating meat, fish, egg, beans, or tofu with every meal were higher in boys than in girls. Sex-adjusted weighted kappa values ranged from 0.23 to 0.47. Of the behavior factors, eating breakfast every day showed the highest proportion for "stable" (83.1%), while eating milk or dairy products every day showed the lowest proportion (49.0%) (Table 4).

Table 2. Multiple regression analysis of the effects of potential factors on dietary pattern at two observation times.

Potential Factor at 7 Years	Dietary Pattern Scores at 7 Years Old						Dietary Pattern Scores at 9 Years Old					
	Healthy Intake		Animal Food Intake		Snack Intake		Healthy Intake		Animal Food Intake		Snack Intake	
	β	S.E.	β	S.E.	β	S.E.	β	S.E.	β	S.E.	β	S.E.
Sex	−0.010	0.06	0.183 [a]	0.06	−0.078	0.10	−0.027	0.10	0.056	0.13	0.127	0.18
Monthly household income	0.023	0.04	0.003	0.04	0.014	0.07	0.037	0.07	0.068	0.09	0.186	0.13
Body mass index (BMI)	−0.007	0.02	−0.0002	0.02	−0.016	0.03	−0.011	0.03	−0.021	0.04	0.005	0.05
Maternal obesity	0.007	0.08	−0.002	0.08	−0.222	0.14	−0.051	0.14	0.022	0.18	0.007	0.24
Watching television (TV)	−0.043	0.04	0.057	0.04	0.152 [a]	0.07	−0.004	0.07	−0.052	0.09	0.015	0.13
Eating breakfast every day	0.242 [a]	0.10	−0.071	0.10	−0.071	0.17	0.091	0.16	0.206	0.20	−0.296	0.28
Healthy dietary habits												
DH1	0.071	0.05	0.036	0.05	0.129	0.08	0.026	0.07	−0.0004	0.09	0.152	0.13
DH2	−0.002	0.05	0.071	0.05	0.016	0.09	−0.048	0.09	0.007	0.11	−0.114	0.16
DH3	0.068	0.05	0.026	0.05	−0.226 [a]	0.08	−0.153	0.08	−0.067	0.10	−0.435 [a]	0.14
DH4	0.048	0.05	−0.043	0.05	0.117	0.09	0.154	0.08	−0.120	0.10	0.028	0.14
DH8	0.075	0.06	0.069	0.06	−0.069	0.11	−0.083	0.10	0.069	0.13	0.063	0.18
DH10	0.190 [a]	0.05	0.047	0.05	0.114	0.08	0.166 [a]	0.07	−0.021	0.09	0.123	0.13
Unhealthy dietary habits												
DH5	0.064	0.05	0.021	0.05	−0.047	0.08	−0.129	0.07	−0.035	0.09	−0.245	0.13
DH6	−0.038	0.05	−0.154 [a]	0.05	−0.105	0.08	−0.047	0.08	−0.048	0.11	0.250	0.15
DH7	−0.005	0.06	−0.127 [a]	0.06	−0.152	0.10	−0.027	0.10	−0.052	0.12	−0.358 [a]	0.17
DH9	0.010	0.04	−0.007	0.04	−0.113	0.07	0.006	0.07	0.024	0.08	−0.160	0.12

[a] $p < 0.05$. S.E. = standard error. DH1: Eating more than two portions of milk or dairy products every day. DH2: Eating meat, fish, eggs, beans, or tofu with every meal. DH3: Eating vegetables other than kimchi with every meal. DH4: Eating one portion of fruit or drinking one portion of fruit juice every day. DH5: Eating more than two portions of fried or stir-fried food every week. DH6: Eating more than two portions of fatty meat (e.g., bacon, ribs, eel) every week. DH7: Generally adding table salt or soy sauce to food. DH8: Eating three regular meals a day. DH9: Eating ice cream, cake, snacks, and soda (e.g., cola, cider) as snacks more than twice a week. DH10: Eating a variety of food every day. The possible responses to dietary habits (DHs) were "always", "generally", or "seldom". The daily TV-watching time was categorized as <1 h, 1–2 h, and >2 h. Eating breakfast everyday was grouped as yes or no.

Table 3. Changes in dietary pattern scores between the two observational times.

Dietary Pattern Scores	Tracking Coefficient [†]	At 7 Years		At 9 Years [‡]		Differences of Dietary Pattern Scores [‡]		Paired *t* Test *p*
		Mean	S.D.	Mean	S.D.	Mean	S.D.	
Healthy intake	0.369 [a]	−0.106	0.498	0.062	0.613	0.176	0.624	<0.001
Animal food intake	0.215 [b]	−0.091	0.479	0.123	0.691	0.204	0.717	<0.001
Snack intake	0.526 [a]	−0.003	0.861	0.213	0.969	0.161	0.864	0.02

[†] The tracking coefficients between the dietary pattern scores at the two time points were estimated by deriving Spearman's correlations. [‡] Results are presented for those who participated in both follow-ups (*n* = 154). [a] *p* < 0.0001, [b] *p* < 0.01. S.D. = standard deviation.

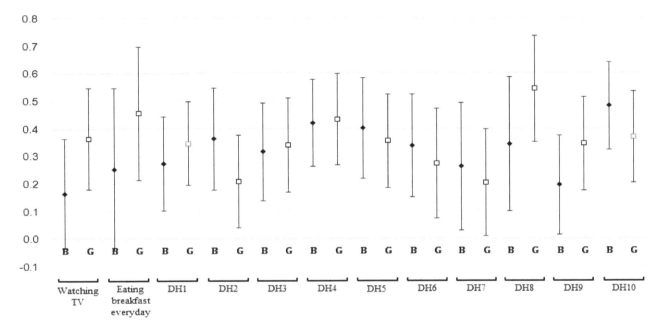

Figure 1. Weighted κ of two repeated measures for behaviors by sex. B: boys (black diamonds), G: girls (white squares), line indicates 95% confidence interval. DH1: Eating more than two portions of milk or dairy products every day. DH2: Eating meat, fish, egg, beans, or tofu with every meal. DH3: Eating vegetables other than kimchi with every meal. DH4: Eating one portion of fruit or drinking one portion of fruit juice every day. DH5: Eating more than two portions of fried or stir-fried food every week. DH6: Eating more than two portions of fatty meat (e.g., bacon, ribs, eel) every week. DH7: Generally adding table salt or soy sauce to food. DH8: Eating three regular meals per day. DH9: Eating ice cream, cake, snacks, and soda (e.g., cola, cider) as snacks more than twice a week. DH10: Eating a variety of food every day. The possible responses to dietary habits (DHs) were "always", "generally", or "seldom". The daily TV-watching time was categorized as <1 h, 1–2 h and >2 h. Eating breakfast everyday was grouped as yes or no.

Table 5 shows the effects of behavioral changes on changes in dietary patterns. Those with improved dietary habits (who ate vegetables other than kimchi with every meal and consumed more than two portions of milk or dairy products every day) exhibited improved healthy intake pattern scores over two years, whereas those with worsening habits (less food variety and more than two portions of fried or stir-fried food every week) exhibited decreased scores. In addition, worsening with regard to eating ice cream, cake, snacks, and soda as snacks increased in the animal food intake patterns. However, other dietary habit changes were not significantly related to dietary pattern changes.

Table 4. Changes in individual's behaviors over two years.

	Sex-Adjusted Weighted Kappa	Stable		Increased		Decreased	
		n	%	*n*	%	*n*	%
Watching TV	0.271	75	56.39	27	20.30	31	23.31
Eating breakfast	0.373	128	83.12	9	5.84	17	11.04
Healthy dietary habits							
DH1	0.314	75	49.02	30	19.61	48	31.37
DH2	0.277	82	53.95	34	22.37	36	23.68
DH3	0.328	83	54.25	39	25.49	31	20.26
DH4	0.427	90	59.21	25	16.45	37	24.34
DH8	0.466	115	75.66	18	11.84	19	12.5
DH10	0.427	88	57.52	42	27.45	23	15.03
Unhealthy dietary habits							
DH5	0.376	90	59.21	27	17.76	35	23.03
DH6	0.307	97	63.4	27	17.65	29	18.95
DH7	0.227	101	66.01	25	16.34	27	17.65
DH9	0.273	74	48.68	41	26.97	37	24.34

DH1: Eating more than two portions of milk or dairy products every day. DH2: Eating meat, fish, egg, beans, or tofu with every meal. DH3: Eating vegetables other than kimchi with every meal. DH4: Eating one portion of fruit or drinking one portion of fruit juice every day. DH5: Eating more than two portions of fried or stir-fried food every week. DH6: Eating more than two portions of fatty meat (e.g., bacon, ribs, eel) every week. DH7: Generally adding table salt or soy sauce to food. DH8: Eating three regular meals per day. DH9: Eating ice cream, cake, snacks, and soda (e.g., cola, cider) as snacks more than twice a week. DH10: Eating a variety of food every day. The possible responses to dietary habits (DHs) were "always", "generally", or "seldom". The daily TV-watching time was categorized as <1 h, 1–2 h, and >2 h. Eating breakfast everyday was grouped as yes or no.

Table 5. Effects of behavioral changes over two years within dietary patterns.

		Difference in Dietary Pattern 1 Score		Difference in Dietary Pattern 2 Score		Difference in Dietary Pattern 3 Score	
		β	S.E.	β	S.E.	β	S.E.
Eating breakfast	increased	−0.057	0.23	−0.483	0.29	0.251	0.35
	decreased	−0.175	0.17	−0.375	0.23	−0.013	0.27
Healthy dietary habits							
DH1	increased	0.374 [a]	0.15	0.122	0.20	0.240	0.23
	decreased	0.143	0.13	0.255	0.17	0.130	0.20
DH2	increased	−0.089	0.14	0.152	0.18	0.060	0.21
	decreased	−0.215	0.14	−0.233	0.17	−0.134	0.21
DH3	increased	0.272 [a]	0.13	−0.136	0.17	0.278	0.20
	decreased	0.167	0.15	0.078	0.19	0.263	0.23
DH4	increased	−0.073	0.15	0.128	0.20	0.021	0.24
	decreased	−0.196	0.13	−0.042	0.17	−0.174	0.20
DH8	increased	−0.108	0.17	0.141	0.23	−0.140	0.26
	decreased	0.037	0.17	0.235	0.22	−0.073	0.25
DH10	increased	0.117	0.13	0.099	0.17	0.090	0.20
	decreased	−0.301 [a]	0.15	0.021	0.20	−0.285	0.23
Unhealthy dietary habits							
DH5	increased	0.153	0.14	0.046	0.19	0.219	0.22
	decreased	−0.310 [a]	0.14	−0.199	0.18	−0.261	0.22
DH6	increased	0.095	0.15	−0.090	0.19	−0.176	0.22
	decreased	−0.070	0.14	0.166	0.19	−0.033	0.22
DH7	increased	−0.137	0.16	−0.287	0.20	−0.081	0.23
	decreased	−0.051	0.14	0.009	0.18	0.047	0.22
DH9	increased	−0.010	0.13	−0.227	0.17	0.019	0.20
	decreased	0.239	0.14	0.390 [a]	0.18	0.348	0.21

[a] $p < 0.05$. DH1: Eating more than two portions of milk or dairy products every day. DH2: Eating meat, fish, egg, beans, or tofu with every meal. DH3: Eating vegetables other than kimchi with every meal. DH4: Eating one portion of fruit or drinking one portion of fruit juice every day. DH5: Eating more than two portions of fried or stir-fried food every week. DH6: Eating more than two portions of fatty meat (e.g., bacon, ribs, eel) every week. DH7: Generally adding table salt or soy sauce to food. DH8: Eating three regular meals per day. DH9: Eating ice cream, cake, snacks, and soda (e.g., cola, cider) as snacks more than twice a week. DH10: Eating a variety of food every day. The possible responses to dietary habits (DHs) were "always", "generally", or "seldom". The daily TV-watching time was categorized as <1 h, 1–2 h, and >2 h. Eating breakfast everyday was grouped as yes or no. All of the results were obtained by multiple regression analyses after adjusting for sex, maternal obesity, body mass index at 7 years of age, and household income.

4. Discussion

We explored the childhood dietary patterns at 7 and 9 years of age and assessed the changes in individual dietary patterns. There were three dietary patterns, namely, "healthy intake", "animal food intake", and "snack intake", the contributions of which differed at each time point. The tracking coefficients ranged from 0.21 for animal food intake to 0.53 for snack intake. Overall, the mean dietary pattern scores tended to increase over time. Moreover, changes in behaviors that improved the consumption of milk and dairy products or vegetables with every meal exhibited improved healthy intake pattern scores over two years, whereas those with worsened habits, such as less food variety and more than two portions of fried or stir-fried food every week, exhibited decreased scores.

Individual dietary patterns change over time, even in childhood [5,21]. As individual diet-related behaviors can also change, the above findings appear reasonable. Supporting evidence from intervention studies is required to improve the dietary habits of children. Repeated measures in cohort design could also be used to assess the effects of natural changes in dietary behaviors. In this study, we examined the effects of changes in diet-related behaviors on changes in pattern scores. The results indicated that improved individual dietary behaviors related to eating vegetables with every meal independently attributed to increased healthier dietary patterns over time. The advantages of eating vegetables have been demonstrated by several systematic review studies with regard to diverse health effects, as well, they reflect the nutritional quality of meals [24–26]. However, interventions involving increasing the vegetable intake among children were unsuccessful [10]. One large study conducted in American teens estimated that within-person correlations for eating behaviors were >0.41 for the intake frequencies of fruit and vegetables, whole grains, soda, and snacks using four sets of repeated-measure data, and time-varying intake frequency of fruit and vegetables was positively associated with time-varying breakfast and family meals and negatively associated with fast food intake using a generalized estimating equations model. However, this previous study did not discuss the intake of various food [6]. In addition, eating a variety of food reflects adequate intake of essential nutrients, and is recommended in most dietary guidelines, including those in South Korea [27]. In addition, milk and dairy products are major sources of calcium for growing children. A national study found that more than half of all Korean children have inadequate calcium intake [28]. Although it is difficult to compare previous findings with ours because different assessment methods were used, we also found that it was beneficial to eat a variety of foods including milk and dairy products. In contrast, fried or stir-fried food was associated with high fat intake. We found that increased consumption of fried or stir-fried food unfavorably influenced a healthy dietary pattern. Thus, our results are meaningful in terms of epidemiological approaches. The unexpected results regarding the association between changes in eating ice cream, cake, snacks, and soda (e.g., cola, cider) as snacks seemed to be influenced by increased food frequency. Unlike other dietary habits, overall intake frequencies were higher for subjects with worsening behaviors regarding eating ice cream, cake, snacks, and soda as snacks compared with those with stable and increased behaviors. Indeed, all dietary pattern scores increased with a decrease of that behavior, as shown in Table 5.

As presented in Table 1, there were some changes in the composition of the three types of dietary patterns over two years. This was not surprising based on the results of previous studies [5,7]. Generally, the traditional diet in South Korea includes high levels of various vegetables and is low in fat [29,30]. These features were similar in our study. A previous study among South Korean adults also showed similar patterns to those in the present study [30], but little evidence was available regarding dietary patterns in South Korean children. For variation during two years, the intakes of most food items increased at 9 years old compared to those at 7 years old, with the exceptions of yellow vegetables, mushrooms, fruit, milk, and seaweed laver. Soda, potatoes, bread, and pizza showed relatively large increases (data not shown). Increased soda intake with increasing age was also observed in a previous growth and health study from the National Heart, Lung, and Blood Institute [31] and the Bogalusa Heart Study [32]. The environmental influences on food choice, preference, and accessibility vary over the lifespan. The opportunity to choose food oneself would increase with increasing age. Consistent with our study, the results regarding dietary pattern derived from the ALSPAC study showed that notable loading factors differed among food groups at 9 years old compared with those at 7 years old [4]. Another two studies using reduced rank regression and cluster analysis of the same cohort data indicated that dietary patterns at 7 years of age was a strong determinant of later dietary patterns [4,21]. Children starting school and participating in various activities are placed in a new environment, which may influence food choice. Therefore, further studies on changes in dietary habits and patterns over longer periods are required.

Several factors potentially related to dietary patterns have been reported, including low maternal education level [14,15,21]; socioeconomic status [15]; passive smoking and watching TV [14]; childhood obesity or maternal obesity [2]; diet-related factors, such as being vegetarian [33]; and TV meals, family meals, and breakfast [6]. However, most of these studies reported effects at a critical time on dietary patterns rather than changes in potential factors as mentioned above. Parental education level and birth- or infancy-related features were considered as time-independent factors. In this study, associations between household income and dietary patterns were more notable than parental education level. These observations may be explained by more highly educated parents having a better understanding of nutritional information and being more likely to restrict their children's intake of unhealthy food [34]. These observations may also be explained by the dependence of the ability to pay for food or groceries on household income, because a nutrient-dense diet is more expensive than an energy-dense diet [35]. However, any independent effects of household income were not significant as determined by multiple regression analyses. Moreover, we found no association with maternal obesity and child BMI.

Several points must be taken into consideration when interpreting the results of our study. Our results were derived from a smaller sample than previous studies. Bias due to follow-up loss would probably have an impact on the results. However, there were no differences in the distribution of demographic factors or dietary habits between subjects who successfully followed up or were lost to follow-up, except in eating a variety of food (p_{chi} = 0.02). Therefore, this did not seem to affect our results. To allow comparison, loading factors were applied to the calculated dietary pattern scores at the older age. This approach also has limitations in that it did not reflect the changes in characteristics of dietary patterns. Healthy intake pattern showed a positive loading factor for eating vegetables at the two time points, but eating fruit showed a higher weighting for a healthy diet at 9 years old. Thus, scores of a change within dietary patterns do not reflect the above-mentioned change. We used the same validated questionnaires at both follow-ups, and all of the data were collected by trained dieticians. Thus, any bias imparted by this procedure would be small. Moreover, there could be residual confounding effects of several factors that were not considered in this study.

This cohort study had several strengths. In this cohort study, we observed behavioral changes within individuals and were able to assess the associated effects, although the observational period was short. This work is the first step towards observationally determining whether behavioral changes in early life can modify dietary patterns, thereby improving health later in life. In addition, our results yield important data from a non-Western country. Future studies are needed to determine if the effects that we observed will persist in the long term.

5. Conclusions

Our results suggest that single measurements of food frequency intake and dietary habits during childhood may be insufficient to determine individual dietary patterns. In addition, diet-related behaviors can change, even in a short period, and such changes can affect dietary patterns.

Acknowledgments: This study was supported by National Research Foundation of Korea Grant funded by the Korean Government (NRF-2014R1A1A1007207). It had no role in the design, analysis or writing of this article.

Author Contributions: H.A.L. wrote the paper and performed the statistical analyses; S.Y.O., H.J.H., E.A.P., S.J.C. and H.S.K. provided advice about writing the paper, and H.P. provided advice about interpreting the data.

References

1. Patterson, E.; Wärnberg, J.; Kearney, J.; Sjöström, M. The tracking of dietary intakes of children and adolescents in Sweden over six years: The European Youth Heart Study. *Int. J. Behav. Nutr. Phys. Act.* **2009**, *6*, 91. [CrossRef] [PubMed]

2. Burke, V.; Beilin, L.J.; Dunbar, D. Family lifestyle and parental body mass index as predictors of body mass index in Australian children: A longitudinal study. *Int. J. Obes. Relat. Metab. Disord.* **2001**, *25*, 147–157. [CrossRef] [PubMed]

3. Wang, Y.; Bentley, M.E.; Zhai, F.; Popkin, B.M. Tracking of dietary intake patterns of Chinese from childhood to adolescence over a six-year follow-up period. *J. Nutr.* **2002**, *132*, 430–438. [PubMed]

4. Emmett, P.M.; Jones, L.R.; Northstone, K. Dietary patterns in the Avon longitudinal study of parents and children. *Nutr. Rev.* **2015**, *73*, 207–230. [CrossRef] [PubMed]

5. Northstone, K.; Emmett, P.M. Are dietary patterns stable throughout early and mid-childhood? A birth cohort study. *Br. J. Nutr.* **2008**, *100*, 1069–1076. [CrossRef] [PubMed]

6. Lipsky, L.M.; Haynie, D.L.; Liu, D.; Chaurasia, A.; Gee, B.; Li, K.; Iannotti, R.J.; Simons-Morton, B. Trajectories of eating behaviors in a nationally representative cohort of U.S. adolescents during the transition to young adulthood. *Int. J. Behav. Nutr. Phys. Act.* **2015**, *12*, 138. [CrossRef] [PubMed]

7. Mikkilä, V.; Räsänen, L.; Raitakari, O.T.; Pietinen, P.; Viikari, J. Consistent dietary patterns identified from childhood to adulthood: The cardiovascular risk in young Finns study. *Br. J. Nutr.* **2005**, *93*, 923–931. [CrossRef] [PubMed]

8. Birch, L.; Savage, J.S.; Ventura, A. Influences on the development of children's eating behaviours: From infancy to adolescence. *Can. J. Diet. Pract. Res.* **2007**, *68*, s1–s56. [PubMed]

9. Racey, M.; O'Brien, C.; Douglas, S.; Marquez, O.; Hendrie, G.; Newton, G. Systematic review of school-based interventions to modify dietary behavior: Does intervention intensity impact effectiveness? *J. Sch. Health* **2016**, *86*, 452–463. [CrossRef] [PubMed]

10. Evans, C.E.; Christian, M.S.; Cleghorn, C.L.; Greenwood, D.C.; Cade, J.E. Systematic review and meta-analysis of school-based interventions to improve daily fruit and vegetable intake in children aged 5 to 12 years. *Am. J. Clin. Nutr.* **2012**, *96*, 889–901. [CrossRef] [PubMed]

11. Hoffmann, K.; Schulze, M.B.; Schienkiewitz, A.; Nöthlings, U.; Boeing, H. Application of a new statistical method to derive dietary patterns in nutritional epidemiology. *Am. J. Epidemiol.* **2004**, *159*, 935–944. [CrossRef] [PubMed]

12. Hu, F.B. Dietary pattern analysis: A new direction in nutritional epidemiology. *Curr. Opin. Lipidol.* **2002**, *13*, 3–9. [CrossRef] [PubMed]

13. Borges, C.A.; Rinaldi, A.E.; Conde, W.L.; Mainardi, G.M.; Behar, D.; Slater, B. Dietary patterns: A literature review of the methodological characteristics of the main step of the multivariate analyzes. *Rev. Bras. Epidemiol.* **2015**, *18*, 837–857. [CrossRef] [PubMed]

14. Leventakou, V.; Sarri, K.; Georgiou, V.; Chatzea, V.; Frouzi, E.; Kastelianou, A.; Gatzou, A.; Kogevinas, M.; Chatzi, L. Early life determinants of dietary patterns in preschool children: Rhea mother-child cohort, Crete, Greece. *Eur. J. Clin. Nutr.* **2016**, *70*, 60–65. [CrossRef] [PubMed]

15. Pisa, P.T.; Pedro, T.M.; Kahn, K.; Tollman, S.M.; Pettifor, J.M.; Norris, S.A. Nutrient patterns and their association with socio-demographic, lifestyle factors and obesity risk in rural South African adolescents. *Nutrients* **2015**, *7*, 3464–3482. [CrossRef] [PubMed]

16. Lee, H.A.; Park, E.A.; Cho, S.J.; Kim, H.S.; Kim, Y.J.; Lee, H.; Gwak, H.S.; Kim, K.N.; Chang, N.; Ha, E.H.; et al. Mendelian randomization analysis of the effect of maternal homocysteine during pregnancy, as represented by maternal MTHFR C677T genotype, on birth weight. *J. Epidemiol.* **2013**, *23*, 371–375. [CrossRef] [PubMed]

17. Lee, H.A.; Kim, Y.J.; Lee, H.; Gwak, H.S.; Hong, Y.S.; Kim, H.S.; Park, E.A.; Cho, S.J.; Ha, E.H.; Park, H. The preventive effect of breast-feeding for longer than 6 months on early pubertal development among children aged 7–9 years in Korea. *Public Health Nutr.* **2015**, *18*, 3300–3307. [CrossRef] [PubMed]

18. Oh, S.Y.; Chung, J.; Kim, M.; Kwon, S.O.; Cho, B. Antioxidant nutrient intakes and corresponding biomarkers associated with the risk of atopic dermatitis in young children. *Eur. J. Clin. Nutr.* **2010**, *64*, 245–252. [CrossRef] [PubMed]

19. Chung, J.; Kwon, S.O.; Ahn, H.; Hwang, H.; Hong, J.S.; Oh, S.Y. Association between dietary patterns and atopic dermatitis in relation to *GSTM1* and *GSTT1* polymorphisms in young children nutrients. *Nutrients* **2015**, *7*, 9440–9452. [CrossRef] [PubMed]

20. Shin, K.O.; Oh, S.Y.; Park, H.S. Empirically derived major dietary patterns and their associations with overweight in Korean preschool children. *Br. J. Nutr.* **2007**, *98*, 416–421. [CrossRef] [PubMed]

21. Ambrosini, G.L.; Emmett, P.M.; Northstone, K.; Jebb, S.A. Tracking a dietary pattern associated with increased adiposity in childhood and adolescence. *Obesity (Silver Spring)* **2014**, *22*, 458–465. [CrossRef] [PubMed]

22. Kim, W.Y.; Cho, M.S.; Lee, H.S. Development and validation of mini dietary assessment index for Koreans. *Korean J. Nutr.* **2003**, *36*, 82–92.

23. Park, S.; Cho, S.C.; Hong, Y.C.; Oh, S.Y.; Kim, J.W.; Shin, M.S.; Kim, B.N.; Yoo, H.J.; Cho, I.H.; Bhang, S.Y. Association between dietary behaviors and attention-deficit/hyperactivity disorder and learning disabilities in school-aged children. *Psychiatry Res.* **2012**, *198*, 468–476. [CrossRef] [PubMed]

24. Gorgulho, B.M.; Pot, G.K.; Sarti, F.M.; Marchioni, D.M. Indices for the assessment of nutritional quality of meals: A systematic review. *Br. J. Nutr.* **2016**, *115*, 2017–2024. [CrossRef] [PubMed]

25. Alissa, E.M.; Ferns, G.A. Dietary fruits and vegetables and cardiovascular diseases risk. *Crit. Rev. Food Sci. Nutr.* **2015**. [CrossRef] [PubMed]

26. Hung, H.C.; Joshipura, K.J.; Jiang, R.; Hu, F.B.; Hunter, D.; Smith-Warner, S.A.; Colditz, G.A.; Rosner, B.; Spiegelman, D.; Willett, W.C. Fruit and vegetable intake and risk of major chronic disease. *JNCI J. Natl. Cancer Inst.* **2004**, *96*, 1577–1584. [CrossRef] [PubMed]

27. Jang, Y.A.; Lee, H.S.; Kim, B.H.; Lee, Y.; Lee, H.J.; Moon, J.J.; Kim, C.I. Revised dietary guidelines for Koreans. *Asia Pac. J. Clin. Nutr.* **2008**, *17*, 55–58.

28. Im, J.G.; Kim, S.H.; Lee, G.Y.; Joung, H.; Park, M.J. Inadequate calcium intake is highly prevalent in Korean children and adolescents: The Korea National Health and Nutrition Examination Survey (KNHANES) 2007–2010. *Public Health Nutr.* **2014**, *17*, 2489–2495. [CrossRef] [PubMed]

29. Kim, S.; Moon, S.; Popkin, B.M. The nutrition transition in South Korea. *Am. J. Clin. Nutr.* **2000**, *71*, 44–53. [PubMed]

30. Woo, H.D.; Shin, A.; Kim, J. Dietary patterns of Korean adults and the prevalence of metabolic syndrome: A cross-sectional study. *PLoS ONE* **2014**, *9*, e111593. [CrossRef] [PubMed]

31. Striegel-Moore, R.H.; Thompson, D.; Affenito, S.G.; Franko, D.L.; Obarzanek, E.; Barton, B.A.; Schreiber, G.B.; Daniels, S.R.; Schmidt, M.; Crawford, P.B. Correlates of beverage intake in adolescent girls: The National Heart, Lung, and Blood Institute Growth and Health Study. *J. Pediatr.* **2006**, *148*, 183–187. [CrossRef] [PubMed]

32. Demory-Luce, D.; Morales, M.; Nicklas, T.; Baranowski, T.; Zakeri, I.; Berenson, G. Changes in food group consumption patterns from childhood to young adulthood: The Bogalusa Heart Study. *J. Am. Diet. Assoc.* **2004**, *104*, 1684–1691. [CrossRef] [PubMed]

33. Northstone, K.; Emmett, P. Multivariate analysis of diet in children at four and seven years of age and associations with socio-demographic characteristics. *Eur. J. Clin. Nutr.* **2005**, *59*, 751–760. [CrossRef] [PubMed]

34. Béghin, L.; Dauchet, L.; De Vriendt, T.; Cuenca-García, M.; Manios, Y.; Toti, E.; Plada, M.; Widhalm, K.; Repasy, J.; Huybrechts, I.; et al. Influence of parental socio-economic status on diet quality of European adolescents: Results from the HELENA study. *Br. J. Nutr.* **2014**, *111*, 1303–1312. [CrossRef] [PubMed]

35. Darmon, N.; Drewnowski, A. Does social class predict diet quality? *Am. J. Clin. Nutr.* **2008**, *87*, 1107–1117. [PubMed]

10

Parents' Qualitative Perspectives on Child Asking for Fruit and Vegetables

Alicia Beltran, Teresia M. O'Connor, Sheryl O. Hughes, Debbe Thompson, Janice Baranowski, Theresa A. Nicklas and Tom Baranowski *

USDA/ARS Children's Nutrition Research Center, Department of Pediatrics, Baylor College of Medicine, Houston, TX 77030, USA; abeltran@bcm.edu (A.B.); teresiao@bcm.edu (T.M.O.); shughes@bcm.edu (S.O.H.); dit@bcm.edu (D.T.); jbaranow@bcm.edu (J.B.); tnicklas@bcm.edu (T.A.N.)
* Correspondence: tbaranow@bcm.edu

Abstract: Children can influence the foods available at home, but some ways of approaching a parent may be better than others; and the best way may vary by type of parent. This study explored how parents with different parenting styles would best receive their 10 to 14 years old child asking for fruits and vegetables (FV). An online parenting style questionnaire was completed and follow-up qualitative telephone interviews assessed home food rules, child influence on home food availability, parents' preferences for being asked for food, and common barriers and reactions to their child's FV requests. Parents ($n = 73$) with a 10 to 14 years old child were grouped into authoritative, authoritarian, permissive, or uninvolved parenting style categories based on responses to questionnaires, and interviewed. Almost no differences in responses were detected by parenting style or ethnicity. Parents reported their children had a voice in what foods were purchased and available at home and were receptive to their child's asking for FV. The most important child asking characteristic was politeness, especially among authoritarian parents. Other important factors were asking in person, helping in the grocery store, writing requests on the grocery shopping list, and showing information they saw in the media. The barrier raising the most concern was FV cost, but FV quality and safety outside the home environment were also considerations.

Keywords: fruit; vegetables; asking skills; parenting style; children

1. Introduction

Fruit and vegetable consumption has been inversely correlated with all-cause mortality, especially cardiovascular disease mortality [1], and with hypertension, coronary heart disease, and stroke [2]. Despite these health benefits, children's FV consumption is below recommended levels [3]. Focusing on children is important because establishing healthy eating behaviors at any child age tracks into adulthood [4]. A determinant of child FV consumption is home availability [5], i.e., having the item in the home (e.g., carrots in the refrigerator) [6].

Parents influence their children's dietary intake [7]. Keeping healthy foods in the home and unhealthy foods out of the home (i.e., home availability) were consistently the most important parental influences on child intake [8]. In addition, parents influence children's eating behavior through their parenting style [9], i.e., the emotional tone set by the parent for the parent–child relationship. Four general types of parenting style have been identified: authoritarian (highly demanding, and controlling; low emotional warmth), authoritative (highly demanding and controlling; high emotional support and responsiveness), permissive/indulgent (low control and non-demanding, high emotional support and responsiveness), and uninvolved (low demanding, low responsiveness) [10,11]. Parenting style was related to the healthfulness of joint parent–child food shopping selections [12]. Uninvolved parenting style moderated the relationship of child emotional eating and BMIz scores [13]. Maternal indulgent feeding style (i.e., parenting style specific to food) and restrictive parenting practices were related to BMIz score increase over an 18 month interval [14]. Ethnic group differences have been detected in parenting style [15].

Parent–child relationships, however, are a two-way interaction [16]. Children have influenced home food availability by expressing their preferences [17,18] and making requests [19]. Children have developed knowledge, skills, and values for decision making to influence purchases for the home [20,21]. One strategy to increase home FV availability is to teach children to effectively ask parents for their favorite FV. Early adolescence (e.g., 10–14 years old) is a time when children are beginning to establish independence [22], and thus an ideal time to learn new ways to relate to parents. A role-playing intervention improved child asking and negotiation skills and showed a positive effect on home FV availability [23], while another reported that a school based intervention increased parent report of child asking for FV [24]. Asking behaviors at baseline among fourth or fifth grade children predicted home FV availability, but small increases in asking behaviors did not increase home FV availability [25]. Children 12–15 years of age expressed reluctance to ask for FV due to the anticipated negative reaction of their parents [26], which may affect how they ask for FV, and depress impact. Furthermore, parents with the alternative parenting styles may respond differently to various ways of child asking.

Given child reluctance to ask parents to increase FV at home [26], more effective asking interventions may be created if nutrition education interventionists understood how parents might respond to their child's FV asking behaviors and whether these responses vary by parenting style. Given ethnic group differences in parenting style [15], it would also be valuable to understand differences in parent responses by ethnic group.

This study explored how parents from different ethnic groups with different parenting styles would best receive asking for FV from their 10–14-year-old child, and thereby provide the basis for an intervention teaching children asking skills to enhance home FV availability.

2. Materials and Methods

2.1. Study Design

This study was conducted in two phases in 2006. Phase I was a cross sectional online survey that assessed parenting styles. Parents were categorized by parenting style (i.e., authoritative, authoritarian, permissive, or uninvolved). Phase II was an intensive telephone interview with the parent primarily responsible for home food purchase and preparation. Participants were stratified by parenting style and ethnic group based on survey responses. While the project was based in Houston, TX, USA, and the more intensive recruitment activities were located in Houston, respondents from across the USA could participate since inclusion required only completing a web-based questionnaire and responding to a telephone interview. Participants were asked in the survey to select the state and city in which they were located.

2.2. Sample and Recruitment

Eligible participants were parents or guardians with a 10–14-year-old child, had Internet access, were English or Spanish speaking, and were the person in the household responsible for home food purchase, preparation, and serving. Participants were excluded if their 10–14-year-old child had a health condition that affected their dietary intake.

Participants were recruited via a national Children's Nutrition Research Center newsletter, the Children's Nutrition Research Center volunteer list and webpage, health related electronic mailing lists; flyers, a health fair, and radio advertisements targeted to the African American population. Since African American children tend to eat fewer FV [27] and are less likely to participate in research [28], an attempt was made to increase participation from this group. This convenience approach to recruitment and enrollment lasted nine months. A total of 537 participants entered the website and consented to participate, 8 participants declined to participate; of these, 198 parent/guardian and child pairs (36.3%) completed the online survey. Twenty-two participants did not qualify because they were not the parent or guardian of the child and one participant did not qualify because the child did not live with the parent. We have no data for why the 316 participants who consented electronically did not complete the survey.

2.3. Procedures

The study website informed parents about the purpose of the study, assured confidentiality and obtained online consent to participate for self and child. The parent then completed a screening and demographic questionnaire, the Children's Report of Parental Behavior Inventory (CRPBI-30) (Schludermann EH & Schludermann SM, 1988, unpublished results) adapted to parents (English or Spanish). After the parent completed the questionnaires, their 10–14-year-old child completed online assent, and answered the CRPBI-30 for children and youth [29].

The parent/guardian–child pairs who met the inclusion criteria were then categorized on parenting style calculated from the child CRPBI-30 responses. The goal was to enroll 100 participants: 40 authoritative and 40 authoritarian participants with 10 African American, White, Hispanic, and Other in each of these categories; and 10 participants each in the permissive and uninvolved cells. In our experience with research on parenting, theoretical saturation is usually attained with 10 or fewer participants, thereby providing an adequate sample for ethnicity differences within parenting style groups. Theoretically, we expected the permissive and uninvolved parenting style parents would be less likely to be responsive to child asking behaviors. For example, permissive parents would be expected to allow any food (healthy or not) the child wanted into the home; and uninvolved parents would not be expected to respond to any entreaty. Also, based on previous experience we knew there would be fewer permissive and uninvolved respondents, likely reflecting their indifference to participating in such projects. We continued enrollment for as long as participants were agreeing to be interviewed. The parent was then contacted for the 45-min telephone interview. Interviews were pilot tested. All interviewed parents were compensated $25. The Institutional Review Board of the Baylor College of Medicine approved the protocol and procedures.

2.4. Measures

The demographic and screening questionnaire included questions about ethnicity, parent education and parent household role. The revised children and youth report of parental behavior inventory questionnaire (CRPBI-30) is a short (30 item) version of the 108-item questionnaire (Schludermann EH & Schludermann SM, 1988, unpublished results), which measures three dimensions: acceptance/rejection, psychological control/autonomy, and firm/lax control. Each item was answered on a three-point scale (1 = not like my parent or guardian, 2 = a little like my parent or guardian, and 3 = a lot like my parent or guardian). In a sample of older adolescents reporting on their mothers, Cronbach's alphas and test–retest correlations were 0.75 and 0.84 for acceptance (10 items), 0.72 and 0.84 for psychological control (10 items), and 0.65 and 0.79 for firm control (10 items), respectively (Schludermann EH & Schludermann SM, 1988, unpublished results) and dimensions were associated with Family Satisfaction as measured by Olson's Family Satisfaction Scale [29].

2.5. Qualitative Interview

A semi-structured interview script was designed by researchers with expertise in child feeding behavior and qualitative interview techniques. The script guided the interview; prompts were used to assess different aspects of the questions while probes were used to expand or clarify the responses (see Table 1). The script explored the family rules about foods eaten at home, participation, and influence of the child in the decision making of the foods available at home, times when parents were willing to talk with the child about foods, ways in which the child could best ask the parent for foods, parent reactions towards specific child FV requests, and barriers to comply with their child's request.

Table 1. Questions used to guide the semi-structured interview

1.   How much say, if any, does your child have about the foods and beverages you buy for home?
2.   If your child wanted to talk with you about the foods they like or don't like, when are the best times or situations for them to talk with you?
3.   If your child wanted to have specific foods available at home, describe the best way for them to ask you.
a.   What other ways, other than asking, could they use to let you know about specific foods they wanted at home?
4.   How likely would you be to buy fruit or vegetables if your child asked for them?
a.   How would your response to your child change: • If no one else in your home would eat the fruit or vegetable? • If you've bought this fruit or vegetable in the past but had to throw it away? • If you personally do not like this fruit or vegetable? • If the fruit or vegetable is expensive? • If the fruit or vegetable cannot be prepared quickly? • If you don't know how to prepare this fruit or vegetable?
5.   How likely would you be to do the following, if your child asked you to: • Buy 100% fruit juice for breakfast? • Buy fruit for an after-school snack? • Buy vegetables and dip for a snack (e.g., carrots and low fat ranch dip)? • Buy a salad for home? • Make a salad for home? • Make their favorite vegetable for dinner? • Add a fruit or vegetable to the grocery list? • Buy fruit at a restaurant? • Buy a salad at a restaurant? • Buy a vegetable at a restaurant?

2.6. Data Analysis

As prescribed by the originators, children's reports on two of the dimensions: acceptance and firm control were used to categorize their parents on the parenting style category based on median splits from the validation studies (Schludermann EH & Schludermann SM, 1988, unpublished results): authoritarian (high control, low acceptance), authoritative (high control, high acceptance), permissive (low control, high acceptance), and uninvolved (low control, low acceptance). Child responses were used to avoid the possible confounding of common response bias of parent report of parenting style with parent responses to the interview.

Audio-recordings were transcribed verbatim and transcriptions checked against audio-recordings prior to analysis to ensure accuracy. Analysis was conducted in phases: first, separate responses were identified on the transcripts, and entered into Excel (version 12, 2007 Microsoft Office Excel, Microsoft Corp, Redmond, WA, USA); coding was performed manually with thematic codes [30,31] reflecting the questions asked. Within questions, codes were derived as the classification proceeded. Interview response codes were grouped by parenting style and ethnicity to assess possible differences. Given the large number of interviews, coding was conducted independently by six staff members and a coordinator. All transcripts were coded by two coders. The coordinator discussed discrepancies with the independent coders until consensus was established; codings were revised based on the consensus opinion. Comparison summary tables were created to assess differences by ethnicity and then by parenting style.

3. Results

Seventy-three participants (36.9% of the 193 completing the web-based questionnaire) were interviewed: 36 authoritative, 30 authoritarian, 5 permissive, and 2 uninvolved parents (Table 2). The majority were mothers (98.6%) with an average 40.0 ± 5.0 years of age. More parents of girls were interviewed (60.3%). Participants were heavily sourced from Houston (55%), but came from across the

US (Table 2). Since no or only slight differences in responses were detected by parenting style, or by ethnicity in the authoritarian and authoritative categories, findings are presented by questions in the script. The few differences by parenting style and ethnicity are noted.

Table 2. Parent–child demographic characteristics.

Characteristic	*n* (%)	M (SD)
Total parent–child interviews	73 (100.0)	
Age of 10–14 yo child (years)		
10	13 (17.8)	
11	13 (17.8)	
12	17 (23.3)	
13	17 (23.3)	
14	13 (17.8)	
Parent Age		39.97 (5.89)
Child gender		
Male	29 (39.7)	
Female	44 (60.3)	
Parent gender		
Male	1 (1.4)	
Female	72 (98.6)	
Child Race/Ethnicity		
White	22 (30.1)	
AA	19 (26.0)	
Hispanic	23 (31.5)	
Other	9 (12.3)	
Parent Race/Ethnicity		
White	27 (37)	
AA	20 (27.4)	
Hispanic	20 (27.4)	
Other	6 (8.2)	
Parenting style		
Authoritative	36 (49.3)	
Authoritarian	30 (41.1)	
Permissive	5 (6.8)	
Uninvolved	2 (2.7)	
Highest Parent Education		
HS Graduate or less	10 (13.7)	
Some college/technical school	22 (30.1)	
College graduate	23 (31.5)	
Post graduate study	18 (24.7)	
Highest Household Education		
HS Graduate or less	11 (15.1)	
Some college/technical school	21 (28.8)	
College graduate	19 (26.0)	
Post graduate study	22 (30.1)	
State of participants		
California	2 (2.7)	
Colorado	1 (1.4)	
Maine	1 (1.4)	
Minnesota	2 (2.7)	
North Carolina	1 (1.4)	
New Mexico	4 (5.4)	
Oklahoma	1 (1.4)	
Oregon	1 (1.4)	
Texas Houston	40 (55)	
Other Cities	18 (24.6)	
Tennessee	1 (1.4)	
Wyoming	1 (1.4)	

Percentages that do not sum to 100% are due to rounding. Legend: AA = African-American; HS = High School.

3.1. Influence of the Child on the Food and Beverages Bought for Home

When asking parents how much influence their child had on the foods and beverages purchased for home, most of the parents (88%) said their child had a lot of, or some, influence. Three ways in which the child influenced the parent included: the child decided the type of food; the parent controlled the situation, but allowed the child some input upon request; and the parent asked what the child wanted to eat. "...somewhat my child has a say, because if he's not going to eat it, it's no use for me buying it. I have to buy something that I know he's going to eat, or he wants." (Interview 380, Authoritarian–African American)

Some parents (23%) said the child influenced them to buy what the child liked, implying they do not have to ask the child. A few parents (11%) reported the child had a say in food purchases depending on the type of food. If the parent considered the food healthy the parent would buy the requested food, but if the parent considered the food unhealthy, the parent would not purchase it. Some parents (37%) said their child had some say by adding food items to the shopping list, while others (52%) said their child went grocery shopping with them.

3.2. Types of Food Requested by the Child and the Parents' Reaction

Children requested a variety of foods; whether parents bought the requested food depended on the type of food. If the food requested was chips or cookies, a small group (11%) would not buy it. Another factor influencing the purchase was budget. A minority (7%) suggested buying a healthier version of the requested food, or buying the food for limited occasions or quantities. Only 14% of parents reported buying the food without any restrictions, in order to please the child. "...if they're saying, ...can we get green grapes and red grapes, ...if it is something healthy and they ask for it, and granted it is affordable, ...and in the budget ...they can have it, because I encourage them to eat good foods." (Interview 286, Authoritarian–White)

3.3. Times or Channels for the Parent and Child to Talk about Foods

Most parents (73%) reported that a good time to discuss purchasing a food was in the car, because they had time to talk, and the family was together as a captive audience. However, a small number of parents (18%) reported talking in the car was not a good time. Most parents (89%) reported mealtimes as a good time, preferring dinnertime, because they are together as a family, and talk about the day with food present. Another good time was while making the grocery list (53% of parents). "Usually ...at dinner, or ...because we spend a lot of time in the car driving to different activities and that's always a very good time for us to talk." (Interview 650, Authoritative–Other Ethnicity)

Some parents (30%) reported anytime was good to talk about food. The grocery store (18%), while cooking (10%), and before or after school (15%) were other times mentioned by small numbers of parents.

3.4. How Parents Liked Their Child to Ask for Food

Some parents (44%) reported a good way was just asking them in person. About 40% thought their child should ask in a polite manner. This was mentioned more often by the authoritarian parents (18/30) than authoritative (7/36) or permissive (2/5) parents. Across all groups, some of the parents (37%) indicated a good way was asking or selecting the food at the grocery store. "... if they ... asked me, "Mom, could you get me something today?" and they said it in a nice tone with a good attitude and they were happy about it". (Interview 722, Uninvolved–White)

Another good way was writing the food on the grocery list (52% of parents). "I keep a list that they can add to. But they pretty much know, ...what's okay to put on there." (Interview 310, Authoritative–White) Some parents (26%) reported another way to ask was showing them information from the TV or child magazine ads.

When asked whether a child could ask too often, a small group (8% of parents) reported they would prefer not having the child ask too often (not further specified). However, other parents (32%) indicated they would get what the child asked for, depending on the type of food and the attitude of the child.

3.5. Common Barriers to Comply with Child Requests

Most parents (84%) said they would buy FV if their child asked; further, they reported that buying only the FV their child ate was not a barrier. However, a small number (15%) indicated they would be careful with the amount of FV purchased, if no one else at home ate that particular FV. " . . . if one liked it and the rest did not, I would just buy less of it, but I would still buy it." (Interview 311, Permissive-White)

Across all groups, some parents (58%) reported being willing to buy the FV even if it had to be thrown away in the past. However, if this was the case they would purchase less of it or less frequently in the future and a few authoritarian parents would remind the child this would be the last time. A small number of parents (26%) reported they were not likely to purchase the FV if it had been thrown away in the past.

Parents' FV preferences were not a barrier to buying FV for their child. Some parents (42% would buy an expensive FV if the child asked. Others (52%) would buy the requested FV depending on their budget and only if the FV were in season. A small number of parents (19%) would limit the quantity purchased. "If it's expensive but still a little reasonable I will buy it as long as it's something healthy and I know they will eat it..." (Interview 436, Authoritative–Hispanic)

Time for FV preparation and lack of knowledge about preparation were not considered barriers for most parents (66%). Some parents (19%) would purchase the FV and prepare them only when they had time to do so. Only a few parents (16%) reported the lack of time and knowledge to prepare FV to be a barrier and therefore not likely to buy them.

3.6. Reactions to Specific FV Requested by Their Child

Most parents (78%) had a positive reaction toward buying 100% fruit juice for breakfast, and F and V and dip for a snack for their child. A few parents (11%) reported not likely buying 100% fruit juice because of the high sugar content and price. A few parents (10%) would not buy V and dip for a snack because they believed their child would not eat it or was not in their budget. Most parents (59%) already bought salad for home, while some parents (11%) would not buy salad for home because of the quality of salad and beliefs their child would not eat it. "Maybe a fruit salad but a vegetable leaf salad, she will not touch it with a ten-foot pole." (Interview 439, Authoritarian–Hispanic)

Many (84%) reported they would make their child's favorite V for dinner when available. Most parents (75%) would add a F or V to the grocery list, if asked, and buy F at a restaurant (59%), even though a few (5%) thought it was expensive. However, some parents (36%) were not likely to buy F at a restaurant because of perceived low quality, high price, and preference to eat F at home. "No, I don't buy fruit or vegetables ...you don't know what they put inside, ...what kind of seasoning. ...how they prepare it." (Interview 146, Authoritative–African American)

Most, but not all, parents (79%) said they would very likely buy salad or a V at a restaurant for their child.

4. Discussion

Availability of FV at home has consistently been shown to be related to child vegetable intake [32], but reticence in child asking to increase FV has been reported [26]. This study explored how parents would best respond to their 10–14-year-old child asking for FV. In general, parents appeared to be receptive, but the receptiveness of some appeared to be tempered by whether the food requested was considered healthy, and the parent retained control over the situation by limiting the quantity purchased. Although differences in parental acceptance of child asking was expected by parenting style and ethnicity, only slight differences were found in parent responses across authoritative and authoritarian styles and ethnicities. Thus, tailoring an intervention to parenting style or ethnicity does not appear to be needed. Alternatively, an intervention should take steps to appeal to all ethnicities or to be ethnic neutral [33].

Most of this literature has emphasized how parents do or can influence children, and so few references exist for comparison on how children can influence parents and the home food environment [26]. Children directly and indirectly had an influence on what foods were available at home. This is the first report of parent receptiveness to child asking. Parents expressed some control over the food available at home, but kept in mind the child's preferences when buying food, or allowing the child to select the food. Similar observations have been reported about how child preferences influence food availability at home [17]. Furthermore, children's influence on food purchases has been fully recognized and successfully used by marketers [19,20]. A community-based gardening intervention showed children influenced the families' decision making [34]. Marketers have identified influence tactics used by the children to persuade their parents to fulfill their needs e.g., consultation, where the child involves a parent in making a decision [19] or ingratiation where the child gets the parent in a good mood, before asking the parent to comply with their request. Thus, teaching a child to state their FV preferences and ask for FV appear to be promising techniques for helping increase availability of FV in the home and thereby its consumption. Future research should investigate these four pathways of child influence in the context of FV asking.

Parents were aware of the importance of having "healthy food" available at home, and limiting availability of unhealthy food. Concern of parents to have healthy food available in the home has been shown in other studies [35]. Thus, since FV are generally considered healthy, most parents would appear to be receptive to FV requests.

The most important child asking characteristic was politeness, especially among authoritarian parents. Another important factor was the channel for asking, whether in person or by helping in the grocery store, writing it on the grocery list or showing parents the information in the media. These factors have been effective at influencing parents' purchases in other settings [19,20]. Any intervention encouraging stating preference or asking for FV should emphasize politeness on the child's part in each of the channels of asking irrespective of parenting style.

Although some parents reported situational barriers, most offered to still purchase FV requested, but in limited quantities or at different times. The barriers that raised more concern were FV costs and the quality and safety of the FV obtained at restaurants. The intervention might teach children to have realistic expectations for parent responses to their asking. Alternatively, this could be an opportunity to combine math training, microeconomics, and nutrition by teaching somewhat older children relative pricing, amounts purchased, and household budgeting.

A limitation of this study was our inability to recruit substantial numbers of parents who practiced permissive and uninvolved parenting, which restricts the comparisons and the generalizability of the findings. Only 36.3% of mothers who completed the online consent also completed the online survey. Mothers lived in diverse locations across the US, and we do not know their reason(s) for participating, or others for not participating, which may bias the results. Thus, the sample may not be representative of all mothers of children this age, thereby limiting generalizability. Since family structure influences food choices in households [36], further research is needed on how the composition of the household affects family negotiations towards foods available at home.

5. Conclusions

Parent–child communication is bidirectional. Parents showed openness to complying with their child FV requests, as long as certain minimal criteria were met. Children need to learn to ask parents for FV in a polite manner. The training should specifically address alternative channels, e.g., during meals, while preparing the grocery list, in the kitchen when the parent is cooking, in the car, or at the grocery store. Strategies should improve the asking skills to overcome some of the parents' perceived barriers like the lack of time to prepare FV, cost of FV, and FV food safety out of the home environment. Tailoring an intervention to parenting style or ethnicity does not appear to be necessary.

Acknowledgments: This work was funded by grant R21 HD058175 from the National Institute of Child Health and Human Development (NICHHD). This work is also a publication of the United States Department of Agriculture (USDA/ARS) Children's Nutrition Research Center, Department of Pediatrics, Baylor College of Medicine, Houston, Texas, and had been funded in part with federal funds from the USDA/ARS under Cooperative Agreement No. 58-6250-0-008.

Author Contributions: Tom Baranowski, Teresia M. O'Connor, Sheryl O. Hughes, Debbe Thompson, Janice Baranowski, and Theresa A. Nicklas conceived and designed the study. Alicia Beltran was involved in the design and planning of the research, conducted the data collection and analysis, and wrote a preliminary draft of the paper. All authors critically reviewed the manuscript and approved the final version submitted for publication.

References

1. Leenders, M.; Sluijs, I.; Ros, M.M.; Boshuizen, H.C.; Siersema, P.D.; Ferrari, P.; Weikert, C.; Tjønneland, A.; Olsen, A.; Boutron-Ruault, M.C.; et al. Fruit and vegetable consumption and mortality: European prospective investigation into cancer and nutrition. *Am. J. Epidemiol.* **2013**, *178*, 590–602. [CrossRef] [PubMed]
2. Boeing, H.; Bechthold, A.; Bub, A.; Ellinger, S.; Haller, D.; Kroke, A.; Leschik-Bonnet, E.; Müller, M.J.; Oberritter, H.; Schulze, M.; et al. Critical review: Vegetables and fruit in the prevention of chronic diseases. *Eur. J. Nutr.* **2012**, *51*, 637–663. [CrossRef] [PubMed]
3. Grimm, K.A.; Kim, S.A.; Yaroch, A.L.; Scanlon, K.S. Fruit and vegetable intake during infancy and early childhood. *Pediatrics* **2014**, *134*, S63–S69. [CrossRef] [PubMed]
4. Craigie, A.M.; Lake, A.A.; Kelly, S.A.; Adamson, A.J.; Mathers, J.C. Tracking of obesity-related behaviours from childhood to adulthood: A systematic review. *Maturitas* **2011**, *70*, 266–284. [CrossRef] [PubMed]
5. Kristiansen, A.L.; Bjelland, M.; Himberg-Sundet, A.; Lien, N.; Andersen, L.F. Associations between physical home environmental factors and vegetable consumption among Norwegian 3–5-year-olds: The BRA-study. *Public Health Nutr.* **2016**, *20*, 1173–1183. [CrossRef] [PubMed]
6. Cullen, K.W.; Baranowski, T.; Owens, E.; Marsh, T.; Rittenberry, L.; de Moor, C. Availability, accessibility and preferences for fruit, 100% juice and vegetables influence children's dietary behavior. *Health Educ. Behav.* **2003**, *30*, 615–626. [CrossRef] [PubMed]
7. Pearson, N.; Biddle, S.J.; Gorely, T. Family correlates of fruit and vegetable consumption in children and adolescents: a systematic review. *Public Health Nutr.* **2009**, *12*, 267–283. [CrossRef] [PubMed]
8. Yee, A.Z.; Lwin, M.O.; Ho, S.S. The influence of parental practices on child promotive and preventive food consumption behaviors: A systematic review and meta-analysis. *Int. J. Behav. Nutr. Phys. Act.* **2017**, *14*, 47. [CrossRef] [PubMed]
9. Gerards, S.M.; Sleddens, E.F.; Dagnelie, P.C.; de Vries, N.K.; Kremers, S.P. Interventions addressing general parenting to prevent or treat childhood obesity. *Int. J. Pediatr. Obes.* **2011**, *6*, e28–e45. [CrossRef] [PubMed]
10. Maccoby, E.; Martin, J. Socialization in the context of the family: Parent–child interaction. In *Handbook of Child Psychology: Socialization, Personality and Social Development*; Hetherington, E.M., Ed.; Wiley: New York, NY, USA, 1983; pp. 1–101.
11. Baumrind, D. Current patterns of parental authority. *Dev. Psychol.* **1971**, *4 1 Pt 2*, 1–103. [CrossRef] [PubMed]
12. Lucas-Thompson, R.G.; Graham, D.J.; Ullrich, E.; MacPhee, D. General and food-selection specific parenting style in relation to the healthfulness of parent–child choices while grocery shopping. *Appetite* **2017**, *108*, 353–360. [CrossRef] [PubMed]
13. Hankey, M.; Williams, N.A.; Dev, D. Uninvolved maternal feeding style moderates the association of emotional overeating to preschoolers' body mass index z-scores. *J. Nutr. Educ. Behav.* **2016**, *48*, 530–537. [CrossRef] [PubMed]
14. Hughes, S.O.; Power, T.G.; O'Connor, T.M.; Fisher, J.O.; Chen, T.A. Maternal feeding styles and food parenting practices as predictors of longitudinal changes in weight status in Hispanic preschoolers from low-income families. *J. Obes.* **2016**, *2016*. [CrossRef] [PubMed]

15. Clark, T.T.; Yang, C.; McClernon, F.J.; Fuemmeler, B.F. Racial differences in parenting style typologies and heavy episodic drinking trajectories. *Health Psychol.* **2015**, *34*, 697–708. [CrossRef] [PubMed]

16. Baranowski, T.; O'Connor, T.; Hughes, S.; Sleddens, E.; Beltran, A.; Frankel, L.; Mendoza, J.A.; Baranowski, J. Houston...We have a problem! Measurement of parenting. *Child Obes.* **2013**, *9*, 1–4. [CrossRef] [PubMed]

17. James, A.; Curtis, P.; Ellis, K. Negotiating family, negotiating food: Children as family participants? In *Children, Food and Identity in Everyday Life*; James, A., Kjørholt, A.T., Tingstad, V., Eds.; Palgrave Macmillan: Hampshire, UK, 2009; pp. 35–51.

18. Story, M.; Neumark-Sztainer, D.; French, S. Individual and environmental influences on adolescent eating behaviors. *J. Am. Diet. Assoc.* **2002**, *102*, S40–S51. [CrossRef]

19. Wimalasiri, J. A cross-national study on children's purchasing behavior and parental response. *J. Consum. Mark.* **2004**, *21*, 274–284. [CrossRef]

20. Kraak, V.; Pelletier, D.L. The influence of commercialism on the food purchasing behavior of children and teenage youth. *Fam. Econ. Nutr. Rev.* **1998**, *11*, 15–24.

21. John, D.R. Consumer socialization of children: A retrospective look at twenty-five years of research. *J. Consum. Res.* **1999**, *26*, 183–213. [CrossRef]

22. Thornburg, H.D. Is early adolescence really a stage of development? *Theory Pract.* **1983**, *22*, 79–84. [CrossRef]

23. Baranowski, T.; Davis, M.; Resnicow, K.; Baranowski, J.; Doyle, C.; Lin, L.S.; Smith, M.; Wang, D.T. Gimme 5 fruit, juice and vegetables for fun and health: Outcome evaluation. *Health Educ. Behav.* **2000**, *27*, 96–111. [CrossRef] [PubMed]

24. Sharma, S.; Helfman, L.; Albus, K.; Pomeroy, M.; Chuang, R.J.; Markham, C. Feasibility and acceptability of Brighter Bites: A food co-op in schools to increase access, continuity and education of fruits and vegetables among low-income populations. *J. Prim. Prev.* **2015**, *36*, 281–286. [CrossRef] [PubMed]

25. DeSmet, A.; Liu, Y.; De Bourdeaudhuij, I.; Baranowski, T.; Thompson, D. The effectiveness of asking behaviors among 9–11 year-old children in increasing home availability and children's intake of fruit and vegetables: Results from the Squire's Quest II self-regulation game intervention. *Int. J. Behav. Nutr. Phys. Act.* **2017**, *14*, 51. [CrossRef] [PubMed]

26. Middlestadt, S.E.; Lederer, A.M.; Smith, N.K.; Doss, D.; Hung, C.L.; Stevenson, L.D.; Fly, A.D. Determinants of middle-school students asking parents for fruits and vegetables: A theory-based salient belief elicitation. *Public Health Nutr.* **2013**, *16*, 1971–1978. [CrossRef] [PubMed]

27. Storey, M.; Anderson, P. Income and race/ethnicity influence dietary fiber intake and vegetable consumption. *Nutr. Res.* **2014**, *34*, 844–850. [CrossRef] [PubMed]

28. Erves, J.C.; Mayo-Gamble, T.L.; Malin-Fair, A.; Boyer, A.; Joosten, Y.; Vaughn, Y.C.; Sherden, L.; Luther, P.; Miller, S.; Wilkins, C.H. Needs, priorities, and recommendations for engaging underrepresented populations in clinical research: A community perspective. *J. Community Health* **2016**, *42*, 472–480. [CrossRef] [PubMed]

29. Olson, D.H.; Wilson, M. Family satisfaction. In *Families: What Makes Them Work*; Olson, D.H., McCubbin, H.I., Barnes, H., Larsen, A., Muxen, M., Wilson, M., Eds.; Sage Publications: Beverly Hills, CA, USA, 1983.

30. Bernard, H.R.; Ryan, G.W. *Analyzing Qualitative Data: Systematic Approaches*; Sage Publications: Thousand Oaks, CA, USA, 2010.

31. Braun, V.; Clarke, V. Using thematic analysis in psychology. *Qual. Res. Psychol.* **2006**, *3*, 77–101. [CrossRef]

32. Johnson, S.L. Developmental and environmental influences on young children's vegetable preferences and consumption. *Adv. Nutr.* **2016**, *7*, 220S–231S. [CrossRef] [PubMed]

33. Resnicow, K.; Baranowski, T.; Ahluwalia, J.S.; Braithwaite, R.L. Cultural sensitivity in public health: Defined and demystified. *Ethn. Dis.* **1999**, *9*, 10–21. [PubMed]

34. Heim, S.; Bauer, K.W.; Stang, J.; Ireland, M. Can a community-based intervention improve the home food environment? Parental perspectives of the influence of the delicious and nutritious garden. *J. Nutr. Educ. Behav.* **2011**, *43*, 130–134. [CrossRef] [PubMed]

35. Nørgaard, M.K.; Brunsø, K. Family conflicts and conflict resolutions regarding food choices. *J. Consum. Behav.* **2011**, *10*, 141–151. [CrossRef]
36. Coveney, J. What does research on families and food tell us? Implications for nutrition and dietetic practice. *Nutr. Diet.* **2002**, *59*, 113–119.

11

Evaluation of the Effect of a Growing up Milk Lite vs. Cow's Milk on Diet Quality and Dietary Intakes in Early Childhood: The Growing up Milk Lite (GUMLi) Randomised Controlled Trial

Amy L. Lovell [1],*, Tania Milne [2], Yannan Jiang [3], Rachel X. Chen [3], Cameron C. Grant [4,5,6] and Clare R. Wall [1]

[1] Discipline of Nutrition and Dietetics, Faculty of Medical and Health Sciences, University of Auckland, Auckland 1142, New Zealand; c.wall@auckland.ac.nz

[2] Faculty of Medical and Health Sciences, University of Auckland, Auckland 1142, New Zealand; t.milne@auckland.ac.nz

[3] Department of Statistics, Faculty of Science, University of Auckland, Auckland 1142, New Zealand; y.jiang@auckland.ac.nz (Y.J.); rachel.chen@auckland.ac.nz (R.X.C.)

[4] Department of Paediatrics: Child and Youth Health, University of Auckland, Grafton 1023, New Zealand; cc.grant@auckland.ac.nz

[5] Centre for Longitudinal Research He Ara ki Mua, University of Auckland, Auckland 1743, New Zealand

[6] General Paediatrics, Starship Children's Hospital, Auckland District Health Board, Auckland, Auckland 1142, New Zealand

* Correspondence: a.lovell@auckland.ac.nz

Abstract: Summary scores provide an alternative approach to measuring dietary quality. The Growing Up Milk-Lite (GUMLi) Trial was a multi-centre, double-blinded, randomised controlled trial of children randomised to receive a reduced protein GUM (GUMLi) or unfortified cow's milk (CM). In a secondary analysis of the GUMLi Trial, we used the Probability of Adequate Nutrient Intake (PANDiet) to determine the nutritional adequacy of the diets of participating children living in Auckland. The PANDiet was adapted to the New Zealand Nutrient Reference Values and data from four 24 h Recalls (24HR) collected at months 7, 8, 10, and 11 post-randomisation were used. Differences between randomised groups (GUMLi vs. CM) of the PANDiet and its components were made. Eighty-three Auckland participants were included in the study (GUMLi $n = 41$ vs. CM $n = 42$). Total PANDiet scores were significantly higher in the GUMLi group ($p < 0.001$), indicating better overall nutrient adequacy and diet quality. Dietary intakes of children in both groups met the recommendations for fat, total carbohydrates and most micronutrients; however, protein intakes exceeded recommendations. Consumption of GUMLi was associated with higher nutritional adequacy, with an increased likelihood of meeting nutrient requirements; however, the impact of the family diet and GUMLi on dietary diversity requires further evaluation.

Keywords: diet quality; PANDiet index; early childhood; nutritional adequacy; nutrient intake quality; growing up milk

1. Introduction

Early food habits, practices, and dietary patterns develop rapidly within the first two years of life [1,2]; with evidence that diet quality may decline as children age [3]. Evaluating diet quality in paediatric populations is of increasing interest, however, due to a paucity of evidence-based dietary guidelines for children under two, combining these multidimensional behaviours into a single meaningful measure remains a challenge [4].

Diet quality can be determined using nutrient, food, or food and nutrient-based indices [5]. Index scores are determined 'a priori', using dietary guidelines, recommended nutrient intakes, or current nutrition knowledge of optimal dietary patterns [6–9]. The resulting numeric representation of dietary quality or nutrient adequacy can be used as a nutritional benchmark in identifying relationships between the whole-of-diet and later health [6,7,10,11]. Nutrient-based measures of diet quality reflect adequacy of nutrient intake, however, require detailed dietary assessment, additional analyses and statistical modelling before a final score is calculated [5,6]. In contrast, food-based indices provide an indirect measure of nutrient and non-nutrient interactions, where a score is easily calculated based on awarding points for fulfilling certain criteria [5,6]. The Probability of Adequate Nutrient Intake (PANDiet) score is a complete, nutrient-based diet quality index, employing probabilistic calculations of nutrient adequacy [12]. The index has been evaluated in French [12], US [12] adult populations and a UK [13] paediatric population and has shown to be a useful tool in assessing diet quality at the population level [12].

There is limited research on the contribution of milk to the diets of children under two [14–16], specifically, whether Growing Up Milks (GUM) provide a nutritional advantage compared to standard cow's milk (CM) [17]. Simulation data have shown that replacing CM with GUM resulted in protein intakes more in line with recommendations, reduced saturated fatty acid (SFA) intake and increased likelihood of adequate intakes of vitamin D and iron [17,18]. We aimed to evaluate the dietary quality of the Auckland children participating in the GUMLi Trial aged 18- to 23-months, using an adapted PANDiet index and determine nutritional adequacy according to intervention allocation.

2. Materials and Methods

2.1. Study Design and Participants

This is a secondary analysis of data collected as part of the GUMLi trial. Briefly, the GUMLi trial was a multi-centre, double blinded, randomised controlled trial performed in Auckland, New Zealand ($n = 108$) and Brisbane, Australia ($n = 52$) from 2015 to 2017. One hundred and sixty healthy children aged one were randomised 1:1 to receive unfortified cow's milk (CM) or a reduced protein GUM (GUMLi), fortified with iron, vitamin D, pre- and probiotics (Danone Pty Ltd., Auckland, New Zealand) until the age of two. GUMLi had a reduced energy and protein content compared to commercial GUM on the market, 60 kcal/100 mL vs. 71 kcal/100 mL and 1.7 g/100 mL protein vs. 2.2 g/100 mL. An energy-matched, non-fortified cow's milk was used as an active control, with a protein content of 3.1 g/100 mL. The primary trial outcome evaluated the effect of consuming GUMLi versus unfortified CM as part of a whole diet for 12-months on body composition at two years of age [19]. Secondary outcomes included dietary intake (food frequency questionnaire or 24 h), micronutrient status, and cognitive development.

The study received ethical approval from the Health and Disability Ethics Committee of the Ministry of Health, New Zealand (14/NTB/152), and the University of Queensland Medical Research Ethics Committee, Brisbane, Australia (2014001318). The GUMLi Trial was registered with the Australian New Zealand Clinical Trials Registry, reference number: ACTRN12614000918628. Written informed consent was obtained from all participants. At month six post-randomisation, primary caregivers were invited to complete four record-assisted twenty-four-hour recalls (24 h). Of the 108 Auckland participants, 83 (77%) completed four 24 h. Four (4%) opted out of the study (but continued with the main trial), eleven (10 %) withdrew from the main trial and nine (8%) took part, but did not complete four 24 h. Only 14 (27%) participants from Brisbane completed four 24 h, therefore, the decision was made not to include them in the analysis.

2.2. Dietary Intakes

A dietitian collected dietary data over the phone using record-assisted 24HRs between months 6 to 11 post-randomisation, according to a standardised procedure [20]. Four 24 h were collected per participant on randomly allocated days (three weekdays and one weekend day). The record-assisted 24HR differed from standard 24HRs, as caregivers recoded their child's intake over the pre-defined 24-h period preceding the phone call. This methodology was used in a pilot validation study for the New Zealand Children's Nutrition Survey [21] and the Australian Children's Nutrition and Physical Activity Survey (CNPAS) [22,23]. A 'Foods fed by other adults' form, adapted from the Feeding Infants and Toddlers study (FITS) [24,25] was used to record intake if the child was in the care of another adult i.e., day-care. Use of dietary supplements, homemade recipes, and portion sizes (household measures or gram weight) were recorded. A food model booklet, reproduced with permission from CNPAS was used to assist with describing serving sizes [22,23]. Breastfeeding was recorded as time (minutes) and quantity estimated using a conversion factor of 10 mL/min, max 10 min [26,27]. All 24HR were double-checked to identify mistakes, missing foods, or clarify recipes. A dietetics student entered the data into Foodworks® (version 9, Xyris Software, Pty Ltd., Australia) and checked for completeness. Nutritional data were derived from the FOODfiles 2016 database [28] and nutritional profiles of commercial toddler foods sourced from companies or nutrient information panels.

2.3. Assessment of Nutrient Intakes with Nutrient Reference Values

Nutrient intakes were compared to the Australian and New Zealand Nutrient Reference Values (NRVs) [29]. Prevalence of inadequate intakes were assessed using the cut-off point method for nutrients with an Estimated Average Requirement (EAR) value [30]. This method has previously been shown to produce realistic estimates of the prevalence of inadequate dietary intakes [30]. The EAR, derived by the Institute of Medicine (IoM) was used for vitamin D (10 µg/day) [31].

2.4. Assessment of Diet Quality Using the PANDiet Score

The development and design of the PANDiet score has been reported in detail elsewhere [12,32]. Briefly, the PANDiet provides a measure of diet quality through the probability of having adequate nutrient intake, ranging from 0–100, where the higher the score, the better the diet quality and nutrient adequacy [12,32]. The PANDiet is an average of the Adequacy and Moderation sub-scores, which rely on the calculation of probability of adequacy for 25 nutrients and consider duration of dietary assessment, day-to-day variability, nutrient reference values, inter-variability of intake, and mean nutrient intakes [12,32]. The Adequacy sub-score calculates the probability that usual nutrient intake is above a reference value and the Moderation sub-score calculates the probability that the usual nutrient intake meets requirements and does not exceed a reference value [12,33]. Using the original methods [12], the PANDiet score calculation for protein and micronutrients was adjusted using the Australian and New Zealand NRVs and inter-variability for children one- to three years of age [29]. There are no recommendations for total fat, poly-unsaturated fatty acids (PUFA) and carbohydrate in children under two. Therefore, as seen in Verger et al. [32], we used the reference values set by the European Food Safety Authority (EFSA) [34], Nordic recommendations for SFA and non-milk extrinsic sugars (NMES) [35] and the IoM upper limit for protein [36]. The risk of excessive intakes were assessed using a penalty value system [12], using the upper limit as a reference [29] (Table S1).

Participants were classified according to their randomisation into the trial and allocation to receive GUMLi or CM. The trial analysis was conducted based on the assumption that the PANDiet index was suitable to use as an outcome measure and the difference between randomised groups, if observed, would indicate an effect of the intervention.

2.5. Statistical Analysis

A sample size of 64 participants in each arm is required to have 80% power at 5% significant level (two-sided) to detect a 0.5 SD difference in body fat percent (primary outcome) between the two arms at the end of the 12-month intervention. Statistical analyses were performed using SAS version 9.4 (SAS Institute Inc., Cary, NC, USA). Baseline characteristics were summarised by treatment group (GUMLi vs. CM) using descriptive statistics. Continuous variables were reported as mean and standard deviation (SD) and categorical variables described as frequencies and percentages. The characteristics of the Auckland sub-group included in this study ($N = 83$) were compared to those in the Auckland cohort who did not participate ($N = 25$). Chi-Square test or Fisher's Exact test were used for categorical variables, and the Kruskal-Wallis test or two-sample t-test was used for continuous variables. The impact of the intervention on energy and nutrient intakes were evaluated at each 24HR time point (month 7, 8, 10, and 11 post-randomisation), using random effect mixed models with an autoregressive covariance structure on repeated measures.

The fixed effects model included participant sex, treatment group, time point and its interaction with the treatment group. Model-adjusted mean differences between nutrient intakes of both groups and 95% confidence intervals (95% CI) were reported at each time point, with associated p-values. The impact of the intervention on the overall PANDiet score, sub-scores and components using all 24 h data were evaluated using linear regression models adjusting for sex. Model-adjusted mean differences between two groups were estimated and tested. All statistical tests were two-sided with a statistical significance of $p < 0.05$. As a secondary analysis, missing data was not imputed and no adjustment for multiple comparisons were considered.

3. Results

One hundred and eight Auckland children participated in the main GUMLi trial. Of these, 83 (77%) were included in this sub-study, with no significant differences between GUMLi and CM groups for any baseline characteristics (Table 1), therefore, it was assumed that any differences in PANDiet scores would be attributed to the intervention milk. No statistical differences were observed between the Auckland participants included in the analysis ($N = 83$) and those excluded ($N = 25$), except for maternal educational attainment (80% vs. 60%; $p = 0.047$) (Table S2). GUMLi and CM composition are presented in Table S3. Both milks were energy-matched per 100 mL, however compared to CM, GUMLi was lower in SFA and protein, with higher carbohydrate and dietary fibre, and nutritionally significant amounts of iron and vitamin D (cholecalciferol).

Table 1. Child and maternal characteristics of the Auckland cohort ($N = 83$) included in the PANDiet cohort.

Baseline Demographics	Study Group Intervention ($N = 41$) n (%)	Control ($N = 42$) n (%)	p-Value *
Child's sex			0.062
Boy	19 (46)	28 (67)	
Girl	22 (54)	14 (33)	
Other children in the family			0.222
No	16 (39)	22 (52)	
Yes	25 (61)	20 (48)	
Day care attendance			0.893
No	25 (61)	25 (60)	
Yes	16 (39)	17 (40)	
Breastfed at baseline			0.415
No	27 (66)	24 (57)	
Yes	14 (34)	18 (43)	
Mother's Ethnicity			0.903
Māori	8 (20)	6 (14)	
Pacific	0 (0)	1 (2)	
Asian	3 (7)	2 (5)	
European	23 (56)	26 (62)	
Other	7 (17)	7 (17)	
Mother's Age, years (mean ± SD)	32 ± 5	32 ± 4	0.874
Mother's BMI, kgm^2 (mean ± SD)	26 ± 5	27 ± 6	0.916

Table 1. *Cont.*

Baseline Demographics	Study Group Intervention (N = 41) n (%)	Control (N = 42) n (%)	p-Value *
Mother's Highest Level of Education			0.589
No school qualifications	0(0)	0(0)	
Primary	2 (5)	0 (0)	
Secondary	5 (12)	7 (17)	
Tertiary	33 (80)	33 (79)	
Other	1 (2)	2 (5)	
Mother's Employment Status			0.082
Full-time caregiver	14 (34)	15 (36)	
Full-time paid employment	5 (12)	13 (31)	
Part-time paid employment	14 (34)	13 (31)	
Receiving a benefit	1 (2)	0 (0)	
Unemployed, no benefit	3 (7)	0 (0)	
Other	4 (10)	1 (2)	
Smoking			
Current smoking	1 (2)	1 (2)	1.000
Smoking before pregnancy	5 (12)	2 (5)	0.432
Smoking during pregnancy	1 (2)	0 (0)	0.494

* Unadjusted *p*-values, Chi-square test or Fisher's Exact test is used to test the difference between groups for categorical variables; the Kruskal-Wallis test or two-sample *t*-test is used to compare the medians/means between groups for continuous variables.

3.1. Evaluation of Nutrient Intakes

Mean (SD) daily nutrient intakes at the four 24HR time points are displayed in Table 2, according to GUMLi or CM group. For the purpose of table length, only nutrients with significant relationships at any time point are displayed. A full table is presented in Table S4. There were no differences between groups at any time point for energy, sodium, PUFA, vitamin A, vitamin B-6, folate, magnesium, and selenium. Children in the GUMLi group had significantly higher intakes of vitamin C and iron across all time points, and children in the CM group had significant higher intakes of riboflavin and potassium.

Table 2. Nutrient intake among Auckland children (N = 83) from 18 and 23 months of age (month 7–11 post randomisation) [1,2].

Nutrients	Usual Intake Values		Adjusted Difference (95%CI)	p *
	Intervention (N = 41) Mean (SD)	Control (N = 42) Mean (SD)		
Energy (kcal)				
Month 07	1135.92 (294.19)	1122.34 (187.51)	36.61 (−93.18, 166.41)	0.579
Month 08	1114.07 (277.52)	1246.07 (378.83)	−108.96 (−238.76, 20.84)	0.100
Month 10	1128.31 (383.78)	1068.61 (291.44)	82.74 (−47.05, 212.54)	0.210
Month 11	1190.24 (288.14)	1118.93 (283.21)	94.34 (−35.45, 224.14)	0.154
Carbohydrate (g)				
Month 07	142.45 (40.53)	127.44 (36.36)	18.26 (−0.25, 36.76)	0.053
Month 08	138.50 (38.12)	144.65 (56.59)	−2.90 (−21.41, 15.61)	0.758
Month 10	138.25 (45.72)	123.41 (41.01)	18.09 (−0.42, 36.59)	0.055
Month 11	145.81 (41.01)	126.61 (43.06)	22.45 (3.94, 40.96)	0.018 *
Total fat (g)				
Month 07	38.49 (13.70)	43.91 (11.34)	−4.69 (−11.04, 1.65)	0.146
Month 08	37.76 (14.79)	46.21 (16.22)	−7.72 (−14.07, −1.37)	0.017 *
Month 10	39.53 (17.61)	40.34 (13.50)	−0.08 (−6.42, 6.27)	0.981
Month 11	43.99 (15.81)	43.75 (13.59)	0.97 (−5.38, 7.32)	0.764
Saturated fat (g)				
Month 07	18.98 (7.37)	21.16 (5.98)	−1.96 (−5.27, 1.34)	0.243
Month 08	18.11 (7.41)	22.16 (8.16)	−3.83 (−7.14, −0.53)	0.023 *
Month 10	19.46 (8.88)	19.73 (7.77)	−0.05 (−3.35, 3.26)	0.977
Month 11	20.93 (8.11)	21.00 (6.84)	0.15 (−3.16, 3.45)	0.930
NMES (g)				
Month 07	45.46 (18.22)	42.02 (17.88)	4.33 (−5.27, 13.93)	0.375
Month 08	45.90 (19.00)	49.01 (30.16)	−2.22 (−11.83, 7.38)	0.649
Month 10	40.13 (23.17)	39.00 (19.24)	2.03 (−7.58, 11.63)	0.678
Month 11	48.53 (25.02)	39.29 (21.47)	10.14 (0.54, 19.74)	0.039 *
Protein (g)				
Month 07	46.07 (17.15)	50.13 (10.13)	−3.26 (−9.65, 3.13)	0.316
Month 08	46.09 (14.01)	56.47 (17.08)	−9.58 (−15.97, −3.19)	0.004 *
Month 10	46.45 (18.34)	44.33 (12.51)	2.92 (−3.47, 9.31)	0.369
Month 11	44.59 (14.36)	47.48 (13.13)	−2.09 (−8.48, 4.30)	0.520

Table 2. *Cont.*

	Usual Intake Values		Adjusted Difference (95%CI)	*p* *
Nutrients	Intervention (*N* = 41) Mean (SD)	Control (*N* = 42) Mean (SD)		
Thiamin (mg)				
Month 07	1.50 (0.63)	1.19 (0.84)	0.34 (0.03, 0.64)	0.030 *
Month 08	1.54 (0.56)	1.29 (0.72)	0.28 (−0.02, 0.59)	0.069
Month 10	1.35 (0.70)	1.03 (0.82)	0.36 (0.05, 0.66)	0.022 *
Month 11	1.36 (0.68)	0.99 (0.64)	0.40 (0.10, 0.71)	0.010 *
Riboflavin (mg)				
Month 07	1.82 (0.64)	2.12 (0.64)	−0.29 (−0.56, −0.02)	0.037 *
Month 08	1.71 (0.54)	2.30 (0.77)	−0.58 (−0.85, −0.30)	<0.0001 *
Month 10	1.66 (0.50)	2.07 (0.67)	−0.39 (−0.66, −0.11)	0.006 *
Month 11	1.63 (0.61)	2.11 (0.57)	−0.47 (−0.74, −0.20)	0.001 *
Niacin (mg)				
Month 07	19.97 (7.25)	17.79 (4.64)	2.49 (−0.12, 5.09)	0.061
Month 08	20.63 (5.18)	20.09 (7.30)	0.85 (−1.75, 3.45)	0.521
Month 10	19.34 (6.64)	15.80 (5.87)	3.84 (1.24, 6.45)	0.004 *
Month 11	19.09 (5.31)	17.28 (5.39)	2.11 (−0.49, 4.71)	0.112
Vitamin B12 (µg)				
Month 07	2.36 (1.12)	2.78 (1.09)	−0.41 (−0.91, 0.09)	0.108
Month 08	2.25 (1.30)	3.17 (1.55)	−0.91 (−1.41, −0.41)	0.0004 *
Month 10	2.14 (0.94)	2.57 (0.93)	−0.42 (−0.92, 0.07)	0.095
Month 11	2.03 (0.91)	2.58 (1.15)	−0.55 (−1.05, −0.05)	0.031 *
Vitamin C (mg)				
Month 07	104.00 (44.39)	45.38 (37.36)	57.38 (35.76, 79.01)	<0.0001 *
Month 08	99.95 (39.44)	50.22 (54.71)	48.48 (26.86, 70.11)	<0.0001 *
Month 10	92.84 (34.62)	50.54 (65.97)	41.05 (19.43, 62.68)	0.0002 *
Month 11	92.51 (48.54)	58.80 (61.49)	32.47 (10.85, 54.10)	0.003 *
Vitamin D (µg)				
Month 07	6.02 (6.57)	3.23 (3.18)	2.80 (1.07, 4.53)	0.002 *
Month 08	4.73 (2.70)	3.59 (4.00)	1.16 (−0.57, 2.89)	0.188
Month 10	5.17 (2.76)	2.92 (2.49)	2.27 (0.54, 4.00)	0.011 *
Month 11	4.86 (3.44)	3.73 (4.75)	1.15 (−0.58, 2.88)	0.194
Calcium (mg)				
Month 07	901.26 (268.15)	898.06 (287.37)	8.15 (−113.76, 130.06)	0.895
Month 08	808.31 (257.94)	943.49 (314.09)	−130.24 (−252.15, −8.33)	0.036 *
Month 10	899.34 (284.54)	836.03 (251.58)	68.25 (−53.65, 190.16)	0.271
Month 11	830.41 (284.29)	891.05 (280.79)	−55.70 (−177.60, 66.21)	0.369
Zinc (mg)				
Month 07	6.75 (2.76)	6.11 (1.51)	0.71 (−0.22, 1.64)	0.133
Month 08	6.64 (2.24)	6.85 (2.65)	−0.13 (−1.07, 0.80)	0.776
Month 10	6.44 (2.45)	5.37 (1.74)	1.14 (0.21, 2.07)	0.017 *
Month 11	6.42 (1.77)	5.45 (1.69)	1.04 (0.11, 1.97)	0.029 *
Phosphorus (mg)				
Month 07	1023.06 (284.32)	1004.05 (202.02)	33.99 (−83.88, 151.87)	0.571
Month 08	966.96 (257.85)	1106.43 (293.65)	−124.49 (−242.36, −6.62)	0.039 *
Month 10	984.67 (335.64)	930.98 (252.54)	68.68 (−49.20, 186.55)	0.252
Month 11	989.53 (278.71)	988.18 (262.19)	16.33 (−101.54, 134.20)	0.785
Potassium (mg)				
Month 07	1666.69 (703.04)	1962.08 (433.28)	−283.10 (−528.37, −37.83)	0.024 *
Month 08	1537.51 (481.42)	2232.75 (761.17)	−682.95 (−928.21, −437.68)	<0.0001 *
Month 10	1406.79 (493.64)	1861.05 (503.26)	−441.97 (−687.24, −196.70)	0.001 *
Month 11	1512.12 (526.22)	1987.09 (511.40)	−462.67 (−707.94, −217.40)	0.000 *
Iron (mg)				
Month 07	10.62 (3.36)	6.23 (2.82)	4.58 (3.31, 5.85)	<0.0001 *
Month 08	10.80 (2.96)	6.90 (2.75)	4.10 (2.83, 5.37)	<0.0001 *
Month 10	9.83 (2.89)	5.64 (3.07)	4.38 (3.11, 5.65)	<0.0001 *
Month 11	10.26 (3.24)	5.24 (2.35)	5.21 (3.93, 6.48)	<0.0001 *
Copper (mg)				
Month 07	0.62 (0.32)	0.6 (0.24)	0.04 (−0.08, 0.15)	0.524
Month 08	0.6 (0.26)	0.68 (0.35)	−0.06 (−0.18, 0.05)	0.255
Month 10	0.63 (0.28)	0.5 (0.21)	0.15 (0.04, 0.26)	0.010 *
Month 11	0.6 (0.18)	0.53 (0.18)	0.09 (−0.02, 0.2)	0.115
Iodine (µg)				
Month 07	64.08 (23.15)	52.65 (24.78)	11.80 (0.49, 23.11)	0.041 *
Month 08	63.58 (29.84)	55.72 (21.88)	8.22 (−3.09, 19.54)	0.154
Month 10	60.53 (27.92)	53.13 (26.95)	7.77 (−3.55, 19.08)	0.178
Month 11	65.92 (30.56)	53.53 (21.06)	12.76 (1.45, 24.07)	0.027

* $p < 0.05$. [1] Repeated measures mixed model with an autoregressive covariance structure, adjusting for sex.
[2] Only nutrients with significant relationships at any of the four time points are displayed.

Compared with New Zealand NRVs [29], intakes of most nutrients were adequate, i.e., median intake (average all four 24 h) ≥ nutrient reference value across both groups Figure 1. Nutrients with median intakes below reference values in both groups were vitamin D, potassium, copper, and iodine.

Group A: Cow's Milk

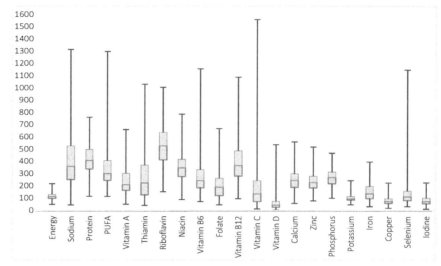

Group B: GUMLi

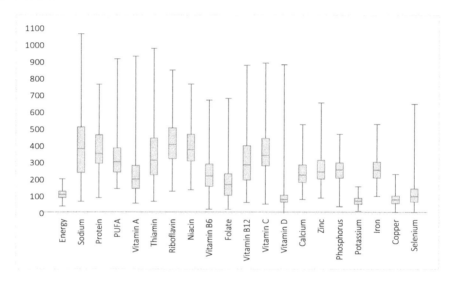

Figure 1. Intake of energy and nutrients as a percentage of New Zealand reference values (28) in 18- to 23-month-old children from the Auckland cohort participating in the GUMLi trial (median (—), interquartile range (box; 25th and 75th percentiles), minimum and maximum value). GUMLi = Growing Up Milk—Lite.

3.2. PANDiet Scores According to Intake of GUMLi or CM

Mean PANDiet score, sub-scores and individual components are displayed in Table 3. After adjusting for sex, children in the GUMLi group had significantly higher PANDiet scores and Adequacy scores compared to the CM group (adjusted mean difference +3.11 and +4.17, respectively). There was no difference in the Moderation sub score and energy intake between groups. Of note, the Adequacy sub-score was 2.5 and 2.6 times greater than the Moderation sub-score in the GUMLi and CM group, respectively, indicating poor adherence to the recommendations for avoiding excessive nutrient intakes.

There were no differences in component of the Moderation sub-score, except for total fat and total carbohydrates, where the CM group had a higher probability of avoiding excessive total fat intake and the GUMLi group had a higher probability of avoiding excessive total carbohydrate intake. The GUMLi group tended to have higher probability of avoiding excessive protein intake (not significant). The mean probabilities for avoiding excessive intakes were low for sodium (≤ 0.03),

SFA ($\leq$0.10) and NMES ($\leq$0.23) in this population. There were no differences between groups in components of the Adequacy sub-score, except for total fat, thiamin, vitamin C, vitamin D, iron, and iodine where the GUMLi group had a higher probability of having adequate intakes for these nutrients, and vitamin B12 where the CM group had a higher probability of having an adequate intake.

Table 3. PANDiet scores, sub-scores, and individual components, among Auckland children (N = 83) from 18 and 23 months of age (month 7–11 post randomisation) [1,2].

Score	Intervention (N = 41) Mean (SD)	Control (N = 42) Mean (SD)	Adjusted Difference (95% CI)	p-Value *
PANDiet [3]	52.9 (3.07)	50.12 (3.97)	3.11 (1.56, 4.67)	0.0001 *
Moderation sub-score	29.82 (6.47)	27.77 (6.58)	2.06 (−0.87, 4.99)	0.1660
Protein	0.41 (0.50)	0.33 (0.48)	0.08 (−0.14, 0.30)	0.4747
Total Fat	0.10 (0.30)	0.48 (0.51)	−0.40 (−0.59, −0.22)	<0001 *
Total Carbohydrate	0.85 (0.36)	0.55 (0.50)	0.33 (0.14, 0.53)	0.0011 *
SFA	0.10 (0.16)	0.06 (0.12)	0.05 (−0.01, 0.11)	0.1231
NMES	0.16 (0.22)	0.23 (0.28)	−0.08 (−0.19, 0.03)	0.1699
Sodium	0.03 (0.14)	0.02 (0.04)	0.01 (−0.03, 0.06)	0.5832
Adequacy sub-score	75.98 (4.98)	72.46 (5.88)	4.17 (1.82, 6.51)	0.0007 *
Protein	0.99 (0.03)	1.00 (0.001)	−0.01 (−0.01, 0.002)	0.1697
Total Carbohydrate	0.98 (0.16)	1.00 (0.00)	−0.02 (−0.07, 0.03)	0.4293
Total Fat	1.00 (0.00)	0.86 (0.35)	0.14 (0.03, 0.26)	0.0140 *
PUFA	0.15 (0.19)	0.18 (0.23)	−0.01 (−0.10, 0.08)	0.7975
Vitamin A	0.96 (0.08)	0.98 (0.02)	−0.02 (−0.05, 0.001)	0.0560
Thiamin	1.00 (0.005)	0.94 (0.09)	0.06 (0.03, 0.09)	0.0001 *
Riboflavin	1.00 (0.001)	1.00 (0.0003)	−0.0003 (−0.001, 0.00)	0.0853
Niacin	1.00 (0.00001)	1.00 (0.0005)	0.0001 (0.00, 0.0002)	0.1819
Vitamin B6	0.00 (0.00)	0.00 (0.00)	0.00 (0.00,0.00)	0.9775
Folate	0.89 (0.18)	0.91 (0.21)	−0.01 (−0.10, 0.07)	0.7717
Vitamin B12	0.99 (0.02)	1.00 (0.01)	−0.01 (−0.02, −0.003)	0.0081 *
Vitamin C	1.00 (0.01)	0.71 (0.32)	0.30 (0.20, 0.40)	<0001 *
Vitamin D	0.43 (0.34)	0.19 (0.31)	0.25 (0.10, 0.39)	0.0011 *
Calcium	0.99 (0.02)	1.00 (0.02)	−0.002 (−0.01, 0.01)	0.7227
Magnesium	0.99 (0.02)	1.00 (0.004)	−0.005 (−0.01, 0.002)	0.1826
Zinc	1.00 (0.003)	0.99 (0.02)	0.01 (−0.0002, 0.01)	0.0585
Phosphorus	1.00 (0.01)	1.00 (0.002)	−0.001 (−0.003, 0.0005)	0.1323
Potassium	1.00 (0.002)	1.00 (1E−6)	−0.0003 (−0.001, 0.0002)	0.1998
Iron	1.00 (0.01)	0.78 (0.32)	0.25 (0.16, 0.35)	<0001 *
Copper	0.34 (0.30)	0.27 (0.27)	0.10 (−0.03, 0.23)	0.1203
Selenium	0.57 (0.37)	0.70 (0.28)	−0.09 (−0.23, 0.06)	0.2314
Iodine	0.46 (0.28)	0.29 (0.24)	0.18 (0.06, 0.30)	0.0035 *

NMES, Non-milk Extrinsic Sugars; PANDiet, The Probability of Adequate Nutrient Intake score; PUFA, Poly0unsaturated Fatty Acids; SFA, Saturated Fatty Acids. * p < 0.05. [1] Linear regression model, adjusting for sex. [2] All the PANDiet component scores range from 0 to 1, where 1 represents a 100% probability that the intake is adequate according to a reference value. [3] Combined data from all four 24HR were used to calculate the overall PANDiet score and adequacy and moderation sub-scores, which ranged from 0 to 100. The higher the score or sub-scores, the better the nutrient adequacy of the diet.

4. Discussion

Using the PANDiet index, we have evaluated the diet quality and nutritional adequacy of 18-to−23-month-old Auckland children participating in the GUMLi Trial, according to GUMLi or CM consumption. This is the first study to use data from a randomised controlled trial to measure the impact of a dietary intervention, such as GUM on diet quality using a nutrient-based index, such as the PANDiet score. Total PANDiet scores were significantly higher in the GUMLi group, indicating better overall nutrient adequacy and diet quality. Nutrient intakes of children in both groups met recommendations for fat, total carbohydrates and most micronutrients; however, protein sodium, NMES, and SFA intakes exceeded recommendations. Whilst average total energy intakes were similar, the children consuming GUMLi had higher probabilities of having adequate intakes of vitamin C, vitamin D and iron, and were less likely to have insufficient intakes of vitamin D. Further analysis of food group consumption, adherence to dietary guidelines, or nutrient densities would elucidate whether the GUMLi intervention had an impact on dietary diversity, as an inverse relationship between dietary diversity and formula intake has previously been reported in 12- to 16-month-old Australian children [16].

4.1. Diet Quality and PANDiet Scores According to GUMLi or CM Allocation

GUM has been shown to improve intakes of iron, vitamin C, vitamin D, and PUFA's during the dietary transition from a milk-based intake to a 'family diet' in cross-sectional, observational studies [14–16,37]. The PANDiet has previously been evaluated in 12- to 18-month-old-children in the U.K. according to GUM or commercial infant foods (CIF) consumption [32]. Consuming GUM was associated with greater nutritional adequacy with a mean PANDiet score of 74.1 compared to children who did not consume GUM or CIF (difference of +7.2 points) [32]. A much smaller difference of +2.78 was observed in our sample, where consuming GUMLi was associated with greater nutritional adequacy. More recently, the difference in PANDiet scores for 'at risk children with Diabetic mothers' and 'not at risk' children in the BABYDIET study was similar at +2.4 points (65.9 and 68.3, respectively) [13].

It is important to note the effect of differences in national nutrient recommendations on PANDiet calculations and resultant scores. In the present study, the PANDiet score calculation was adjusted according to Australia and New Zealand NRVs where available [29], and if not, the reference values determined by Verger et al. [32] who used nutrient recommendations for UK children 12- to 36-months-of-age [34,35,38]. The greatest variation in recommendations were for selenium and folate, where the New Zealand NRVs are 1.7–2.4 times higher than the UK, (folate: 120 µg vs. 50 µg and selenium: 20 µg vs. 11.5 µg). The probability of adequate would be higher than the current calculation if we used the UK recommendations in our sub-score calculation. As all probabilities of adequacy are equally weighted, higher component scores will contribute to a higher total Adequacy sub-score and resultant PANDiet score [12].

In this population, the quality of both fat and carbohydrates are of concern. Children had low probabilities for avoiding excessive intakes for SFA ($\leq$0.10) and low probabilities for having adequate PUFA intakes (<0.20). An altered ratio of total and SFA has been described in two other studies, and is an important consideration, given the role of PUFA's in cognitive and visual development [37,39]. At each time point in the study, NMES exceeded the recommendations (>11% EI). Similar intakes were observed in a nationally representative sample of one- to four-year-old Irish children, where mean NMES intakes exceeded recommendations at 12% energy intake (EI) and increased with age [40].

4.2. Strengths and Limitations

The PANDiet provides an accurate measure of diet quality at an individual and population level through assessing global nutrient adequacy, and is strengthened by the use of a probabilistic calculation of nutrient adequacy, as previously described [12]. The index was designed to be as exhaustive as possible, and describes the role that different foods/food groups have in contributing to diet quality, at the nutrient level [12]. Our analysis is strengthened by the use of New Zealand NRVs to assess nutrient adequacy in the New Zealand context, however, because of this, cross-national comparisons of the PANDiet score are limited. Previous studies have used large, observational cohorts, where each subject has one PANDiet score calculated at a single time point, using multiple measures of dietary assessment [12,32,33]. For the present study, dietary data were collected on one day per month, over four months; therefore, month-to-month variation was considered in the PANDiet calculation. Using a record-assisted 24HR, allowed inclusion of children in the care of other adults (i.e., at day care), however, the reliance on parent and other adult-reported measures may lead to an increase in misreporting or social desirability bias. Mother's in our sample were older and highly educated, which may have affected total PANDiet scores. The ethnicity distribution in our sample was not considered representative of the Auckland population; therefore, no differences between ethnicities were evaluated. The validity of the PANDiet index was not evaluated for RCT data, therefore, further evaluation of the PANDiet in a larger, more representative cohort of New Zealand children under two is recommended to determine whether the PANDiet has predictive validity with respect to longitudinal health outcomes.

5. Conclusions

The consumption of GUMLi was associated with higher nutritional adequacy of the diets of children 18- to 23-months-of-age defined by PANDiet score, with increased likelihood of meeting nutrient requirements. However, consumption of GUMLi did not guarantee 100% nutrient adequacy. GUMLi consumers still had excessive protein intakes, but were more likely to have carbohydrate and SFA intakes that were in line with recommendations and improved iron and vitamin D intakes. Although GUMLi had a positive effect on index scores, consumption toward the latter half of the second year of life may not have the same impact as during early childhood as previously reported in younger children according to GUM consumption [32]. This may be because in the latter part of the second year of life, children are more likely to be following a family diet of varying quality, with a reduced reliance on fortified milks. Suggesting that other dietary strategies to promote a healthy diet through optimising nutrient intake could also result in more favourable dietary intake profiles, rather than solely concentrating on milk [41], however, further research is required on the consequences of consuming GUMLi on overall dietary diversity.

Supplementary Materials:
Table S1. PANDiet for Australian and New Zealand children aged from 18 to 23 months: components, reference values and inter-individual variability, Table S2. Nutritional composition of CM and GUMLi per 100 mL of prepared product, Table S3. Characteristics of the Auckland cohort included versus excluded in the PANDiet analysis, Table S4. Nutrient intake among Auckland children ($N = 83$) from 18 to 23 months of age (month 7–11 post randomisation)

Author Contributions: Conceptualisation: C.R.W. and C.C.G.; methodology: A.L.L. and C.R.W.; formal analysis: Y.J. and R.X.C.; data curation: A.L.L. and T.M.; writing—original draft preparation: A.L.L.; writing—review and editing: A.L.L., C.R.W., and C.C.G.; project administration: A.L.L. and T.M.; funding acquisition: C.R.W. and C.C.G.

Acknowledgments: The authors thank E.O. Verger for his assistance in calculating and interpreting the PANDiet index.

References

1. Northstone, K.; Emmett, P.M. Are dietary patterns stable throughout early and mid-childhood? A birth cohort study. *Br. J. Nutr.* **2008**, *100*, 1069–1076. [CrossRef] [PubMed]
2. Morgan, J. Nutrition for toddlers: The foundation for good health—2. Current problems and ways to overcome them. *J. Fam. Health Care* **2005**, *15*, 85–88. [PubMed]
3. Golley, R.K.; Hendrie, G.A.; McNaughton, S.A. Scores on the Dietary Guideline Index for Children and Adolescents Are Associated with Nutrient Intake and Socio-Economic Position but Not Adiposity—3. *J. Nutr.* **2011**, *141*, 1340–1347. [CrossRef] [PubMed]
4. Ruel, M.T.; Menon, P. Child feeding practices are associated with child nutritional status in Latin America: Innovative uses of the demographic and health surveys. *J. Nutr.* **2002**, *132*, 1180–1187. [CrossRef] [PubMed]
5. Kant, A.K. Indexes of overall diet quality: A review. *J. Am. Diet. Assoc.* **1996**, *96*, 785–791. [CrossRef]
6. Marshall, S.; Burrows, T.; Collins, C.E. Systematic review of diet quality indices and their associations with health-related outcomes in children and adolescents. *J. Hum. Nutr. Diet.* **2014**, *27*, 577–598. [CrossRef]
7. Wirt, A.; Collins, C.E. Diet quality—What is it and does it matter? *Public Health Nutr.* **2009**, *12*, 2473–2492. [CrossRef]
8. Waijers, P.M.; Feskens, E.J.; Ocké, M.C. A critical review of predefined diet quality scores. *Br. J. Nutr.* **2007**, *97*, 219–231. [CrossRef]

9. Hu, F.B. Dietary pattern analysis: A new direction in nutritional epidemiology. *Curr. Opin. Lipidol.* **2002**, *13*, 3–9. [CrossRef]

10. Lazarou, C.; Newby, P.K. Use of dietary indexes among children in developed countries. *Adv. Nutr.* **2011**, *2*, 295–303. [CrossRef]

11. Smithers, L.G.; Golley, R.K.; Brazionis, L.; Emmett, P.; Northstone, K.; Lynch, J.W. Dietary patterns of infants and toddlers are associated with nutrient intakes. *Nutrients* **2012**, *4*, 935–948. [CrossRef] [PubMed]

12. Verger, E.O.; Mariotti, F.; Holmes, B.A.; Paineau, D.; Huneau, J. Evaluation of a diet quality index based on the probability of adequate nutrient intake (PANDiet) using national French and US dietary surveys. *PLoS ONE* **2012**, *7*, e42155. [CrossRef] [PubMed]

13. Schoen, S.; Jergens, S.; Barbaresko, J.; Nöthlings, U.; Kersting, M.; Remer, T.; Stelmach-Mardas, M.; Ziegler, A.G.; Hummel, S. Diet quality during infancy and early childhood in children with and without risk of type 1 diabetes: A DEDIPAC study. *Nutrients* **2017**, *9*, 48. [CrossRef] [PubMed]

14. Ghisolfi, J.; Fantino, M.; Turck, D.; de Courcy, G.P.; Vidailhet, M. Nutrient intakes of children aged 1–2 years as a function of milk consumption, cows' milk or growing-up milk. *Public Health Nutr.* **2013**, *16*, 524–534. [CrossRef]

15. Walton, J.; Flynn, A. Nutritional adequacy of diets containing growing up milks or unfortified cow's milk in Irish children (aged 12–24 months). *Food Nutr. Res.* **2013**, *57*, 21836. [CrossRef] [PubMed]

16. Byrne, R.; Magarey, A.; Daniels, L. Food and beverage intake in Australian children aged 12–16 months participating in the NOURISH and SAIDI studies. *Aust. N. Z. J. Public Health* **2014**, *38*, 326–331. [CrossRef] [PubMed]

17. Vandenplas, Y.; De Ronne, N.; Van De Sompel, A.; Huysentruyt, K.; Robert, M.; Rigo, J.; Scheers, I.; Brasseur, D.; Goyens, P. A Belgian consensus-statement on growing-up milks for children 12–36 months old. *Eur. J. Pediatr.* **2014**, *173*, 1365–1371. [CrossRef]

18. Eussen, S.R.; Pean, J.; Olivier, L.; Delaere, F.; Lluch, A. Theoretical impact of replacing whole cow's milk by young-child formula on nutrient intakes of UK young children: Results of a simulation study. *Ann. Nutr. Metab.* **2015**, *67*, 247–256. [CrossRef] [PubMed]

19. Wall, C.R.; Hill, R.J.; Lovell, A.L.; Matsuyama, M.; Milne, T.; Grant, C.C. A Multi-Centre, Double Blind, Randomised, Placebo Controlled Trial to Evaluate the Effect of Consuming Growing Up Milk. 'Lite' on Body Composition in Children Aged 12–23 Months. Available online: https://www.anzctr.org.au/Trial/Registration/TrialReview.aspx?id=366785 (accessed on 29 December 2018).

20. Blanton, C.A.; Moshfegh, A.J.; Baer, D.J.; Kretsch, M.J. The USDA Automated Multiple-Pass Method accurately estimates group total energy and nutrient intake. *J. Nutr.* **2006**, *136*, 2594–2599. [CrossRef]

21. Watson, P. *Development & Pretesting of Methodologies for the Children's Nutrition Survey: Validation Report: A Report to the Ministry of Health. Report Three*; Institute of Food, Nutrition and Human Health, Massey University: Palmerston North, NZ, USA, 2003.

22. Coblac, L.; Bowen, J.; Burnett, J.; Syrette, J.; Dempsey, J.; Balle, S.; Wilson, C.; Flight, I.; Good, N.; Saunders, I. *Australian National Children's Nutrition and Physical Activity Survey: Main Findings*; Australian Bureau of Statistics: Canberra, Australia, 2008.

23. User Guide. *Australian National Children's Nutrition and Physical Activity Survey*; Commonwealth Scientific Industrial Research Organisation: Canberra, Australia, 2010.

24. Briefel, R.R.; Reidy, K.; Karwe, V.; Devaney, B. Feeding infants and toddlers study: Improvements needed in meeting infant feeding recommendations. *J. Am. Diet. Assoc.* **2004**, *104* (Suppl. 1), 31. [CrossRef]

25. Devaney, B.; Kalb, L.; Briefel, R.; Zavitsky-Novak, T.; Clusen, N.; Ziegler, P. Feeding infants and toddlers study: Overview of the study design. *J. Am. Diet. Assoc.* **2004**, *104* (Suppl. 1), 8. [CrossRef] [PubMed]

26. Emmett, P.; North, K.; Noble, S. Types of drinks consumed by infants at 4 and 8 months of age: A descriptive study. *Public Health Nutr.* **2000**, *3*, 211–217. [CrossRef] [PubMed]

27. Lennox, A.; Sommerville, J.; Ong, K.; Henderson, H.; Allen, R. *Diet and Nutrition Survey of Infants and Young Children*; Department of Health and Food Standards Agency: London, UK, 2013.

28. Institute for Plant & Food Research Limited, Ministry of Health. *New Zealand Food composition Database: New Zealand FOODfiles*; Institute for Plant & Food Research Limited, Ministry of Health: Wellington, New Zealand, 2016.

29.   National Health and Medical Research Council. *Nutrient Reference Values for Australia and New Zealand Including Recommended Dietary Intakes*; National Health and Medical Research Council: Canberra, Australia, 2006.

30.   Carriquiry, A.L. Assessing the prevalence of nutrient inadequacy. *Public Health Nutr.* **1999**, *2*, 23–34. [CrossRef] [PubMed]

31.   Institute of Medicine. *Dietary Reference Itakes for Calcium and Vitamin, D*; Institute of Medicine: Washington, DC, USA, 2011.

32.   Verger, E.O.; Eussen, S.; Holmes, B.A. Evaluation of a nutrient-based diet quality index in UK young children and investigation into the diet quality of consumers of formula and infant foods. *Public Health Nutr.* **2016**, *19*, 1785–1794. [CrossRef] [PubMed]

33.   Verger, E.O.; Eussen, S.; Holmes, B.A. Diet quality and nutritional adequacy of young children in the UK according to their consumption of young child formula and commercial infant food. *Proc. Nutr. Soc.* **2015**, *74*, E250. [CrossRef]

34.   Agostoni, C.V.; Berni Canani, R.; Fairweather Tait, S.; Heinonen, M.; Korhonen, H.; La Vieille, S.; Marchelli, R.; Martin, A.; Naska, A.; Neuhäuser Berthold, M.; et al. Scientific Opinion on nutrient requirements and dietary intakes of infants and young children in the European Union: EFSA Panel on Dietetic Products, Nutrition and Allergies (NDA). *EFSA J.* **2013**, *11*, 1–103.

35.   Nordic Council of Ministers. *Nordic Nutrition Recommendations 2012: Integrating Nutrition and Physical Activity*; Nordic Council of Ministers: Copenhagen, Denmark, 2014.

36.   Institute of Medicine (US); Panel on Macronutrients, Institute of Medicine (US). *Standing Committee on the Scientific Evaluation of Dietary Reference Intakes. Dietary Reference Intakes for Energy, Carbohydrate, Fiber, Fat, Fatty Acids, Cholesterol, Protein, and Amino Acids*; Institute of Medicine: Washington, DC, USA, 2005.

37.   Hilbig, A.; Drossard, C.; Kersting, M.; Alexy, U. Nutrient adequacy and associated factors in a nationwide sample of German toddlers. *J. Pediatr. Gastroenterol. Nutr.* **2015**, *61*, 130–137. [CrossRef] [PubMed]

38.   Panel on Dietary Reference Values of the Committee on Medical Aspects of Food Policy. *Dietary Reference Values for Food Energy and Nutrients for the United Kingdom: Report of the Panel on Dietary Reference Values of the committee On Medical Aspects of Food Policy*; HM Stationery Office: Richmond, UK, 1991.

39.   Butte, N.F.; Fox, M.K.; Briefel, R.R.; Siega-Riz, A.M.; Dwyer, J.T.; Deming, D.M.; Reidy, K.C. Nutrient intakes of US infants, toddlers, and preschoolers meet or exceed dietary reference intakes. *J. Am. Diet. Assoc.* **2010**, *110*, S37. [CrossRef] [PubMed]

40.   Walton, J.; Kehoe, L.; McNulty, B.A.; Nugent, A.P.; Flynn, A. Nutrient intakes and compliance with nutrient recommendations in children aged 1–4 years in Ireland. *J. Hum. Nutr. Diet.* **2017**, *30*, 665–676. [CrossRef] [PubMed]

41.   Hojsak, I.; Bronsky, J.; Campoy, C.; Domellöf, M.; Embleton, N.; Fidler Mis, N.; Hulst, J.; Indrio, F.; Lapillonne, A.; Mølgaard, C.; et al. Young Child Formula: A Position Paper by the ESPGHAN Committee on Nutrition. *J. Pediatr. Gastroenterol. Nutr.* **2018**, *66*, 177–185. [CrossRef] [PubMed]

12

Different Socio-Demographic and Lifestyle Factors can Determine the Dietary Supplement Use in Children and Adolescents in Central-Eastern Poland

Ewa Sicińska *, Barbara Pietruszka, Olga Januszko and Joanna Kałuża

Department of Human Nutrition, Faculty of Human Nutrition and Consumer Sciences, Warsaw University of Life Sciences (WULS—SGGW), 159c Nowoursynowska str., 02-776 Warsaw, Poland; barbara_pietruszka@sggw.pl (B.P.); olga_januszko@sggw.pl (O.J.); joanna_kaluza@sggw.pl (J.K.)
* Correspondence: ewa_sicinska@sggw.pl

Abstract: Vitamin/mineral supplement (VMS) use has become increasingly popular in children and adolescents; however, different predictors may be associated with their usage. Therefore, the aim of this study was to compare determinants of VMS use in 1578 children and adolescents. Data was collected among parents of children ($\leq$12 years old) and among adolescents (>12 years old) who attended public schools by a self-administered questionnaire. Multivariate-adjusted logistic regression models were used to estimate odds ratios (ORs) and 95% confidence intervals (95% CIs) for determining the predictors of VMS use. In children, the following determinants of VMS use were indicated: socioeconomic status (average vs. very good/good; OR: 1.69, 95% CI: 1.16–2.48), physical activity (1–5 vs. <1 h/week; OR: 1.44, 95% CI: 1.02–2.04), BMI ($\geq$25 vs. 18.5–24.9 kg/m^2; OR: 0.67, 95% CI: 0.46–0.98), and presence of chronic diseases (yes vs. no; OR: 2.32, 95% CI: 1.46–3.69). In adolescents, gender (male vs. female; OR: 0.56, 95% CI: 0.37–0.87), residential area (rural vs. urban; OR: 0.63, 95% CI: 0.40–0.99), BMI (<18.5 vs. 18.5–24.9 kg/m^2; OR: 0.35, 95% CI: 0.17–0.73), and health status (average/poor vs. at least good; OR: 1.96, 95% CI: 1.13–3.39) were factors of VMS use. In both groups, the mother's higher educational level, fortified food consumption and diet modification towards better food choices were predictors of VMS use. In conclusion, most of the predictors of VMS use were different in children and adolescents.

Keywords: adolescents; children; determinants; dietary supplements; food choice

---

1. Introduction

Dietary supplement use, especially containing vitamin/mineral supplements (VMSs), has become increasingly popular in developed countries. About half of the US adult population [1] and more than 30% of children and adolescences (<18 years old) [2] are users of these products. In Europe, depending on the country and gender, supplement use ranges from 2% to 66% in adults [3], and from 16% to 45% in children and adolescents in England, Scotland, Germany, Slovenia, and Finland [4–6]. Evidence of the benefits of using VMSs among those who eat properly are insufficient and conflicting [7]; studies have shown that the use of VMSs is usually associated with better dietary habits; however, knowledge on using supplements by adults as well as children and adolescents is insufficient [8,9]. Socio-demographic and lifestyle factors like age, sex, income, education level, health status, or physical activity may associate with dietary supplement usage [8]. Surveys on the determinants of VMS use focus mostly on adults [8], while the number of studies conducted in children (aged 2–10) [10,11] and adolescents (aged 11–19) [5,12,13] is limited, and often combine both age groups together [2,14–18]. Moreover, most of them were carried out in the US population [2,11–16]. Taking into the consideration that, in the case of children, parents decide whether to give a child a dietary supplement, while adolescents often make this decision by themselves based on advertisements, peers' or coach' recommendation [6], factors which determine the usage of dietary supplements may be different in both groups. The aim of the study was to compare socio-demographic and lifestyle determinants of VMS use in school children and adolescents in Central-Eastern Poland.

2. Materials and Methods

2.1. Study Design

The cross-sectional study was conducted in school students who attended public primary and secondary schools. The schools were selected randomly in Central-Eastern Poland based on a list of public schools in this area. The survey was conducted only in those schools of which headmasters gave consent to it. The following inclusion criteria of the students participating in the study were used: attendance to a public primary or secondary school in Central-Eastern Poland and the age of participants from 5–20 years. The exclusion criteria constituted: occurrence of a disease requiring a special diet, pregnancy or lactation (it concerned adolescents only) and incorrectly or incompletely filling in a health and lifestyle questionnaire.

The survey was conducted in accordance with the guidelines laid down by the Declaration of Helsinki. The study design and protocol were approved by the Department of Human Nutrition, Warsaw University of Life Sciences (WULS-SGGW), Poland.

2.2. Study Population and Data Collection

For the study 1200 parents of children (age 5–12 years) and 1200 adolescents (age 13–20 years) were invited to participate (Figure 1). The data was collected using the health and lifestyle questionnaire, which was distributed to parents at school meetings and to adolescents during classroom sessions. Completed questionnaires were verified by trained interviewers. A total of 1624 respondents returned the questionnaires (67.7%); however, due to incorrectly or incompletely filled in questionnaires, 46 were excluded. Finally, 1578 school students were included in the study. By completing the questionnaire, the respondents agreed to participate in the study.

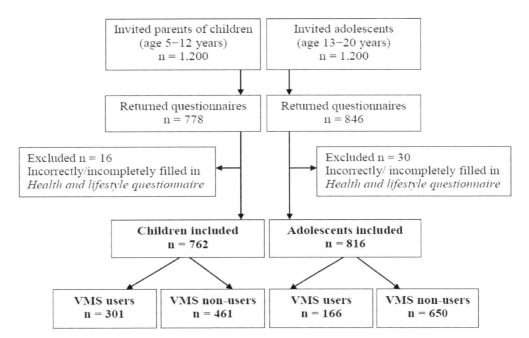

Figure 1. Flow chart of the study population. VMS: vitamin/mineral supplements. Notes: cream colour indicates study groups.

The questionnaire contained 27 questions and was composed of the following sections: socio-demographic characteristics (age, gender, place of living, mother's educational level, economic status of family); health and lifestyle status (health status, occurrence of chronic diseases, use and type of special diet, type and time spent on being physically active); eating habits (number of meals/day consumed habitually, regularity of main meal consumption, diet modification); dietary supplement usage; and voluntarily fortified foods usage. Self-reported height and weight of participants were collected and used to calculate the Body Mass Index (BMI) [19,20]. Details of the study methods have been enumerated elsewhere [21]. The questionnaire was developed and verified in an earlier study among students at the Department of Human Nutrition, WULS-SGGW, Poland [22,23].

2.3. Assessment of VMS Use

The respondents were asked about VMS taken during the year before the study as well as on the test day, about the name, and brand of dietary supplements, the usage form (i.e., pills, powder, drops etc.), and the period of application. As supplement users were considered those participants who used one or more VMSs over the 12 months before the survey. The study included short-term VMS users (from at least seven consecutive days to less than one month), medium-term users (1–3 months) and long-term users (>3 months). VMSs were categorised into: single vitamin; single mineral; multivitamin and/or mineral(s); and multicomponent supplement containing vitamin(s) and/or mineral(s) plus other ingredients including herbs or other.

When the respondents have declared VMS use, they were asked to give the reason for including these products in the diet by marking one or more predefined reasons: "Respondent's diet is poor in nutrients", "VMSs improve overall health", "VMSs are necessary when medicines are used", "VMSs were recommended by a physician", as well as they could list their own reason. When the respondents have declared not using VMSs, they were asked about the reason by marking one or more of the following statements: "Lack of effect on health improvement", "No need to use such products because of proper nutrition", "The use of VMSs can be harmful", "VMSs are too expensive", as well as they could list their own reason.

2.4. Statistical Analysis

All results were presented separately for children (≤12 years) and adolescents (>12 years). The statistically significant differences between categorical variables and VMS usage were determined using the Chi-square test. To examine the associations between VMS usage and parameters that might constitute the determinants of VMS use, the univariate (crude data) as well as multivariate-adjusted odds ratios (ORs) with 95% confidence intervals (95% CIs) were calculated using logistic regression models. The Hosmer-Lemeshow criterion was used to evaluate the models' goodness-of-fit.

The multivariate-adjusted models included potential determinants of VMS usage, i.e., age (continuous variable, years), gender (female or male), residential area (urban or rural), mother's education level (primary, high school, or university), socioeconomic status (very good/good, average, or poor), time spent on being physically active (<1, 1–5, or ≥6 h/week; not including gymnastic classes in school), BMI (<18.5, 18.5–24.9, or ≥25 kg/m^2), self-reported health status (at least good, or average or poor), presence of chronic diseases (no or yes), using a special diet (no or yes), number of meals consumed per day (≤3, 4, or ≥5), consumption of fortified foods (no or yes), and intentional diet modification towards better food choices (lack of modification, excluding or including some food products, or simultaneously excluding and including some food products). Supplement non-users were the referent category for the logistic regression models. Missing data on socio-demographic and lifestyle determinants were modelled as separate categories. The statistical analyses were performed using SPSS version 23.0, and p-values ≤ 0.05 were considered statistically significant.

3. Results

3.1. Characteristics of the Study Population

Over the past 12 months, 29.6% of participants used VMSs, while 15.1% used VMSs on the test day. A statistically significantly higher number of children (mean age 8.6 ± 1.4 years) compared to adolescents (mean age 17.1 ± 2.1 years) used these products during the last year (39.5% vs. 20.3%, respectively; p-value < 0.001). In both groups, significantly more mothers of VMS users compared to non-users had a university education (Table S1). Compared to non-users, children classified as supplement users spent more time on being physically active and suffered from chronic diseases; the same tendencies were observed in adolescents. In both groups, VMS users vs. non-users declared the consumption of fortified foods more frequently, as well as modified their diet towards better food choices by intentionally including (e.g., vegetables, fruits) or/and excluding (e.g., sweets, crisps) some foods. It was observed that significantly more children who were VMS non-users than users were overweight or obese (BMI $\geq$ 25 kg/m^2; 33.1% vs. 23.6%, respectively); in contrast, in adolescents, more VMS non-users than users were underweight (BMI < 18.5 kg/m^2; 14.4% vs. 6.0%, respectively). A description of selected factors associated with the dietary supplement use by a part of the younger respondents, i.e., group of children aged 6–12, was also presented elsewhere [24].

3.2. Types and Duration of VMS Use and Reason for Using/Non-Using

In both groups, the most frequently used type of VMSs were multicomponent supplements containing multivitamin and/or mineral supplements with or without other ingredients, while single vitamin and single mineral were used less commonly (Table 1). As the main reasons for VMS use, parents of children and adolescents pointed out improving overall health, diet poor in nutrients, and physician recommendations. VMS non-users indicated that they did not need them because of proper nutrition. Moreover, parents of children more often than adolescents indicated as a reason not to use VMS a lack of effect on health improvement, harmful impact on health and too high of a price.

The distribution of children and adolescents using specific nutrients with vitamin/mineral supplements (VMSs) stratified by duration of use are presented in Table 2. Compared to adolescents, the number of children using vitamin supplements (A, E, D, C, B$_1$, B$_2$, niacin, B$_6$, folic acid, B$_{12}$, biotin, and pantothenic acid) was statistically significantly higher, whereas magnesium and iron supplements were consumed by a significantly lower number of children. Amongst children and adolescents, the largest number of respondents used vitamin C supplements (83.7% and 65.7%, respectively). The majority of respondents were classified as medium-term VMS users (45.8%), followed by short-term users (31.5%) and lastly long-term users (22.7%). Generally, more adolescents than children were classified as medium-term users of specific nutrients with VMSs, while children respondents were more often classified as short-term and long-term users with statistically significant differences found for vitamins C, B$_1$, B$_2$, niacin, B$_6$, B$_{12}$, and zinc.

3.3. Determinants of VMS Use in Children and Adolescents

Multivariate-adjusted odds ratios (ORs) of VMS use by socio-demographic and lifestyle factors in children and adolescents are presented in Table 3. There was found an association between mother's education level and usage of supplements in children. Compared to children of mothers with primary education, those whose mothers had high school or university education had a higher probability of dietary supplement use (OR: 2.17, 95% CI: 1.17–4.01 and OR: 2.16, 95% CI: 1.14–4.07, respectively). In comparison to respondents who assessed a familiar socioeconomic status as very good or good, children living in families with an average socioeconomic status had significantly higher odds ratios of VMS use (OR: 1.69, 95% CI: 1.16–2.48). Respondents who spent 1 to 5 h/week on being physically active (not including gymnastic classes at school) were 1.44-fold (95% CI: 1.02–2.04) more likely to be VMS users than those being physically active <1 h/week. Moreover, overweight and obese children (BMI $\geq$ 25 kg/m^2) were less likely to be supplement users (OR: 0.67, 95% CI: 0.46–0.98) than those with a normal BMI range (18.5–24.9 kg/m^2). An inverse statistically significant trend between BMI and usage of VMSs was observed, each 1 kg/m^2 increment in BMI was associated with a 7% (95% CI: 2–12%; p-trend = 0.008) lower probability of VMS use. Moreover, children who suffer from chronic diseases were more likely to be supplement users (OR: 2.32, 95% CI: 1.46–3.69) than those without chronic diseases. The prevalence of VMS usage was 3.79-fold (95% CI: 2.54–5.63) higher among those who were fortified product consumers vs. non-consumers. Children who intentionally modified their diet by including or excluding some food products had a 1.60-fold (95% CI: 1.01–2.53) higher probability of usage of VMS and those who simultaneously included and excluded food products had a 2.22-fold (95% CI: 1.29–3.81) higher probability of usage of VMS compared to non-consumers.

Table 1. Prevalence of specific types of vitamin/mineral supplement (VMS) use and reasons for using or non-using them by children (n = 762) and adolescents (n = 816).

Parameters	Children ≤12 years	Adolescents >12 years
	Users [a]	Users [a]
	n = 301 %	n = 166 %
Type of VMS		
Single vitamin	20.2	25.9
Single mineral [b]	4.3	16.9
Multivitamin and/or mineral(s)	39.9	33.1
Vitamin(s)/mineral(s) + other ingredient [b]	72.1	42.8
Usage more than one VMS	13.3	12.0
Reason for using VMSs [c]		
Improve overall health	77.4	76.5
Diet poor in nutrients [b]	45.2	20.5
Physician recommendation [b]	32.2	26.5
Necessary when medicines are used [b]	10.6	4.8
Other	15.0	9.0
	Non-users	Non-users
	n = 461 %	n = 650 %
Reason for avoidance VMSs [c]		
No need to use because of proper nutrition [b]	62.3	44.2
Lack effect on health improvement [b]	24.7	7.8
It can be harmful [b]	22.3	7.2
Too high price [b]	20.8	13.1
Other [c]	9.1	3.4

[a] supplement user—a person who used one or more VMSs over the 12 months before the survey; [b] a statistically significant difference between the group of children and adolescents; chi-square test, p-value < 0.05; [c] each respondent could select one or more answers.

Table 2. The distribution of respondents using specific nutrients with vitamin/mineral supplements (VMSs) stratified by duration of use (n = 467).

VMS Using		n (%) *	p-value	Short-Term Users 7 days–<1 month n = 147 % **	Medium-Term Users 1–3 months n = 214 % **	Long-Term Users >3 months n = 106 % **	p-value
Total [b,c]	children	301 (100)	0.012	29.9	43.9	26.2	0.048
	adolescents	166 (100)		34.3	49.4	16.3	
Vitamin A	children	215 (71.4)	<0.001	22.3	48.4	29.3	0.131
	adolescents	50 (30.1)		14.0	64.0	22.0	
Vitamin E	children	192 (63.8)	<0.001	26.0	47.4	26.6	0.236
	adolescents	51 (30.7)		19.6	60.8	19.6	
Vitamin D	children	217 (72.1)	<0.001	22.6	47.9	29.5	0.279
	adolescents	46 (27.7)		13.0	58.7	28.3	
Vitamin C [c]	children	252 (83.7)	<0.001	30.5	43.3	26.2	0.049
	adolescents	109 (65.7)		29.4	55.0	15.6	
Vitamin B$_1$ [a,c]	children	174 (57.8)	<0.001	24.1	46.0	29.9	0.010
	adolescents	40 (24.1)		12.5	72.5	15.0	
Vitamin B$_2$ [a,c]	children	189 (62.8)	<0.001	27.5	44.4	28.1	0.021
	adolescents	41 (24.7)		17.1	68.3	14.6	
Niacin [a]	children	197 (65.4)	<0.001	25.4	46.7	27.9	0.041
	adolescents	41 (24.7)		14.6	68.3	17.1	
Vitamin B$_6$ [a,c]	children	202 (67.1)	<0.001	26.7	46.6	26.7	0.003
	adolescents	55 (33.1)		12.7	72.7	14.6	

Table 2. *Cont.*

VMS Using		n (%) *	p-value	Short-Term Users 7 days–<1 month n = 147 % **	Medium-Term Users 1–3 months n = 214 % **	Long-Term Users >3 months n = 106 % **	p-value
Folic acid	children	138 (45.8)	<0.001	19.6	50.0	30.4	0.064
	adolescents	41 (24.7)		12.2	70.7	17.1	
Vitamin B$_{12}$ [a,c]	children	167 (55.5)	<0.001	22.8	47.3	29.9	0.016
	adolescents	40 (24.1)		12.5	72.5	15.0	
Biotin	children	127 (42.2)	<0.001	18.9	52.8	28.3	0.328
	adolescents	28 (16.9)		10.7	67.9	21.4	
Pantothenic acid	children	135 (44.9)	<0.001	25.9	48.2	25.9	0.061
	adolescents	39 (23.5)		12.8	69.2	18.0	
Calcium	children	76 (25.2)	0.900	18.4	55.3	26.3	0.828
	adolescents	41 (24.7)		21.9	56.2	21.9	
Magnesium	children	27 (9.0)	<0.001	29.6	48.1	22.3	0.532
	adolescents	44 (26.5)		18.2	56.8	25.0	
Iron	children	35 (11.6)	0.010	22.9	51.4	25.7	0.616
	adolescents	34 (20.5)		14.7	61.8	23.5	
Zinc [a,c]	children	87 (28.9)	0.210	23.0	41.4	35.6	0.015
	adolescents	39 (23.5)		12.8	69.2	18.0	

p-value was determined using the chi-square test; different letters in superscript indicate statistically significant differences between: [a] short-term and medium-term users, [b] short-term and long-term users, [c] medium-term and long-term users; * the percentage of subjects using specific nutrients was given in relation to total VMS users in children (*n* = 301) and adolescents (*n* = 166); ** percentages were calculated in relation to children or adolescents who used supplements containing specific nutrients (percentages are summarized in rows).

Table 3. Logistic regression of vitamin/mineral supplement (VMS) use by socio-demographic and lifestyle determinants in school children and adolescents.

Study Factors	Children ≤12 years (n = 762)		Adolescents >12 years (n = 816)	
	Crude	Multivariate-Adjusted	Crude	Multivariate-Adjusted
	OR (95% CI)	OR (95% CI)	OR (95% CI)	OR (95% CI)
Age (years)	0.96 (0.87–1.06)	1.01 (0.90–1.14)	0.93 (0.86–1.01)	1.15 (0.95–1.39)
P for trend	0.39	0.86	0.09	0.15
Gender				
Female	1.00	1.00	1.00	1.00
Male	0.96 (0.72–1.28)	0.94 (0.68–1.30)	0.75 (0.51–1.09)	**0.56 (0.37–0.87)**
Residential area				
Urban	1.00	1.00	1.00	1.00
Rural	1.04 (0.70–1.57)	1.43 (0.88–2.35)	0.94 (0.67–1.33)	**0.63 (0.40–0.99)**
Mother's education level				
Primary	1.00	1.00	1.00	1.00
High school	1.87 (1.10–3.18)	**2.17 (1.17–4.01)**	2.10 (0.92–4.78)	2.02 (0.85–4.79)
University	2.05 (1.23–3.40)	**2.16 (1.14–4.07)**	6.07 (2.20–16.8)	**5.19 (1.72–15.6)**
Socioeconomic status				
Very good or good	1.00	1.00	1.00	1.00
Average	1.38 (0.99–1.91)	**1.69 (1.16–2.48)**	0.76 (0.52–1.11)	0.75 (0.49–1.15)
Poor	0.64 (0.32–1.32)	1.12 (0.49–2.54)	0.59 (0.33–1.04)	0.83 (0.44–1.56)
Physical activity (h/week)				
<1	1.00	1.00	1.00	1.00
1–5	1.72 (1.26–2.36)	**1.44 (1.02–2.04)**	1.52 (1.07–2.17)	1.26 (0.85–1.86)
≥6	1.35 (0.76–2.41)	1.21 (0.63–2.32)	1.10 (0.49–2.48)	0.87 (0.36–2.13)
Body Mass Index (kg/m^2)				
<18.5	0.99 (0.64–1.52)	1.10 (0.69–1.76)	0.39 (0.20–0.77)	**0.35 (0.17–0.73)**
18.5–24.9	1.00	1.00	1.00	1.00
≥25	**0.62 (0.44–0.88)**	**0.67 (0.46–0.98)**	1.14 (0.71–1.84)	0.99 (0.58–1.70)
P for trend	0.003	0.008	0.19	0.22

Table 3. *Cont.*

Study Factors	Children ≤12 years (n = 762)		Adolescents >12 years (n = 816)	
	Crude	Multivariate-Adjusted	Crude	Multivariate-Adjusted
	OR (95% CI)	OR (95% CI)	OR (95% CI)	OR (95% CI)
Health status				
At least good	1.00	1.00	1.00	1.00
Average or poor	0.70 (0.37–1.32)	0.56 (0.27–1.17)	1.41 (0.89–2.24)	**1.96 (1.13–3.39)**
Current chronic diseases				
No	1.00	1.00	1.00	1.00
Yes	2.24 (1.52–3.31)	**2.32 (1.46–3.69)**	1.90 (0.99–3.68)	1.27 (0.61–2.66)
Special diet				
No	1.00	1.00	1.00	1.00
Yes	1.58 (0.88–2.83)	0.82 (0.40–1.66)	1.57 (0.96–2.58)	1.02 (0.56–1.85)
Number of meals/day				
≤3	1.00	1.00	1.00	1.00
4	1.38 (0.86–2.20)	1.16 (0.69–1.96)	1.52 (1.04–2.22)	1.46 (0.95–2.25)
≥5	1.82 (1.09–3.01)	1.68 (0.96–2.95)	1.47 (0.90–2.41)	1.51 (0.86–2.65)
Fortified food consumption				
No	1.00	1.00	1.00	1.00
Yes	3.39 (2.35–4.89)	**3.79 (2.54–5.63)**	3.12 (2.04–4.77)	**2.54 (1.62–4.00)**
Diet modification				
Lack of modification	1.00	1.00	1.00	1.00
Excluding or including some foods	1.76 (1.17–2.64)	**1.60 (1.01–2.53)**	2.36 (1.51–3.70)	**2.09 (1.24–3.52)**
Simultaneously excluding and including some foods	2.95 (1.83–4.75)	**2.22 (1.29–3.81)**	3.00 (1.85–4.87)	**3.02 (1.71–5.35)**

Supplement user—a person who used one or more VMSs over the 12 months before the survey. Notes: bold font indicates the statistical significant results in the multivariate-adjusted analysis.

Compared to children, in adolescents, some different factors like gender or residential area were associated with VMS usage; however, some of them, like mother's education level, fortified food consumption, or diet modification towards better food choices, were overlapped with those determined for children (Table 3). VMS users vs. non-users were less likely to be male (OR: 0.56, 95% CI: 0.37–0.87) and live in rural areas (OR: 0.63, 95% CI: 0.40–0.99). In comparison to adolescents whose mothers had primary education, those with university mothers' education had a higher probability of VMS use (OR: 5.19, 95% CI: 1.72–15.6). Adolescent who were underweight (BMI < 18.5 kg/m^2) were less likely to be supplement users (OR: 0.35, 95% CI: 0.17–0.73) than those with a normal BMI (18.5–24.9 kg/m^2). In contrast to children, each 1 kg/m^2 increment in BMI was associated with a non-significant 4% (95% CI: −2–10%; p-trend = 0.22) higher probability of VMS usage. It was found that adolescents who declared average or poor health status vs. those who declared at least a good health status were more likely to be supplement users (OR: 1.96, 95% CI: 1.13–3.39). Moreover, the prevalence of VMS use was 2.54-fold (95% CI: 1.62–4.00) higher among those who were fortified food consumers vs. non-consumers; 2.09-fold (95% CI: 1.24–3.52) higher among those who intentionally included or excluded some food products; and 3.02-fold (95% CI: 1.71–5.35) higher among those who simultaneously included and excluded some food products vs. those who not modified their diet.

4. Discussion

The study showed that the majority of significant predictors of VMS use were different in children and adolescents. In children, socioeconomic status, physical activity level, BMI, and presence of chronic disease were determinants of dietary supplement use; while in adolescents, it was gender, residential area, BMI (in opposite trend compared to children), and health status. Notwithstanding, some determinants such as higher mothers' education, consumption of fortified foods, and declaration of diet modifications overlapped in both groups.

In our study, a significantly higher number of children (39.5%) compared to adolescents (20.3%) used VMSs. Similarly, in the National Health Interview Survey 2007 [2] and the National Health and Nutrition Examination Survey (NHANES) 1999–2004 [16], these products were used by more children (aged 5–11) (38.9% and 37.4%, respectively) than adolescents (12–17 years) (23.0% and 26.6%, respectively).

A higher family income was associated with a higher use of dietary supplement in studies conducted among American children and adolescent [2,10,15,16,18]. In our study, children with an average socioeconomic status compared with those with very good/good socioeconomic status had a higher probability of VMS use; however, our study was based on a self-assessment of socioeconomic status, not on exact income, which was reported in other surveys [2,10,15,18].

A higher level of parents' education was associated with an increased probability of supplement use in both examined groups. Similar observations have been reported from studies conducted in the US children and adolescent populations [2,10]. It could be explained by the increased awareness of a healthy lifestyle in people with higher education and by the fact that supplement usage is commonly considered as a pro-healthy behaviour. In fact, dietary supplements are not routinely recommended for children and adolescents who consume a varied diet. NHANES 2003–2006 results suggested that it is a controversial strategy to improve nutrient intakes [25]. Furthermore, the results of some studies indicate that unjustified supplementation may increase the total mortality risk in the population as well as incidence of specific diseases [7,26,27]. However, for certain groups, for example, children with nutritional deficiencies (e.g., vitamin D supplementation during low sunlight exposure), malabsorption or obese children in weight loss programs, VMS use could be recommended [28].

In this study, children who spent 1–5 h per week compared to those who spent <1 h/week of free time being physically active (swimming, playing football, dancing, playing tennis or other sports) had a higher probability of VMS use. Similarly, in studies conducted among American children and adolescents [11,12,14], Finnish [5] and Slovenian [6] adolescents, supplement users vs. non-users were more frequently physically active as well as less likely to watch television or video/computer games [14,15]. In American [14,15] and Korean [17] studies, overweight and obese children and adults were less likely to be supplement users. In our study, the usage of VMSs was associated with a normal BMI; children who were overweight and obese, and adolescents who were underweight had a lower probability to be supplement users.

Adolescents who declared average or poor health status and children suffering from chronic diseases compared to healthy respondents were more likely to consume VMSs. In some studies, dietary supplement use was more common in children and adolescents who used prescribed medication and among those who suffered from chronic diseases or were complaining about health [5,17]. On the contrary, in large American studies, children and adolescents who were supplement users compared to non-users more frequently declared very good or excellent health status [2,13].

Children and adolescents who were VMS users more often consumed fortified food and modified their diet towards better food choices. It was consistent with the results of other studies conducted in children and adolescents, where supplement use was associated with more healthful food choices [11], with higher diet quality score, regular consumption of some meals, low-fat foods [12,17] as well as more healthful food patterns such as higher intakes of whole grains, fruit, vegetables, and lower intakes of soft drinks, fried food, and meat [11,12,14].

We hypothesise that the differences in the determinants of dietary supplements may be a result of motivation for using these products. Parents make this decision in order to improve the nutritional habits of children, because of poor appetite or frequently occurring colds [10]; while adolescents are buying supplements by themselves, expecting a variety of effects, such as increased energy, building muscle mass or decreased weight and enhanced physical appearance, which often reflected the extensive marketing of specific dietary supplements [29]. In our study, as the main reasons for VMS use, parents of children pointed out improving children's overall health and a diet poor in nutrients; while adolescents declared improving overall health and physician recommendations. Similarly, in the American population, the main motivation of children and adolescents to use VMSs was improving overall health and preventing nutrient deficiencies [2,30].

The strengths of the present study include a large number of respondents as well as VMS users, and the detailed characteristics of participants by socio-demographic and lifestyle factors. It provided an opportunity to use the logistic regression models to determine factors significantly associated with VMS use separately in children and adolescents as well as allowed to show differences in the determinants of VMS usage between both groups. As in all observational studies, unmeasured or residual confounding cannot be disregarded. In the study, a limited number of determinants was examined; it is highly probable that some of the important factors of VMS use were not taken into account. Another limitation of this study was that the survey might not be representative for all primary and secondary school students from Central-Eastern Poland, since the study was carried out only in those schools in which the headmasters gave consent to it. Moreover, it is possible that respondents with a more health-oriented lifestyle are more likely to participate in the study. Furthermore, the methodology was not uniform; in children (5–12 years), the survey was completed by parents, while in adolescents (13–20 years) by the students themselves; this could have an effect on the outcomes.

5. Conclusions

Socio-demographic and lifestyle factors associated with VMS use may vary by age groups among school students. Children with an average socioeconomic status, who spent more free time on being physically active, with a normal body weight, and who suffered from chronic diseases, were more likely to use supplements. In adolescents, VMS users compared with non-users more often were female and lived in urban areas, less likely were underweight and assessed their health status as average or poor. In both groups, higher mothers' education, consumption of fortified food, and declaration of diet modifications towards better food choices were predictors of VMS use. Since the age of the respondents may determine different behaviours associated with the use of dietary supplements, further research should be conducted also among other age groups. Understanding the determinants affecting the use of dietary supplements in children and adolescents may identify the risk to subgroup populations of the incorrect use of dietary supplements, as well as allow the planning of appropriate public health education; therefore, further research is warranted.

Author Contributions: Conceptualization: E.S., B.P., and J.K.; data curation: E.S. and O.J.; formal analysis: E.S. and J.K.; investigation: B.P. and J.K.; methodology: E.S. and J.K.; supervision: B.P. and J.K.; writing—original draft: E.S.; writing—review and editing: B.P. and J.K.

Acknowledgments: The authors thank Katarzyna Rolf for technical support with creating the database.

References

1. Bailey, R.L.; Gahche, J.J.; Lentino, C.V.; Dwyer, J.T.; Engel, J.S.; Thomas, P.R.; Betz, J.M.; Sempos, C.T.; Picciano, M.F. Dietary supplement use in the United States, 2003–2006. *J. Nutr.* **2011**, *141*, 261–266. [CrossRef] [PubMed]

2. Dwyer, J.; Nahin, R.L.; Rogers, G.T.; Barnes, P.M.; Jacques, P.M.; Sempos, C.T.; Bailey, R. Prevalence and predictors of children's dietary supplement use: The 2007 National Health Interview Survey. *Am. J. Clin. Nutr.* **2013**, *97*, 1331–1337. [CrossRef] [PubMed]

3. Skeie, G.; Braaten, T.; Hjartaker, A.; Lentjes, M.; Amiano, P.; Jakszyn, P.; Pala, V.; Palanca, A.; Niekerk, E.M.; Verhagen, H.; et al. Use of dietary supplements in the European Prospective Investigation into Cancer and Nutrition calibration study. *Eur. J. Clin. Nutr.* **2009**, *63*, S226–S238. [CrossRef] [PubMed]

4. Bristow, A.; Qureshi, S.; Rona, R.J.; Chinn, S. The use of nutritional supplements by 4–12 year olds in England and Scotland. *Eur. J. Clin. Nutr.* **1997**, *51*, 366–369. [CrossRef] [PubMed]

5. Mattila, V.M.; Parkkari, J.; Laakso, L.; Pihlajamaki, H.; Rimpela, A. Use of dietary supplements and anabolic-androgenic steroids among Finnish adolescents in 1991–2005. *Eur. J. Public Health* **2010**, *20*, 306–311. [CrossRef] [PubMed]

6. Sterlinko Grm, H.; Stubelj Ars, M.; Besednjak-Kocijancic, L.; Golja, P. Nutritional supplement use among Slovenian adolescents. *Public Health Nutr.* **2012**, *15*, 587–593. [CrossRef]

7. Fortmann, S.P.; Burda, B.U.; Senger, C.A.; Lin, J.S.; Whitlock, E.P. Vitamin and mineral supplements in the primary prevention of cardiovascular disease and cancer: An updated systematic evidence review for the U.S. Preventive Services Task Force. *Ann. Intern. Med.* **2013**, *159*, 824–834. [CrossRef] [PubMed]

8. Dickinson, A.; MacKay, D. Health habits and other characteristics of dietary supplement users: A review. *Nutr. J.* **2014**, *13*, 14. [CrossRef]

9. Dickinson, A.; MacKay, D.; Wong, A. Consumer attitudes about the role of multivitamins and other dietary supplements: Report of a survey. *Nutr. J.* **2015**, *14*, 66. [CrossRef]

10. Yu, S.M.; Kogan, M.D.; Gergen, P. Vitamin-mineral supplement use among preschool children in the United States. *Pediatrics* **1997**, *100*, E4. [CrossRef]

11. George, G.C.; Hoelscher, D.M.; Nicklas, T.A.; Kelder, S.H. Diet- and body size-related attitudes and behaviors associated with vitamin supplement use in a representative sample of fourth-grade students in Texas. *J. Nutr. Educ. Behav.* **2009**, *41*, 95–102. [CrossRef]

12. George, G.C.; Springer, A.E.; Forman, M.R.; Hoelscher, D.M. Associations among dietary supplement use and dietary and activity behaviors by sex and race/ethnicity in a representative multiethnic sample of 11th-grade students in Texas. *J. Am. Diet. Assoc.* **2011**, *111*, 385–393. [CrossRef]

13. Gardiner, P.; Buettner, C.; Davis, R.B.; Phillips, R.S.; Kemper, K.J. Factors and common conditions associated with adolescent dietary supplement use: An analysis of the National Health and Nutrition Examination Survey (NHANES). *BMC Complement. Altern. Med.* **2008**, *8*, 9. [CrossRef] [PubMed]

14. Reaves, L.; Steffen, L.M.; Dwyer, J.T.; Webber, L.S.; Lytle, L.A.; Feldman, H.A.; Hoelscher, D.M.; Zive, M.M.; Osganian, S.K. Vitamin supplement intake is related to dietary intake and physical activity: The Child and Adolescent Trial for Cardiovascular Health (CATCH). *J. Am. Diet. Assoc.* **2006**, *106*, 2018–2023. [CrossRef]

15. Picciano, M.F.; Dwyer, J.T.; Radimer, K.L.; Wilson, D.H.; Fisher, K.D.; Thomas, P.R.; Yetley, E.A.; Moshfegh, A.J.; Levy, P.S.; Nielsen, S.J.; et al. Dietary supplement use among infants, children, and adolescents in the United States, 1999–2002. *Arch. Pediatr. Adolesc. Med.* **2007**, *161*, 978–985. [CrossRef]

16. Shaikh, U.; Byrd, R.S.; Auinger, P. Vitamin and mineral supplement use by children and adolescents in the 1999–2004 National Health and Nutrition Examination Survey: Relationship with nutrition, food security, physical activity, and health care access. *Arch. Pediatr. Adolesc. Med.* **2009**, *163*, 150–157. [CrossRef]

17. Yoon, J.Y.; Park, H.A.; Kang, J.H.; Kim, K.W.; Hur, Y.I.; Park, J.J.; Lee, R.; Lee, H.H. Prevalence of dietary supplement use in Korean children and adolescents: Insights from Korea National Health and Nutrition Examination Survey 2007–2009. *J. Korean Med. Sci.* **2012**, *27*, 512–517. [CrossRef]

18. Jun, S.; Cowan, A.E.; Tooze, J.A.; Gahche, J.J.; Dwyer, J.T.; Eicher-Miller, H.A.; Bhadra, A.; Guenther, P.M.; Potischman, N.; Dodd, K.W.; et al. Dietary Supplement Use among U.S. Children by Family Income, Food Security Level, and Nutrition Assistance Program Participation Status in 2011–2014. *Nutrients* **2018**, *10*, 1212. [CrossRef]

19. Cole, T.J.; Bellizzi, M.C.; Flegal, K.M.; Dietz, W.H. Establishing a standard definition for child overweight and obesity worldwide: International survey. *BMJ* **2000**, *320*, 1240–1243. [CrossRef]

20. Cole, T.J.; Flegal, K.M.; Nicholls, D.; Jackson, A.A. Body mass index cut offs to define thinness in children and adolescents: International survey. *BMJ* **2007**, *335*, 194. [CrossRef]

21. Sicińska, E.; Kałuża, J.; Januszko, O.; Pietruszka, B. Comparison of factors determining voluntarily fortified food consumption between children and adolescents in Central-Eastern Poland. *J. Food Nutr. Res.* **2018**, *57*, 284–294.

22. Pietruszka, B.; Brzozowska, A. Homocysteine Serum Level in Relation to Intake of Folate, Vitamins B12, B1, B2, and B6 and MTHFR c.665C→T Polymorphism among Young Women. *Austin J. Nutr. Food Sci.* **2014**, *2*, 1052–1059.

23. Pietruszka, B. *The Effectiveness of Diet Supplementation with Folates Relative to Risk Factors for Folate Deficiencies in Young Women*; Warsaw University of Life Sciences: Warsaw, Poland, 2007; pp. 1–182.

24. Bylinowska, J.; Januszko, O.; Rolf, K.; Sicinska, E.; Kaluza, J.; Pietruszka, B. Factors influenced vitamin or mineral supplements use in a chosen group of children aged 6–12. *Rocz. Panstw. Zakl. Hig.* **2012**, *63*, 59–66. [PubMed]

25. Bailey, R.L.; Fulgoni, V.L., 3rd; Keast, D.R.; Lentino, C.V.; Dwyer, J.T. Do dietary supplements improve micronutrient sufficiency in children and adolescents? *J. Pediatr.* **2012**, *161*, 837–842. [CrossRef] [PubMed]

26. Brzozowska, A.; Kaluza, J.; Knoops, K.T.; de Groot, L.C. Supplement use and mortality: The SENECA study. *Eur. J. Nutr.* **2008**, *47*, 131–137. [CrossRef] [PubMed]

27. Kaluza, J.; Januszko, O.; Trybalska, E.; Wadolowska, L.; Slowinska, M.A.; Brzozowska, A. Vitamin and mineral supplement use and mortality among group of older people. *Przegl. Epidemiol.* **2010**, *64*, 557–563. [PubMed]

28. Kleinman, R.E. Current Approaches to Standards of Care for Children: How Does the Pediatric Community Currently Approach This Issue? *Nutr. Today* **2002**, *37*, 177–179. [CrossRef] [PubMed]

29. Dorsch, K.D.; Bell, A. Dietary supplement use in adolescents. *Curr. Opin. Pediatr.* **2005**, *17*, 653–657. [CrossRef]

30. Bailey, R.L.; Gahche, J.J.; Thomas, P.R.; Dwyer, J.T. Why US children use dietary supplements. *Pediatr. Res.* **2013**, *74*, 737–741. [CrossRef] [PubMed]

13

Association between Picky Eating Behaviors and Nutritional Status in Early Childhood: Performance of a Picky Eating Behavior Questionnaire

Kyung Min Kwon [1], Jae Eun Shim [2,3,*], Minji Kang [4] and Hee-Young Paik [1,4]

[1]   Department of Food and Nutrition, College of Human Ecology, Seoul National University, 1 Gwanak-ro, Gwanak-gu, Seoul 08826, Korea; ckyme@snu.ac.kr (K.M.K.); hypaik@snu.ac.kr (H.-Y.P.)

[2]   Department of Food and Nutrition, Daejeon University, 62 Daehak-ro, Dong-gu, Daejeon 34520, Korea

[3]   Daejeon Dong-gu Center for Children's Food Service Management, Daejeon University, 62 Daehak-ro, Dong-gu, Daejeon 34520, Korea

[4]   Research Institute of Human Ecology, College of Human Ecology, Seoul National University, 1 Gwanak-ro, Gwanak-gu, Seoul 08826, Korea; mjkang@snu.ac.kr

*   Correspondence: jshim@dju.kr

Abstract: Picky eating behaviors are frequently observed in childhood, leading to concern that an unbalanced and inadequate diet will result in unfavorable growth outcomes. However, the association between picky eating behaviors and nutritional status has not been investigated in detail. This study was conducted to assess eating behaviors and growth of children aged 1–5 years from the Seoul Metropolitan area. Primary caregivers completed self-administered questionnaires and 3-day diet records. Differences in the nutrient intake and growth indices between picky and non-picky eaters were tested by analysis of covariance. Children "eating small amounts" consumed less energy and micronutrients (with the exception of calcium intake), but picky behaviors related to a "limited variety" resulted in a significant difference regarding nutrient density for some micronutrients. Children with the behavior of "eating small amounts" had a lower weight-for-age than that of non-picky eaters; especially, the older children with the behaviors of "eating small amounts" or "refusal of specific food groups" had lower height-for-age compared with non-picky eaters. These results suggest that specific picky eating behaviors are related to different nutrient intake and unfavorable growth patterns in early childhood. Thus, exploration of potential interventions according to specific aspects of picky eating and their efficacy is required.

Keywords: picky eating; early childhood; diet; growth

1. Introduction

Picky eating is a frequent eating problem in childhood that concerns many parents [1–4]. In young children, picky eating can contribute to a poor dietary intake and growth status [2,4–6] and may have long-term effects [7–10]. A recent review presented conflicting reports on dietary intake patterns in picky eating children: some studies reported an increased intake of energy or energy-dense foods including snacks and sweets, while most studies reported a limited variety of food intake with reduced energy consumption [11]. Both patterns could cause inappropriate changes in the nutrient composition of the diet and are related to unfavorable growth (i.e., poor growth and overweight) and subsequent health problems [11–14].

However, previous approaches to evaluating picky eaters are insufficient to explain the conflicting reports on dietary intake patterns, and investigate the association with growth outcomes. In previous studies, caregivers of picky-eating children reported various problems with feeding them: eating insufficient amounts, avoiding new foods, preferring foods prepared in specific ways, or having a strong preference for particular foods [2,4,6,8,15–18]. Picky eating is a complex concept composed of several types of eating behaviors [19]; nevertheless, picky eating has generally been measured by a single simple question based on parents' perceptions of feeding difficulty or pickiness [2,18], or by a list of questions about eating behaviors and feeding practices [4,7,16,20,21]. The differences in measurements regarding picky eating focusing on one aspect or approaches using measurement tools consisting of mixed concepts leads to confusion and problems in interpretation [22].

Two recent studies have tried to present a clear definition of picky eating, and have characterized children's picky eating behaviors with two attributes based on previously-reported aspects of picky eating behaviors: eating small amounts of food, and eating a limited variety of foods [19,23]. In the studies, "limited variety" consisted of three sub-constructs of "unwillingness to try new food", "rejection of specific food groups" (i.e., fruits, vegetables, meats, and fish), and "preference for specific food preparation methods". To find critical behaviors in child growth, the association of the four aspects of picky behaviors and growth in young children was examined at a medical clinic for picky eaters [23]. The medical clinic study measured the level of the four aspects of picky eating behaviors using similar questions to the present study (i.e., the same questions for the measurement of "eating small amounts" and "neophobic behavior", 9 vs. 12 food groups for "refusal of specific food groups", and 7 vs. 9 food groups for preference for specific food preparation method). In the study, negative association between "eating small amounts" and height-for-age was observed. Difference in nutrient intake and the relations with growth outcomes in a community setting have not yet been examined.

Thus, the present study investigated the picky eating behaviors of the four constructs in children aged 1 to 5 years at the community level. Further, the performance using the four-construct scale was evaluated qualitatively by examining how the four different aspects of picky eating were associated with dietary intake and growth. It is hypothesized that each aspect would have a specific pattern in dietary intake and growth.

2. Materials and Methods

2.1. Study Participants

This study is a cross-sectional survey targeting children aged 1 to 5 years from the Seoul Metropolitan Area of Korea. Participants were recruited between September 2014 and July 2015. Convenience sampling was employed to recruit volunteers by using flyers, public announcements, and online announcements at Community Health centers, a pharmacy, and an online caregiver's community. Voluntarily participating primary caregivers of the children were asked to complete the survey questionnaire. Participants were enrolled after the caregivers were given a full explanation of the purpose and protocols of the research in person. The Seoul National University Institutional Review Board approved the study protocol (IRB No. 1407/001-034), and all primary caregivers provided written informed consent.

2.2. Measurements

2.2.1. Picky Eating Behaviors

Picky eating behaviors were assessed using survey questions from previous studies [19,23]. Caregivers were asked to respond to the frequency of each question using a five-point response scale of 1 (almost never) to 5 (almost always). The higher scores demonstrated greater picky eating behavior, so the reverse-described questions were transposed. Self-administered surveys were reviewed by a trained dietitian and confirmed by interview. The four specific picky eating behaviors and the related questions were:

- Eating small amounts, with the question of "How often do you attempt to persuade your child to eat a food?", and two reversed-described questions: "In general, at the end of a meal how often has your child eaten the amount you think he/she should eat?" and "Does your child have a good appetite?"

- Neophobic behavior, with two reverse-described questions: "How often does your child try new and unfamiliar foods at home?", and "How willing is your child to enjoy new and unfamiliar food when offered?"
- Refusal to eat specific food groups, using the question on 12 food groups: "How often does your child refuse the following foods: beans, vegetables, mushrooms, seaweeds, meat, fish, shrimp, shellfish, eggs, fruits, milk, and yogurt?"
- Preference for a specific food preparation method, with the question on nine food groups: "Does your child eat any of the following foods only if prepared in a specific way: beans, vegetables, mushrooms, seaweeds, meat, fish, shrimp, shellfish, and eggs?"

It was assumed that the children have potential picky eating characters if the response score to each question was higher than neutral. "Eating small amounts" and "neophobic behavior" were summated rating scales. Therefore, the children whose mean score of responses was >3 were classified as "picky eaters" for "eating small amounts" and "neophobic behavior". The internal consistency of items on these constructs was measured using the Cronbach's coefficient α ($\alpha = 0.80$ for "eating small amounts" and $\alpha = 0.73$ for "neophobic behavior"). Whether children refused a food group or whether children had preference for a specific preparation method to a food group was also determined by a response score > 3. However, "refusal to eat specific food groups" and "preference for a specific food preparation method" were not summated rating scales. The constructs consisted of multiple questions about behaviors to different food groups. Therefore, "refusal to eat specific food groups" and "preference for a specific food preparation method" were evaluated based on the number of foods refused and number of foods with specific preparation method preferred, respectively. The cut-off number was set based on the mean numbers of food groups with responses more than neutral (1.8 for refused food groups and 1.2 for preference for a specific food preparation method). Therefore, children who refused more than two food groups were classified as picky eaters of "refusal to eat specific food groups" and children with a preference for a specific food preparation method in any food group were categorized as picky eaters of "preference for a specific food preparation method". If certain food groups had never been tried, the food groups were not counted when "refusal to eat specific food groups" or "preference for a specific food preparation method" was evaluated. Children who had any one of the sub-constructs, "neophobic behavior", "refusal to eat specific food groups", and "preference for a specific food preparation method" were defined as children with 'limited variety'. Children who had any one of the picky eating main constructs, "eating small amounts" and "limited variety", were classified as picky eaters.

2.2.2. Dietary Intakes

Non-consecutive 3-day diet records were used to collect the dietary intake data of each subject. To minimize errors in portion size, the caregivers were asked to record the intake amount by using two-dimensional measurement tools. The protocol for coding diet records was prepared by a research dietitian supervisor. Based on the protocol, trained dietitian interviewers reviewed the data by telephone interview. For children who were still being breastfed, the intake of breastmilk was assessed according to the reported feeding time; the amount being fed was considered to be 1 fl. oz. (29.6 mL) for every 5 min [24]. All dietary data were converted to nutrient intake values using the DES-KOREA (Diet Evaluation System, 2011, Human Nutrition Lab at Seoul National University, Republic of Korea), which is a web-based dietary assessment program [25,26]. The DES incorporates a recipe and nutrient database. The recipe database contains 3916 recipes for common Korean dishes, and the nutrient database contains 4222 food items [27,28]. The mean daily intake, the energy distribution for macronutrients, the nutrient density (intake/1000 kcal of energy) for micronutrients, and the total dietary fiber were evaluated.

2.2.3. Growth Indices

Primary caregivers were asked to measure the weight and height of their children at the local hospital or community health center and report the values to the research dietitian by mail. Confirmation was made through telephone interviews. The height data for children aged ≤24 months were converted into lengths by adding 0.7 cm, following the WHO (World Health Organization) child growth standards [29]. The height/length and weight values were converted into z-scores for weight-for-age, height-for-age (length-for-age), and BMI (body mass index)-for-age, compared with the WHO child growth standards for 0–60 months [29] and the WHO growth reference data for 61–228 months [30].

2.2.4. Covariates

A questionnaire investigating the children's eating behaviors, feeding practices, and care environment was administered, and data were obtained by self-reporting via the caregivers of the participating children. The sociodemographic characteristics included information pertaining to the caregivers, such as age, education level of both parents (≤high school, college graduate, graduate school), and monthly household income (≤$2800, $2800 to $3900, and ≥$3900), and information pertaining to the children, such as age and sex. In addition, Nutrition Plus participation (a nutrition supplemental program for women, infants and children in Korea) and infant feeding practices were investigated. Infant feeding practice was evaluated according to the duration of breastfeeding, the introduction of formula or milk, and the introduction of supplementary foods. This information was transformed into binary variables, including breastfeeding initiation, exclusive breastfeeding during the first 3 months and 6 months of life, and early introduction of supplementary foods before 6 months of age [31].

2.3. Statistical Analysis

The data of sociodemographic characteristics and the prevalence of picky eating habits were presented as numbers and proportions for categorical variables or as means and standard deviations for numeric variables. The differences in nutrient intake and z-scores of growth indices between picky eaters and non-picky eaters in each construct were tested by analysis of covariance to adjust for the child's age and sex and the education level of both parents, after examination of covariates as potential confounders [32]. All the statistical analyses were performed using SAS (version 9.3, 2011, SAS Institute Inc., Cary, NC, USA), and the statistical significance was determined at 0.05.

3. Results

3.1. Sociodemographic Characteristics of Study Participants

Among the 221 children of the caregivers who initially volunteered and were eligible for the study, 14 with missing data from their diet records and 1 who had consecutive food records were excluded. An additional 22 participants were excluded because of food restrictions due to food allergies, a vegetarian diet, or religious beliefs, leaving 184 children with complete data.

As shown in Table 1, participants generally lived in well-educated middle-class families. Approximately 39% of children participated in Nutrition Plus. The growth indices of all participants were within the normal ranges.

Table 1. Selected characteristics of children aged 1 to 5 years and their caregivers ($n = 184$).

Variables	
Characteristics of children	
Age (year), mean ± SD	2.8 ± 1.4
Sex, % boy	48.9
	n (%)
Infant feeding practice	
Breastfeeding initiation	177 (96.2)
Exclusive breastfeeding under 3 months of life	166 (90.2)
Exclusive breastfeeding under 6 months of life	93 (50.5)
Introduction of complementary foods [a] before 6 months of age	55 (29.9)
Nutrition Plus [b] participation	
Yes	72 (39.1)
No	112 (60.9)
Picky eating behavior [c]	129 (70.1)
Eating small amount	55 (29.9)
Limited variety [d]	123 (66.9)
Neophobic behavior	60 (32.6)
Refusal of specific food groups	81 (44.0)
Preference for a specific food preparation method	91 (49.5)
	mean ± SD
Growth status (z-score)	
Weight for age	0.1 ± 0.8
Height for age	−0.3 ± 1.1
BMI for age	0.3 ± 1.0
Characteristics of caregivers and the household	
Age (year), mean ± SD	34.9 ± 3.8
	n (%)
Education level of father	
≤High school	18 (9.8)
University	137 (74.5)
Graduate school	29 (15.8)
Education level of mother	
≤High school	29 (15.8)
University	135 (73.4)
Graduate school	20 (10.9)
Household income	
≤$2800	76 (41.3)
$2800 to $3900	58 (31.5)
≥$3900	50 (27.2)

[a] All foods except breast milk and formula; [b] A Nutrition supplemental program for women, infant, and children in Korea; [c] Children who had any one of the picky eating constructs: 'eating small amounts' and 'limited variety'; [d] Children who had any one of the sub- constructs of limited variety: 'neophobic behavior', 'refusal to eat specific food groups', and 'preference for a specific food preparation method'.

3.2. Proportion of Picky Eaters

The proportion of participants with the behavior of "eating small amounts" was 29.9% and with the "limited variety" was 66.9%; with the "preference for a specific food-preparation method" was 49.5%, with the "refusal to eat specific food groups" was 44.0%, with the "neophobic behavior" was 32.6% (Table 1). In addition, compared with the younger children, the older children aged 4 to 5 years showed higher rates of eating behaviors related to a variety of foods, especially "neophobic behavior" (47.5% vs. 25.6%, p = 0.0032). Most children showed more than one kind of picky behavior: of the children with the behavior of "eating small amounts", 67.3% also displayed a "refusal to eat specific food groups" and 43.6% "neophobic behavior"; of the children with "neophobic behavior", 40.0% exhibited "eating small amounts" and 75.0% a "refusal to eat specific food groups"; of the children with a "refusal to eat specific food groups", 45.7% exhibited "eating small amounts" and 55.6% "neophobic behavior"; of the children with "preference for a specific food-preparation method", 63.7% exhibited a "refusal to eat specific food groups"; 9.8% of the children exhibited all of these picky eating behaviors, while 29.9% had none of the picky eating behaviors (data not shown).

The proportions of children who refused each food groups and who preferred specific preparation for each food groups are shown in Figures 1 and 2. The three most frequently refused food groups were shellfish, beans, and vegetables, and the three least refused food groups were fish, fruits, and eggs. Children required foods to be prepared in a certain way—mainly for shellfish and beans. Only 3% of children required eggs to be prepared in a certain way. Fish was not likely to be refused; however, it was required to be prepared in a certain way.

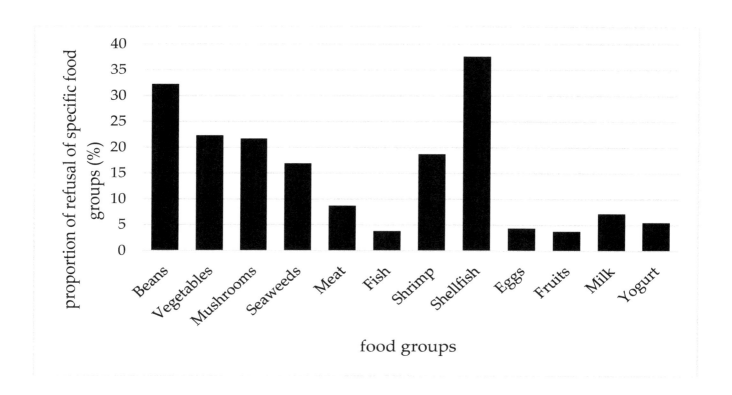

Figure 1. The proportion of children who usually refused a specific food group. The descriptive statistics for the distribution of number of food groups refused as follows: mean $\pm$ SD = 1.8 $\pm$ 1.9, Q_1 = 0, median = 1, and Q_3 = 3.

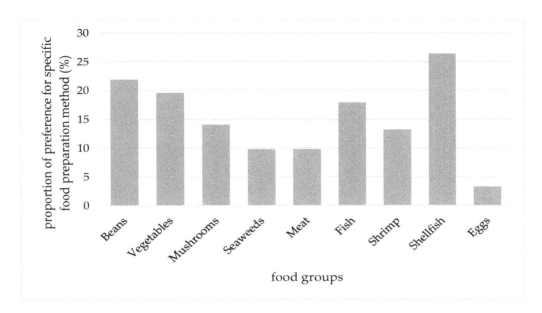

Figure 2. The proportion of children who usually requested food preparation in a certain way for each food group. The descriptive statistics for the distribution of number of food groups with specific preparation as follows: mean ± SD = 1.2 ± 1.8, $Q_1 = 0$, median = 0, and $Q_3 = 1$.

3.3. Comparison of the Dietary Intake and Growth Indices between Picky Eaters and Non-Picky Eaters

3.3.1. Dietary Intake

The characteristics of the dietary intake of picky eaters—as compared to non-picky eaters—varied with each eating behavior (Table 2). Children considered to be "eating small amounts" had a significantly lower intake of energy and all micronutrients, with the exception of calcium intake. With respect to the picky eating behavior of a limited variety, there was no significant difference in energy intake between picky and non-picky eaters. The children with "neophobic behavior" consumed less dietary fiber per 1000 kcal of energy intake than did their counterparts. Picky eaters with a "refusal of specific food groups" consumed less micronutrients, with the exception of calcium and niacin intake. There was also a significant difference in nutrient density with some micronutrients. The "preference for a specific food preparation method" was related to lower intakes of iron and vitamin A.

3.3.2. Growth Indices

The comparison of growth indices between picky eaters and non-picky eaters are presented in Table 3. Picky eaters "eating small amounts" had lower z-scores for weight-for-age ($p = 0.0010$) and BMI-for-age ($p = 0.0278$) but lower scores for height-for-age, with marginal significance ($p = 0.054$). Picky eaters "eating small amounts" aged 4 to 5 years had significantly lower z-scores for all three growth indices. Picky eaters with "refusal of specific food groups" were related with lower height-for-age in this age group.

Table 2. Comparison of nutrient intakes between picky eaters and non-picky eaters according to specific picky eating behaviors (n = 184).

	Eating Small Amounts			Neophobic Behavior			Refusal of Specific Food Groups			Preference for Specific Food Preparation Method		
	Yes (n = 55)	No (n = 129)	p^a	Yes (n = 60)	No (n = 124)	p^a	≥2 (n = 81)	0–1 (n = 103)	p^a	≥1 (n = 91)	0 (n = 93)	p^a
	mean ± standard deviation											
Mean daily dietary intake												
Energy (kcal)	1155 ± 340	1340 ± 348	0.0005	1299 ± 393	1278 ± 336	0.6959	1261 ± 364	1304 ± 348	0.2210	1265 ± 361	1304 ± 350	0.1273
Protein (% Energy)	16 ± 3	16 ± 2	0.8880	16 ± 2	16 ± 2	0.0745	16 ± 2	16 ± 2	0.8004	16 ± 2	16 ± 2	0.4553
Lipid (% Energy)	24 ± 5	24 ± 5	0.4794	24 ± 6	24 ± 5	0.4390	24 ± 5	24 ± 5	0.6578	23 ± 5	24 ± 5	0.8095
Carbohydrate (% Energy)	60 ± 6	61 ± 6	0.5902	60 ± 6	61 ± 6	0.1876	60 ± 6	61 ± 6	0.7830	61 ± 6	60 ± 5	0.9370
Calcium (mg)	416 ± 146	449 ± 217	0.2252	440 ± 209	438 ± 194	0.3546	404 ± 157	466 ± 223	0.0919	411 ± 162	466 ± 227	0.0705
Iron (mg)	8 ± 3	10 ± 4	0.0073	9 ± 3	10 ± 4	0.0938	9 ± 3	10 ± 5	0.0198	9 ± 3	10 ± 5	0.0146
Vit. A (μg RE)	393 ± 205	460 ± 239	0.0370	382 ± 187	468 ± 245	0.0859	386 ± 187	483 ± 252	0.0064	404 ± 199	475 ± 254	0.0231
Thiamin (mg)	0.66 ± 0.24	0.78 ± 0.26	0.0116	0.78 ± 0.29	0.72 ± 0.25	0.5680	0.71 ± 0.27	0.76 ± 0.25	0.0367	0.74 ± 0.26	0.75 ± 0.26	0.1562
Riboflavin (mg)	0.9 ± 0.3	1.0 ± 0.3	0.0072	1.0 ± 0.3	1.0 ± 0.3	0.6564	0.9 ± 0.3	1.0 ± 0.3	0.0444	0.9 ± 0.3	1.0 ± 0.3	0.1868
Niacin (mg)	8 ± 3	9 ± 3	0.0018	9 ± 4	9 ± 3	0.2177	9 ± 3	9 ± 3	0.1640	9 ± 3	9 ± 3	0.1754
Vit. C (mg)	77 ± 55	94 ± 61	0.0380	83 ± 64	92 ± 57	0.1119	82 ± 57	95 ± 61	0.0274	89 ± 67	90 ± 52	0.4510
Total Dietary Fiber (g)	11 ± 4	13 ± 5	0.0122	12 ± 5	12 ± 4	0.1032	12 ± 5	13 ± 5	0.0110	12 ± 5	13 ± 5	0.0980
Nutrient density (intake/1000 kcal)												
Calcium (mg)	371 ± 113	332 ± 111	0.2044	336 ± 102	347 ± 117	0.2556	327 ± 103	357 ± 118	0.3166	328 ± 93	359 ± 127	0.1935
Iron (mg)	7 ± 2	7 ± 3	0.2711	7 ± 1	7 ± 3	0.1159	7 ± 1	8 ± 3	0.0524	7 ± 2	8 ± 3	0.0696
Vit. A (μg RE)	349 ± 172	348 ± 172	0.4670	301 ± 151	371 ± 177	0.1554	315 ± 154	375 ± 181	0.0514	325 ± 146	371 ± 192	0.1247
Thiamin (mg)	0.56 ± 0.12	0.58 ± 0.12	0.3715	0.60 ± 0.13	0.56 ± 0.11	0.1805	0.56 ± 0.13	0.58 ± 0.11	0.0335	0.58 ± 0.11	0.57 ± 0.12	0.6568
Riboflavin (mg)	0.8 ± 0.2	0.8 ± 0.2	0.6383	0.8 ± 0.1	0.8 ± 0.2	0.2690	0.8 ± 0.2	0.8 ± 0.2	0.1702	0.7 ± 0.1	0.8 ± 0.2	0.6353
Niacin (mg)	7 ± 1	7 ± 2	0.0758	7 ± 1	7 ± 1	0.0683	7 ± 1	7 ± 1	0.3064	7 ± 1	7 ± 2	0.7212
Vit. C (mg)	68 ± 35	71 ± 42	0.2579	64 ± 42	72 ± 39	0.1617	65 ± 38	73 ± 42	0.0769	69 ± 42	70 ± 38	0.6559
Total Dietary Fiber (g)	9 ± 3	10 ± 2	0.4781	9 ± 2	10 ± 3	0.0167	9 ± 2	10 ± 3	0.0074	10 ± 2	10 ± 3	0.3655

^a P-value adjusted for age, sex, and education level of both parents. RE: retinol equivalent.

Table 3. Comparison of growth indices between picky eaters and non-picky eaters according to specific picky eating behaviors ($n = 184$).

	Eating Small Amounts			Neophobic Behavior			Refusal of Specific Food Groups			Preference for Specific Food Preparation Method		
Total subjects ($n = 184$)	Yes ($n = 55$)	No ($n = 129$)	p^a	Yes ($n = 60$)	No ($n = 124$)	p^a	≥ 2 ($n = 81$)	0–1 ($n = 103$)	p^a	≥ 1 ($n = 91$)	0 ($n = 93$)	p^a
Growth status (z-score)												
Weight-for-age	−0.2 ± 0.9	0.2 ± 0.8	0.0010	0.1 ± 0.9	0.1 ± 0.8	0.9797	0.0 ± 0.9	0.1 ± 0.7	0.4137	0.1 ± 0.8	0.0 ± 0.8	0.2268
Height-for-age	−0.5 ± 1.1	−0.2 ± 1.1	0.0545	−0.5 ± 1.3	−0.2 ± 1.0	0.1057	−0.3 ± 1.1	−0.2 ± 1.1	0.8774	−0.1 ± 1.1	−0.4 ± 1.1	0.0275
BMI-for-age	0.0 ± 1.3	0.4 ± 0.9	0.0278	0.5 ± 1.1	0.2 ± 1.0	0.1329	0.2 ± 0.9	0.3 ± 1.1	0.4653	0.2 ± 0.9	0.3 ± 1.2	0.4831
Children aged 1 to 3 years ($n = 125$)	Yes ($n = 42$)	No ($n = 83$)	p^a	Yes ($n = 32$)	No ($n = 93$)	p^a	≥ 2 ($n = 52$)	0–1 ($n = 73$)	p^a	≥ 1 ($n = 61$)	0 ($n = 64$)	p^a
Growth status (z-score)												
Weight-for-age	−0.1 ± 0.9	0.2 ± 0.8	0.0911	0.0 ± 1.0	0.1 ± 0.8	0.8962	0.1 ± 1.0	0.1 ± 0.7	0.6288	0.1 ± 0.9	0.0 ± 0.8	0.5295
Height-for-age	−0.4 ± 1.2	−0.2 ± 1.2	0.3665	−0.7 ± 1.5	−0.1 ± 1.0	0.0657	−0.2 ± 1.2	−0.3 ± 1.2	0.3806	−0.1 ± 1.2	−0.4 ± 1.2	0.1739
BMI-for-age	0.1 ± 1.3	0.3 ± 0.9	0.2833	0.6 ± 1.2	0.1 ± 1.0	0.0575	0.2 ± 0.8	0.2 ± 1.2	0.8383	0.2 ± 0.9	0.3 ± 1.3	0.6564
Children aged 4 to 5 years ($n = 59$)	Yes ($n = 13$)	No ($n = 46$)	p^a	Yes ($n = 28$)	No ($n = 31$)	p^a	≥ 2 ($n = 29$)	0–1 ($n = 30$)	p^a	≥ 1 ($n = 30$)	0 ($n = 29$)	p^a
Growth status (z-score)												
Weight-for-age	−0.6 ± 0.7	0.2 ± 0.7	0.0007	0.1 ± 0.8	0.0 ± 0.8	0.9373	−0.2 ± 0.8	0.2 ± 0.8	0.0750	0.1 ± 0.8	0.0 ± 0.8	0.3427
Height-for-age	−0.8 ± 0.7	−0.1 ± 0.8	0.0049	−0.2 ± 0.9	−0.3 ± 0.7	0.8754	−0.5 ± 0.9	−0.1 ± 0.7	0.0450	−0.1 ± 0.8	−0.4 ± 0.8	0.1434
BMI-for-age	−0.2 ± 0.9	0.4 ± 0.9	0.0194	0.3 ± 0.9	0.3 ± 0.9	0.9966	0.2 ± 0.9	0.4 ± 0.9	0.8184	0.2 ± 1.0	0.4 ± 0.9	0.7406

^{a} P-value adjusted for age, sex, and education level of both parents. BMI: body mass index.

4. Discussion

Research on picky eating faces difficulties due to a lack of widely-accepted definitions and appropriate measurement tools. Different definitions used by different researchers may indicate that picky eating behavior is not simple, but rather has complex characteristics that cannot be defined by one single aspect. Thus, in the present study, different aspects of picky eating were clarified and then measured and evaluated separately for their associations with nutritional status. The results suggested that picky eating behavior consists of different constructs showing specific nutrient intake and growth patterns, and the measurement tool could be used to investigate picky eating behaviors and the associated outcomes.

The present study adopted the previous approach to measure the two main constructs of "eating small amounts" and "limited variety" in picky eating behaviors, and the three sub-constructs of "neophobic behavior", "refusal of specific food groups", and "preference for a specific preparation method" in "limited variety" [19,23]. "Eating small amounts" refers to consuming insufficient food, and "limited variety" includes "neophobic behavior", which refers to avoiding new foods and a "refusal of specific food groups" as well as a "preference for a specific preparation method", which refers to children's likes and dislikes of specific foods and certain recipes for each food [19,23]. While children show more than one construct behavior simultaneously and the classification of children overlapped, this approach could find a specific association between children's eating behaviors and diet and growth.

Children "eating small amounts" consumed less energy and nutrients and had lower scores for growth indices compared with non-picky eaters in the present study. The frequently reported behaviors of picky eating children were spitting food out, eating avoidance, or throwing food, which may lead to "eating small amounts" [33]. Additionally, caregivers who experienced feeding difficulties reported that their children had a low appetite [34]. These fussy behaviors—which lead to consuming less food—were related to dietary problems in the present study. In previous studies, children classified as picky eaters had lower intakes of energy and nutrients, such as vitamin E, folate, and dietary fiber [2,4,5,17], and the children had slower growth rates and gained less weight [2,6,12]. However, the previous studies did not try to identify which specific picky eating behaviors were associated with the nutrient intakes and the growth outcomes.

A longitudinal study reported that children who are picky eaters are more likely to have a low BMI-for-age [12]. The risk was likely to increase when the picky eating problem continued as the children became older [30]. In the present study, it was observed that association between growth indices and picky eating behaviors was more prominent in the older children than in the younger children. Moreover, in the present study, the children with picky eating habits in the older age group had shorter heights and lower BMIs than those in the younger age group, indicating the need for further examination whether unfavorable long-term growth outcomes would be induced by picky eating behaviors.

In other studies, food neophobia and food rejection were related with limited preference for all food groups—especially vegetables and fruits [35,36]. In the present study, picky eaters with behaviors related to choosing a limited variety of foods had a lower quality of diet for some micronutrients, but not energy. However, the "refusal of some food groups" was related to lower height-for-age among children aged 4 to 5 years in this study. This suggests the necessity for further investigation on long-term problems induced by food avoidance, in terms of the negative influence of micronutrient deficiency on linear growth. Younger picky eaters with "neophobic behavior" were likely to have a lower z-score for height-for-age ($p = 0.0657$) and a higher z-score for BMI-for-age ($p = 0.0575$). If food neophobia is not appropriately countered at the period of introduction of complementary food, some food groups may remain refused throughout the life. Thus, in younger children, food neophobia and the long-term impact on growth may be concerns, even though energy consumption is not compromised.

It has been reported that the main reason for rejecting foods is distaste and dislike of color [37,38]. Cooking changes the color, taste, and texture of foods. Many of the children with "preference for a specific food preparation" had the picky eating behavior of "refusal of some food groups", while their dietary intake and growth indices were not compromised. The most dramatic change of children's food choice was fish. It indicated that if children could find an appropriate preparation for disliked foods then they might choose to eat the foods with the preparation. These findings imply that an appropriate food preparation method that positively influences food intake would be helpful for the prevention of poor growth. The impact of "preference for a specific food preparation method" needs to be assessed in further studies.

However, there are some limitations to this study. It was conducted as a cross-sectional study of a well-educated, small-scale sample living in a metropolitan area. Thus, this study was not free from counter causality (i.e., smaller children with less appetite behaving in a way to be classified as picky eaters), and generalizability of the results is limited. Potential confounders were not fully evaluated and controlled for; a few socio-demographic characteristics were controlled for, but other potential covariates such as the child's characteristics and child feeding practices were not. The study variables were measured by the caregiver's report, which represented personal values and expectations. Additionally, separate evaluation of "refusal to eat specific food groups" and "preference for a specific food preparation method" was a novel approach in this area. Therefore, evidence for relevant question forms and response cut-off criteria was scarce. Mean numbers of food groups were adopted as cut-off values, but might seem to be arbitrary. Currently, the two sub-constructs were not absolutely diagnosed, but relatively; nevertheless, association with growth status was observed. Especially strength of the association was dependent on the duration of picky eating behaviors. Further examinations in various populations and exploration of the association with growth outcome through a relevant study design (i.e., a cohort study) could accumulate evidence for more relevant criteria. In addition, the dietary intake of the children was estimated by parents, and the influence of childcare was not considered. Finally, analysis of the association between picky eating behaviors and the adequacy of nutrient intake and growth was stratified by age group; however, the significance of the association was marginal due to the small sample size.

Despite these limitations, the findings from this study should enhance understanding of the association between eating and growth patterns in children. A child's picky eating behavior has several aspects, although they tend to overlap somewhat. Moreover, different aspects of the behaviors seemed to have a different meaning in terms of a child's nutritional status. Further study is required to confirm the causality of the observed associations. Investigations of the development of specific picky eating behaviors and long-term outcomes induced by the specific picky eating behaviors are also required. In addition, various attempts to improve the accuracy of classification of the picky eating behaviors are also required.

5. Conclusions

This study established concepts for—and measurement of—picky eating behaviors, and assessed the association of picky eating with diet and growth in early childhood. The specific measurement—which consisted of the categories "eating small amounts", "neophobic behavior", "refusal of specific food groups", and "preference for a specific food preparation method"—properly explained the characteristics of various picky eating problems in early childhood. The results of this study suggest that picky eating behaviors—especially eating small amounts of food—are related to insufficient nutrient intake, creating an unfavorable growth pattern. However, the long-term impacts of a diet with limited variety need to be identified.

Acknowledgments: This research was supported by Basic Science Research Program through the National Research Foundation of Korea (NRF) funded by the Ministry of Science, ICT & Future Planning (NRF-2013R1A1A2057600 and NRF-2016R1D1A1B03931820).

Author Contributions: J.S. conceived and designed the research; K.K. and M.K. performed the research; K.K., N.K., H.P. and J.S. analyzed the data; H.P. contributed reagents/materials/analysis tools; K.M.K. and J.S. wrote the paper.

Appendix A. Children's Picky Eating Behavior Questionnaire

Eating Small Amounts

1. In general, at the end of a meal how often has your child eaten the amount you think he/she should eat?

Almost Never				Almost Always
1	2	3	4	5

2. How often do you attempt to persuade your child to eat a food?

Almost Never				Almost Always
1	2	3	4	5

3. Does your child have a good appetite?

Very Bad				Very Good
1	2	3	4	5

Limited Variety

Neophobic Behavior

4. How often does your child try new and unfamiliar foods at home?

Almost Never				Almost Always
1	2	3	4	5

5. How willing is your child to enjoy new and unfamiliar food when offered?

Very Unwilling				Very Willing
1	2	3	4	5

Refusal of Specific Food Groups

6. How often does your child refuse the following foods: beans, vegetables, mushrooms, seaweeds, meat, fish, shrimp, shellfish, eggs, fruits, milk, and yogurt?

Food	Almost Never 1	2	3	4	Almost Always 5	Not Applicable
Beans	☐	☐	☐	☐	☐	☐
Vegetables	☐	☐	☐	☐	☐	☐
Mushrooms	☐	☐	☐	☐	☐	☐
Seaweeds	☐	☐	☐	☐	☐	☐
Meat	☐	☐	☐	☐	☐	☐
Fish	☐	☐	☐	☐	☐	☐
Shrimp	☐	☐	☐	☐	☐	☐
Shellfish	☐	☐	☐	☐	☐	☐
Eggs	☐	☐	☐	☐	☐	☐
Fruits	☐	☐	☐	☐	☐	☐
Milk	☐	☐	☐	☐	☐	☐
Yogurt	☐	☐	☐	☐	☐	☐

Preference for a Specific Food Preparation Method

7. Does your child eat any of the following foods only if prepared in a specific way: beans, vegetables, mushrooms, seaweeds, meat, fish, shrimp, shellfish, and eggs?

Food	Almost Never 1	2	3	4	Almost Always 5	Not Applicable
Beans	☐	☐	☐	☐	☐	☐
Vegetables	☐	☐	☐	☐	☐	☐
Mushrooms	☐	☐	☐	☐	☐	☐
Seaweeds	☐	☐	☐	☐	☐	☐
Meat	☐	☐	☐	☐	☐	☐
Fish	☐	☐	☐	☐	☐	☐
Shrimp	☐	☐	☐	☐	☐	☐
Shellfish	☐	☐	☐	☐	☐	☐
Eggs	☐	☐	☐	☐	☐	☐

References

1. Jacobi, C.; Schmitz, G.; Agras, W.S. Is picky eating an eating disorder? *Int. J. Eat. Disord.* **2008**, *41*, 626–634. [CrossRef] [PubMed]
2. Carruth, B.R.; Ziegler, P.J.; Gordon, A.; Barr, S.I. Prevalence of picky eaters among infants and toddlers and their caregivers' decisions about offering a new food. *J. Am. Diet. Assoc.* **2004**, *104*, S57–S64. [CrossRef] [PubMed]
3. Li, Y.; Shi, A.P.; Wan, Y.; Hotta, M.; Ushijima, H. Child behavior problems: Prevalence and correlates in rural minority areas of China. *Pediatr. Int.* **2001**, *43*, 651–661. [CrossRef] [PubMed]
4. Galloway, A.T.; Fiorito, L.; Lee, Y.; Birch, L.L. Parental pressure, dietary patterns, and weight status among girls who are "picky eaters". *J. Am. Diet. Assoc.* **2005**, *105*, 541–548. [CrossRef] [PubMed]
5. Dubois, L.; Farmer, A.P.; Girard, M.; Peterson, K. Preschool children's eating behaviours are related to dietary adequacy and body weight. *Eur. J. Clin. Nutr.* **2007**, *61*, 846–855. [CrossRef] [PubMed]
6. Wright, C.M.; Parkinson, K.N.; Shipton, D.; Drewett, R.F. How do toddler eating problems relate to their eating behavior, food preferences, and growth? *Pediatrics* **2007**, *120*, e1069–e1075. [CrossRef] [PubMed]
7. Ashcroft, J.; Semmler, C.; Carnell, S.; van Jaarsveld, C.H.M.; Wardle, J. Continuity and stability of eating behaviour traits in children. *Eur. J. Clin. Nutr.* **2008**, *62*, 985–990. [CrossRef] [PubMed]
8. Mascola, A.J.; Bryson, S.W.; Agras, W.S. Picky eating during childhood: a longitudinal study to age 11 years. *Eat. Behav.* **2010**, *11*, 253–257. [CrossRef] [PubMed]
9. Kotler, L.A.; Cohen, P.; Davies, M.; Pine, D.S.; Walsh, B.T. Longitudinal relationships between childhood, adolescent, and adult eating disorders. *J. Am. Acad. Child. Adolesc. Psychiatry* **2001**, *40*, 1434–1440. [CrossRef] [PubMed]
10. Taylor, C.M.; Northstone, K.; Wernimont, S.M.; Emmett, P.M. Macro-and micronutrient intakes in picky eaters: A cause for concern? *Am. J. Clin. Nutr.* **2016**, *104*, 1647–1656. [CrossRef] [PubMed]
11. Taylor, C.M.; Wernimont, S.M.; Northstone, K.; Emmett, P.M. Picky/fussy eating in children: Review of definitions, assessment, prevalence and dietary intakes. *Appetite* **2015**, *95*, 349–359. [CrossRef] [PubMed]
12. Dubois, L.; Farmer, A.; Girard, M.; Peterson, K.; Tatone-Tokuda, F. Problem eating behaviors related to social factors and body weight in preschool children: A longitudinal study. *Int. J. Behav. Nutr. Phys. Act.* **2007**, *4*, 9. [CrossRef] [PubMed]
13. Rivera, J.A.; Hotz, C.; Gonzalez-Cossio, T.; Neufeld, L.; Garcia-Guerra, A. The effect of micronutrient deficiencies on child growth: A review of results from community-based supplementation trials. *J. Nutr.* **2003**, *133*, 4010S–4020S. [PubMed]
14. Nicklas, T.A.; Baranowski, T.; Cullen, K.W.; Berenson, G. Eating Patterns, Dietary Quality and Obesity. *J. Am. Coll. Nutr.* **2001**, *20*, 599–608. [CrossRef] [PubMed]
15. Wardle, J.; Guthrie, C.A.; Sanderson, S.; Rapoport, L. Development of the Children's Eating Behaviour Questionnaire. *J. Child Psychol. Psychiatry* **2001**, *42*, 963–970. [CrossRef] [PubMed]

16. Davies, W.H.; Ackerman, L.K.; Davies, C.M.; Vannatta, K.; Noll, R.B. About Your Child's Eating: Factor structure and psychometric properties of a feeding relationship measure. *Eat. Behav.* **2007**, *8*, 457–463. [CrossRef] [PubMed]

17. Carruth, B.R.; Skinner, J.; Houck, K.; Moran, J.; Coletta, F.; Ott, D. The Phenomenon of "Picky Eater": A Behavioral Marker in Eating Patterns of Toddlers. *J. Am. Coll. Nutr.* **1998**, *17*, 180–186. [CrossRef] [PubMed]

18. Jacobi, C.; Agras, W.S.; Bryson, S.; Hammer, L.D. Behavioral validation, precursors, and concomitants of picky eating in childhood. *J. Am. Acad. Child. Adolesc. Psychiatry* **2003**, *42*, 76–84. [CrossRef] [PubMed]

19. Shim, J.E.; Kim, J.; Mathai, R.A.; Team, S.K.R. Associations of infant feeding practices and picky eating behaviors of preschool children. *J. Am. Diet. Assoc.* **2011**, *111*, 1363–1368. [CrossRef] [PubMed]

20. Galloway, A.T.; Lee, Y.; Birch, L.L. Predictors and consequences of food neophobia and pickiness in young girls. *J. Am. Diet. Assoc.* **2003**, *103*, 692–698. [CrossRef] [PubMed]

21. Van der Horst, K. Overcoming picky eating. Eating enjoyment as a central aspect of children's eating behaviors. *Appetite* **2012**, *58*, 567–574. [CrossRef] [PubMed]

22. Dovey, T.M.; Staples, P.A.; Gibson, E.L.; Halford, J.C. Food neophobia and "picky/fussy" eating in children: A review. *Appetite* **2008**, *50*, 181–193. [CrossRef] [PubMed]

23. Shim, J.E.; Yoon, J.H.; Kim, K.; Paik, H.Y. Association between picky eating behaviors and growth in preschool children. *J. Nutr. Health* **2013**, *46*, 418. [CrossRef]

24. Fisher, J.O.; Butte, N.F.; Mendoza, P.M.; Wilson, T.A.; Hodges, E.A.; Reidy, K.C.; Deming, D. Overestimation of infant and toddler energy intake by 24-h recall compared with weighed food records. *Am. J. Clin. Nutr.* **2008**, *88*, 407–415. [PubMed]

25. Jung, H.J.; Han, S.N.; Song, S.; Paik, H.Y.; Baik, H.W.; Joung, H. Association between adherence to the Korean Food Guidance System and the risk of metabolic abnormalities in Koreans. *Nutr. Res. Pract.* **2011**, *5*, 560–568. [CrossRef] [PubMed]

26. Jung, H.J.; Lee, S.N.; Kim, D.; Noh, H.; Song, S.; Kang, M.; Song, Y.J.; Paik, H.Y. Improvement in the technological feasibility of a web-based dietary survey system in local settings. *Asia Pac. J. Clin. Nutr.* **2015**, *24*, 308–315. [PubMed]

27. Rural Development Administration. *Studies on Developing the Software Program for Dietary Evaluation in Rural Area*; Rural Development Administration: Suwon, Korea, 2000; pp. 383–454. (In Korean)

28. Korea Centers for Disease Control and Prevention. *Development of Open-Ended Dietary Assessment System for Korean Genetic Epidemiological Cohorts*; Korea Centers for Disease Control and Prevention: Suwon, Korea, 2008. (In Korean)

29. Group WHOMGRS. WHO Child Growth Standards based on length/height, weight and age. *Acta Paediatr.* **2006**, *95*, 76–85.

30. De Onis, M.; Onyango, A.W.; Borghi, E.; Siyam, A.; Nishida, C.; Siekmann, J. Development of a WHO growth reference for school-aged children and adolescents. *Bull. World Health Org.* **2007**, *85*, 660–667. [CrossRef] [PubMed]

31. Gartner, L.M.; Morton, J.; Lawrence, R.A; Naylor, A.J.; O'Hare, D.; Schanler, R.J.; Eidelman, A.I. American Academy of Pediatrics Section on Breastfeeding. Breastfeeding and the use of human milk. *Pediatrics* **2005**, *115*, 496–506. [PubMed]

32. Margetts, B.M.; Nelson, M. Overview of the principles of nutritional epidemiology. In *Design Concepts in Nutritional Epidemiology*; Margetts, B.M., Nelson, M., Eds.; Oxford University Press: New York, NY, USA, 1997; pp. 3–38.

33. Lewinsohn, P.M.; Holm-Denoma, J.M.; Gau, J.M.; Joiner, T.E.; Striegel-Moore, R.; Bear, P.; Lamoureux, B. Problematic eating and feeding behaviors of 36-month-old children. *Int. J. Eat. Disord.* **2005**, *38*, 208–219. [CrossRef] [PubMed]

34. Wright, C.M.; Parkinson, K.N.; Drewett, R.F. How does maternal and child feeding behavior relate to weight gain and failure to thrive? Data from a prospective birth cohort. *Pediatrics* **2006**, *117*, 1262–1269. [CrossRef] [PubMed]

35. Russell, C.G.; Worsley, A. A population-based study of preschoolers' food neophobia and its associations with food preferences. *J. Nutr. Educ. Behav.* **2008**, *40*, 11–19. [CrossRef] [PubMed]

36. Cooke, L.; Wardle, J.; Gibson, E.L. Relationship between parental report of food neophobia and everyday food consumption in 2–6-year-old children. *Appetite* **2003**, *41*, 205–206. [CrossRef]

37.　Addessi, E.; Galloway, A.T.; Visalberghi, E.; Birch, L.L. Specific social influences on the acceptance of novel foods in 2–5-year-old children. *Appetite* **2005**, *45*, 264–271. [CrossRef] [PubMed]

38.　Koivisto, U.K.; Sjoden, P.G. Reasons for rejection of food items in Swedish families with children aged 2–17. *Appetite* **1996**, *26*, 89–103. [CrossRef] [PubMed]

14

Advising Consumption of Green Vegetables, Beef and Full-Fat Dairy Products has no Adverse Effects on the Lipid Profiles in Children

Ellen José van der Gaag [1,*], **Romy Wieffer** [2] **and Judith van der Kraats** [1]

[1]   Ziekenhuisgroep Twente, Hengelo, Geerdinksweg 141, Hengelo 7555 DL, The Netherlands;
      e.gaagvander@zgt.nl (E.J.v.d.G.); judithvanderkraats@hotmail.com (J.v.d.K.)
[2]   Isala Zwolle, Dokter van Heesweg 2, Zwolle 8025 AB, The Netherlands; romywieffer@gmail.com
*   Correspondence: e.gaagvander@zgt.nl

Abstract: In children, little is known about lipid profiles and the influence of dietary habits. In the past, we developed a dietary advice for optimizing the immune system, which comprised green vegetables, beef, whole milk, and full-fat butter. However, there are concerns about a possible negative influence of the full-fat dairy products of the diet on the lipid profile. We investigated the effect of the developed dietary advice on the lipid profile and BMI (body mass index)/BMI-z-score of children. In this retrospective cohort study, we included children aged 1–16 years, of whom a lipid profile was determined in the period between June 2011 and November 2013 in our hospital. Children who adhered to the dietary advice were assigned to the exposed group and the remaining children were assigned to the unexposed group. After following the dietary advice for at least three months, there was a statistically significant reduction in the cholesterol/HDL (high-density lipoproteins) ratio ($p < 0.001$) and non-HDL-cholesterol ($p = 0.044$) and a statistically significant increase in the HDL-cholesterol ($p = 0.009$) in the exposed group, while there was no difference in the BMI and BMI z-scores. The dietary advice has no adverse effect on the lipid profile, BMI, and BMI z-scores in children, but has a significant beneficial effect on the cholesterol/HDL ratio, non-HDL-cholesterol, and the HDL-cholesterol.

Keywords: children; dietary advice; full-fat dairy products; green vegetables; beef; cholesterol; lipid profile; BMI; cardiovascular risk factors

1. Introduction

Little is known about cholesterol and lipid profiles in children, except from children known to have familiar dyslipidemia. However, concerns about the cholesterol levels are troubling parents when doctors advise to give full-fat dairy products to their children. Are these concerns realistic or not? At this moment, adult recommendations are also used for children.

There are circumstances when full-fat dairy products are investigated for their possible positive contribution to different health aspects in children. One aspect is the functioning of the immune system, which is partly dependent on the nutritional status. Nutrients, such as vitamins and minerals, play an important role in the strengthening of the immune system. As a consequence, an adequate nutritional status, and thereby a strong immune system, might prevent infections [1–7].

In a previous study, we compared the dietary intake of children with recurrent respiratory infection (without immunological disorders) and healthy children [8]. These children usually have respiratory complaints without an adequate explanation, like immunological deficiencies. The outcomes showed that the group of children with recurrent infections eats less beef, natural milk, and green vegetables compared to the healthy children.

Following this study, a nutrient-rich diet has been developed as a possible intervention for recurrent infections using the NEVO (Nederlands Voedingsstoffenbestand) tables, a Dutch nutrient database containing information about the nutrients of each food [9]. There are more international databases containing macro and micronutrients. We choose this database because this database contains the most information about the regular food that is eaten and sold in The Netherlands.

The diet is based on foods high in nutrients that could support the immune system, namely green vegetables, beef, whole milk, and butter (Table 1). This are also the food groups that are not frequently consumed by children with recurrent infections. Compared to other vegetables, green vegetables contain more zinc, vitamin A, and vitamin C. Beef contains more iron, zinc, vitamin A and vitamin E compared with other types of meat [9]. These nutrients have immune supporting effects and play a role in the antiviral mechanisms, which could positively affect recurrent upper respiratory tract infections [2–7]. Looking at the full-fat dairy products, whole milk, and butter are a source of lipids, vitamins, and essential fatty acids, such as linoleic acid and alpha-linolenic acid [9]. The lipids can act as a carrier for vitamins A, D, E, and K, [10] which can have a positive effect on the immune system [9,10]. In addition, the extra fats in whole milk have anti-microbial properties and can act as bacteriostatics [9,11].

Table 1. Nutrients in food products of the dietary advice compared to other food products (according to the NEVO tables [9]).

Food Product	Nutrients per 100 Grams									
	Vitamin A (ug)	Vitamin D (ug)	Vitamin E (mg)	Iron (mg)	Zinc (mg)	Calorie (kcal)	Saturated Fats (g)	Total Unsaturated Fats (g)	N-3 Fats (g)	Linoleic Acid (N-6 fat) (g)
Spinach cooked	652	-	3.5	2.4	1.20	25	0.1	0.7	0.5	0.1
Broccoli cooked	116	-	2.5	0.9	0.62	27	0.1	0.2	0.1	-
Cauliflower cooked	0	-	0.1	0.3	0.26	23	0.1	0.2	0.2	-
Chicory cooked	1	-	0.2	0.2	0.17	17	-	0.1	-	0.1
Beef > 10% fat	68	0.5	2.4	2.8	5.84	277	6.2	10.5	0.2	2.9
Chicken breast	18	0.1	1.1	0.7	0.74	158	1.4	1.8	0.1	0.8
Pork 10%–19% fat	25	0.6	1.1	1.0	2.65	378	5.4	10.1	0.2	3.2
Butter	903	1.2	2.5	0.1	0.09	737	52.9	19.9	0.5	1.3
Margarine	800	7.5	9.5	0.1	-	349	8.5	34.5	5.9	19
Whole milk	36	-	0.1	-	0.46	62	2.2	0.8	-	0.1
Skimmed milk	1	-	-	-	0.46	35	0.1	-	-	-
Adequate intake or recommended dietary allowance/day for children [12,13]	♂/♀ 2–5 years: 350 ug	♂/♀ 4–8 years: 10 ug	♂/♀ 2–5 years: 5 mg	♂/♀ 2–5 years: 8 mg	♂/♀ 2–5 years: 6 mg	4–8 years: ♂1720 kcal ♀1552 kcal	♂/♀ 4–8 years: 10 En%	♂/♀ all ages: 8–38 En%	♂/♀ 4–8 years: 0.15–0.2 g	♂/♀ 4–8 years: 2 En%

This previous study showed that the dietary advice had significant positive effects on the length and gravity of respiratory tract infections in children [14]. Furthermore, another study showed that the same dietary advice decreases some symptoms of medically unresolved fatigue in children [1,15].

Strengthening the immune system just by changing food habits might be a solution for many patients with recurrent infections but without an immunological disorder or for patients with medically unresolved fatigue. However, there are thoughts that the saturated fats in the recommended whole milk and butter could have a negative influence on the lipid profile and/or the risk of cardiovascular disease. The National Heart Foundation of Australia states that the intake of saturated fatty acids is highly associated with an increased risk of coronary heart disease due to elevated LDL-cholesterol (low-density lipoproteins cholesterol) and serum cholesterol levels [16]. The American Heart Association (AHA) and American Academy of Pediatrics advise the use of dairy products that are fat-free or low in fat, in order to minimize the intake of saturated fat. They mention that a decline in saturated fat and cholesterol intake has been associated with a reduction in cardiovascular disease [17]. The Dutch Centre of Food recommends replacing saturated fats with unsaturated fats, which should lower the risk of cardiovascular disease [18].

Recently, conflicting findings have been reported regarding the association of saturated fats and the risk of cardiovascular disease. Several studies show no evidence for the assumed association and some even describe an inverse association [19–21].

The aim of our study was to determine whether the developed dietary advice—relatively high in saturated fats—has an influence on the BMI (body mass index) of children and on risk factors of cardiovascular disease. The total cholesterol/HDL (high-density lipoproteins) ratio is an important predictor of later risk of cardiovascular disease [22,23]. Additionally, the American Academy of Pediatrics recommends non-HDL concentration as an important benchmark for the screening of cardiovascular risk in children [24]. Therefore, we used the lipid profile of children in order to determine whether the dietary advice with its beneficial effect on at least respiratory tract infections in children can be safely used.

2. Materials and Methods

The present study is a non-randomized retrospective cohort study. The determination of the lipid profile of the children was executed by blinded laboratory workers. The measurements of weight and height were not blindly executed.

We performed a laboratory search in our laboratory database for patient blood samples. Included in the search were children aged from 1 to 16 years with at least two measurements of a lipid profile in the period between June 2011 and November 2013 at hospital ZGT (Hospital Group Twente) Hengelo/Almelo in the Netherlands. Patient charts were hand-searched for dietary habits/advice. If no details were given in the patient charts, dietary habits were addressed as unknown. When no abnormalities were noted, we assumed it was according to the Dutch dietary guidelines [12]. Children who had followed the dietary advice were assigned to the exposed group and the remaining children were assigned to the unexposed group. A schematic overview of the data collection is shown in Figure 1.

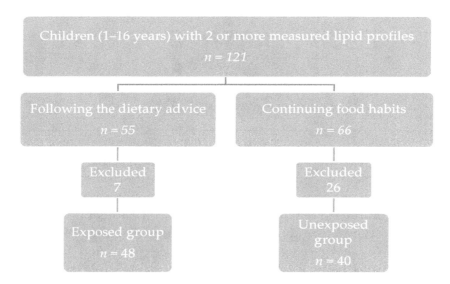

Figure 1. Schematic overview of the data collection.

We excluded all children with a disorder that might influence the lipid profile, such as familiar hypercholesterolemia, hypothyroidism, diabetes mellitus type I and II, obesity, metabolic disorders, and medication which influences the lipid profile (according to [25]). As shown in Table 2, in the exposed group six patients were excluded based on the exclusion criteria described above, and one patient withdrew informed consent. Following the exclusion criteria, 26 patients were excluded in the unexposed group.

Table 2. Overview of the excluded patients.

Exposed Group	(n = 55)	Unexposed Group	(n = 66)
Incomplete lipid profile	2	Incomplete lipid profile	5
Familiar hypercholesterolemia	2	Familiar hypercholesterolemia	3
Obesity	1	Obesity	13
Age < 1 year or > 16 years	1	Age < 1 year or > 16 years	1
Diabetes mellitus	0	Diabetes mellitus	3
Metabolic disorder	0	Metabolic disorder	1
Medication	0	Medication	0
Dropouts	1	Dropouts	0
Exposed group	(n = 48)	Unexposed group	(n = 40)

The children visited the pediatric outpatient clinic for several complaints. In the exposed group, most of them suffered from recurrent infections, subclinical hypothyroidism or tiredness. The unexposed group consisted of children with recurrent infections, abdominal complaints, epilepsy, failure to thrive, behavioral disorders.

The dietary advice, based on the NEVO tables [9], consists of eating beef three times a week, green vegetables five times a week (both age-related portions, according to the Dutch Center of Food), at least one glass (200 mL) of full-fat milk (3.4% fat) each day, and the use of five grams per slice of bread of natural butter (80% fat) for at least three months. Each item of the advice counted for 25% and children had to score at least 75% to meet the criteria of the exposed group. All other dietary habits remained unchanged. The children who did not follow the dietary advice were included in the unexposed group. For ethical reasons we were not allowed to approach them and had to assume that there were no large changes in their food habits during the period of follow-up.

We recorded information of all children from both groups: gender, age, weight, height, duration, and degree of following the dietary advice, lipid profile at the time of presentation, and follow-up.

The height of the children was measured with a vertical ruler. The children were weighed in underwear and all measurements were performed by a pediatrician. The children's BMI was calculated by dividing their weight in kilograms by the square of their height in meters. The BMI z-score is calculated on the basis of gender, age, height, and weight [26]. The BMI z-score can be calculated only from the age of 24 months. This means that no BMI z-score was calculated in children younger than two years. These data were calculated, but not added in the tables, due to lacking data in the younger children.

Both for the start of the dietary advice, and at the end of the follow-up, the lipid profile was determined in all children. At the time of blood collection by venapuncture the children had an empty stomach, as nutrition can affect LDL and triglyceride concentrations [27]. The lipids from the lipid profile are total cholesterol, high-density lipoprotein cholesterol (HDL-C), cholesterol/HDL ratio, low-density lipoprotein cholesterol (LDL-C), triglycerides (TG), and non-HDL. The lipid profile was measured by enzymatic colorimetric techniques with the COBAS 6000 (Roche Diagnostics, Almere, The Netherlands). The LDL was calculated with Friedewald's formula: LDL = total cholesterol − HDL − (0.45 × TG). The primary outcome of this study, the cholesterol/HDL ratio, was calculated by dividing the total cholesterol by HDL cholesterol [23]. The non-HDL can be calculated by the following formula: total cholesterol − HDL cholesterol = non-HDL cholesterol (non-HDL).

We used SPSS Statistics 20 (SPSS Inc., Chicago, IL, USA) to execute our data analysis. Normality was checked by visual expectation of histograms and Shapiro-Wilk test. Continuous variables were expressed as the mean with the standard deviation (SD) or the median with the interquartile range (IQR); categorical variables were expressed as counts with corresponding percentages. Differences in baseline characteristics between groups was tested using an independent t-test or Mann-Whitney (continuous variables) or Pearson's chi-square (categorical). To test changes of the lipid profile between measurements within each group a paired T-test or Wilcoxon was used. Concerning the BMI and

BMI z-score, several data were lacking. Therefore, the BMI and BMI z-scores were tested using mixed models analysis. For all comparisons, a p-value ≤ 0.05 was regarded as significant.

3. Results

3.1. Baseline Data

The baseline data of the unexposed and exposed group are presented in Table 3. The demographic characteristics, period of follow-up, the lipid profiles, and the BMI characteristics did not differ significantly at the start of this study.

Table 3. Baseline characteristics of the unexposed and exposed group.

Characteristic	Unexposed Group $n = 40$	Exposed Group $n = 48$	p-Value
Gender (n, %)MenWomen	24 (60%) 16 (40%)	25 (52%) 23 (48%)	0.457
Age (years) (median, IQR)	4.7 (2.3–9.0)	2.6 (1.6–8.0)	0.102
Follow-up (months)(median, IQR)	5.0 (4.0–8.0)	4.5 (4.0–8.8)	0.744
BMI (median, IQR)	15.9 (15.1–17.5)	16.7 (15.4–18.5)	0.408

IQR (interquartile range); SD (standard deviation).

3.2. Changes within Groups

The baseline, follow up and differences in lipid profile within the two groups between the start and follow-up are shown in Table 4. In the exposed group, the HDL-cholesterol increased significantly with 0.14 mmol/L ($p = 0.009$), 95% CI (-0.24 to -0.04) (confidence interval). The cholesterol/HDL ratio was significantly reduced ($p < 0.001$), 95% CI (0.35–0.84), as was the non-HDL ($p = 0.044$), 95% CI (0.01–0.34). The decrease in the cholesterol/HDL is caused by the significant increase in the HDL-cholesterol. The total cholesterol did not change significantly and barely affects the cholesterol/HDL ratio. No significant changes occurred in the BMI and BMI z-score (a change of -0.06) in the exposed group. There were no significant changes of the lipid profile or BMI and BMI z-score (change of 0.09) in the unexposed group.

Table 4. Changes in lipid profile and BMI of both groups between the start and end of follow-up.

Measurements	Unexposed Group $n = 40$				Exposed Group $n = 48$			
	Baseline	Follow-up	Change (95%-CI/IQR))	p-Value	Baseline	Follow-up	Change (95%-CI)	p-Value
Total cholesterol (mmol/L) (median, IQR)	4.05 (3.83–4.70)	4.20 (3.70–4.68)	-0.06 [a] (-0.11–0.22)	0.581 [d]	4.20 (3.5–5.0)	4.35 (3.7–4.7)	-0.03 [a] (-0.25–0.18)	0.738 [c]
HDL-cholesterol (mmol/L) (median, IQR)	1.35 (0.93–1.59)	1.30 (0.95–1.57)	-0.01 [b] (-0.19–0.12)	0.842 [c]	1.17 (0.88–1.48)	1.35 (1.12–1.53)	0.14 [a] (0.04–0.24)	0.009 [d]
Cholesterol/HDL (mmol/L) (median, IQR)	3.45 (2.57–4.70)	3.40 (2.53–4.45)	0,00 [b] (-0.35–0.38)	0.883 [d]	3.75 (3.00–4.95)	3.15 (2.80–4.95)	-0.30 [b] (-1.2–0.17)	< 0.001 [c]
Triglycerides (mmol/L) (median, IQR)	0.96 (0.70–1.93)	1.00 (0.80–1.47)	0.05 [b] (-0.38–0.30)	0.821 [d]	1.10 (0.80–1.67)	1.05 (0.80–1.50)	-0.07 [a] (-0.31–0.16)	0.469 [d]
LDL-cholesterol (mmol/L) (median, IQR)	2.30 (2.00–2.80)	2.30 (1.90–2.88)	0.00 [a] (-0.15–0.13)	0.852 [c]	2.55 (1.70–3.00)	2.40 (1.93–2.80)	-0.10 [b] (-0.60–0.30)	0.384 [c]
Non-HDL cholesterol (mmol/L) (median, IQR)	3.01 (2.54–3.49)	2.83 (2.40–3.39)	-0.06 [a] (-0.21–0.08)	0.384 [c]	3.14 (2.56–3.61)	2.98 (2.45–3.28)	-0.17 [a] (-0.34–-0.01)	0.044 [d]
BMI (median, IQR)	15.9 (15.1–17.5)	15.8 (15.1–17.5)	0.24 [a] (-0.05-0.54)	0.178 [d]	16.7 (15.4–18.5)	16.0 (14.9–18.0)	0.00 [b] (-0.63–0.30)	0.719 [d]

[a] Normally distributed (mean, 95% CI); [b] non-normally distributed (median, IQR); [c] paired t-test; [d] Wilcoxon signed rank test.

4. Discussion

Our research shows that consumption of green vegetables, beef, whole milk, and butter has no adverse effect on the lipid profile in children. The dietary advice, no advice with respect to carbohydrate intake, but relatively high in saturated fats is even shown to have a favorable effect on the lipid profile: it gave a significant increase in HDL cholesterol, and a decrease in non-HDL cholesterol and the cholesterol/HDL ratio.

In a previous study the dietary advice has been shown to have a significant improving effect on the incidence and duration of recurrent respiratory tract infections [15]. This nutritional advice will probably be discouraged by major national and international organizations since the idea exists that saturated fats have a negative effect on the lipid profile and/or the cholesterol/HDL ratio and, thus, increases the risk of cardiovascular disease.

The American Heart Association and the American Academy of Pediatrics recommend not offering any whole-milk products to children, because of the higher concentrations of saturated fats and, therefore, the increased risk of later cardiovascular disease [17]. The Dutch Nutrition Centre recommends that children should not eat full-fat products at all, due to the relatively high concentration of saturated fats. According to the nutrition center the intake of saturated fats has a negative impact on the cholesterol/HDL ratio and, therefore, increases the risk of cardiovascular disease [18].

Over the years, various studies have been published discussing the relationship between saturated fatty acids and cardiovascular disease. The idea that consuming saturated fats can lead to death from cardiovascular disease has certainly not been confirmed by all studies. A meta-analysis of randomized trials showed that saturated fat has an increasing effect on HDL cholesterol. The increase in the HDL-cholesterol is greater when consuming saturated fats, compared to consuming unsaturated fats [28], which can contribute to a decrease in total cholesterol/HDL cholesterol ratio [29]. *The Lancet* published a systematic review of 61 prospective studies, which showed that higher HDL cholesterol levels reduce the risk of death from cardiovascular disease [30].

Contrary to expectations, a large meta-analysis by Siri-Tarino and colleagues shows that there is no significant link between the consumption of saturated fats and an increased risk of cardiovascular disease in general and coronary heart disease in particular [20]. In line with this, a meta-analysis by Skeaf and Miller commissioned by the World Health Organization concluded that the amount of saturated fats in a diet does not have an impact on the risk of coronary heart disease [31]. The American Heart Association claims that replacing saturated fat with carbohydrates lowers the risk of cardiovascular disease. In contrast, a meta-analysis of prospective studies shows that replacing saturated fat with carbohydrates leads to a significantly increased risk of cardiovascular disease [32]. This is supported by Musunuru, who concluded that it is not the saturated fats, but the carbohydrates in a diet that cause atherogenic dyslipidemia [33].

Next to the inconsistent data about dairy fats and cardiovascular risk factors, there are also inconsistent data about the risk of dairy fat on developing diabetes mellitus. A recent study from the Nurses' Health Study and the Health Professionals Follow-Up Study show a protective effect of high plasma dairy fatty acid concentrations and lower incidence of diabetes mellitus [34].

As an alternative to butter with its saturated fats, margarine was developed. This "skinny" dairy product is enriched with "healthy" omega-6 fatty acids. However, the replacement of saturated fatty acids and trans-fatty acids by omega-6 fatty acids is associated with an increased risk of coronary heart disease and overall mortality [35]. We now know that omega-6 fatty acids have pro-inflammatory characteristics while omega-3 fatty acids have anti-inflammatory ones. A diet with a large amount of omega-6 fatty acids and a high omega-6/omega-3 ratio enhances the development of diseases such as cancer, cardiovascular disease, inflammatory and autoimmune diseases. In contrast, high levels of omega-3 fatty acids have suppressive effects on those diseases [36]. The investigated dietary advice contributes to a good fatty-acid balance due to its green vegetables, which contain a relatively high amount of omega-3 fatty acids and are low in omega-6 fatty acids [9]. Recently, a study showed that people who eat a lot of green leafy vegetables have a 32% lower risk of myocardial infarction [37]. In addition, green vegetables have other positive effects concerning health, such as reducing the risk of many forms of cancer [38,39]. Additionally, the dietary advice contributes to the inhibition of oxidation of LDL cholesterol, a crucial step in atherosclerosis, with its relatively high levels of Vitamin A and E in beef, compared to other types of meat [40].

The BMI and BMI z-scores in the exposed group did not significantly change during the months of follow-up. If we calculate the caloric intake of the dietary advice, using age-adequate quantities advised by the Dutch Food Center [12], the diet contains 94 more calories compared to a diet with identical quantities of low-fat milk and margarine [9]. By contrast, beef contains 1.5 times fewer calories compared to, for example, pork, which has 82 calories per serving [9,41]. This almost neutralizes the extra calories ingested by a child with the intake of whole milk and butter. Additionally, whole milk has a favorable glycemic control and, thereby, possibly an inhibitory effect on appetite and food intake [42]. Several investigations show that a higher intake of dairy products does not increase body weight, results that are consistent with the results of our study [43,44].

This study suggests that diet quality can have some benefits for children. However, one of the limitations of this study is the retrospective design. Adherence to the dietary advice was retrospectively controlled through evaluative questions during the consultation with the pediatrician. A more reliable way of checking the nutritional advice is to let patients fill out a daily food questionnaire.

Due to the retrospective design the food habits of the unexposed group could not all be traced. In this case we had to assume that they did not consume full fat dairy (in The Netherlands semi-skimmed milk and low-fat butter are advised) and no changes in diet occurred during follow-up. In a research design such as a randomized controlled trial, the unexposed group could also fill out a food questionnaire so that any changes in diet can be detected.

Following the retrospective design of this study the unexposed and exposed group could not be randomized. A probable advantage is that the patients (and/or their parents) in the exposed group were possibly more motivated to follow the diet given the fact that they chose to follow the diet themselves.

There were missing values in the BMI and, thereby, the BMI z-scores of the children, so that the conclusions of BMI and BMI z-score are based on a smaller number of patients than we included. Furthermore, the mean period of follow-up was 4.4 months, which means that we cannot draw conclusions about these outcomes in the long term. We require long-term follow-up studies to evaluate the course of the lipid profile.

5. Conclusions

This retrospective study shows diet quality in childhood can have some useful benefits. Earlier, it was shown that a dietary advice of green vegetables, beef, whole milk, and full-fat butter reduces the number of days with a respiratory tract infection in children. In this study we have shown that the dietary advice has no adverse effect on the lipid profile, BMI, and BMI z-score in children. Conversely, the dietary advice has a significant beneficial effect on the HDL-cholesterol, cholesterol/HDL ratio, and non-HDL-cholesterol. The dietary advice can, therefore, be safely recommended and might be beneficial for children with recurrent respiratory tract infections. However, the findings of this retrospective study should be further investigated in randomized controlled trials.

Acknowledgments: The authors would like to thank van der Palen (epidemiologist) and Josien Timmerman with their help with the statistical analysis.

Author Contributions: Ellen van der Gaag was responsible for the study design, implementation of the study and writing. Romy Wieffer conducted the data interpretation, literature research, and writing. Judith van der Kraats collected and analyzed the data and performed the literature research. All authors designed the approach, commented, edited, and approved the paper, and are responsible for the final version of the paper.

References

1. Field, C.J.; Johnson, I.R.; Schley, P.D. Nutrients and their role in host resistance to infection. *J. Leukocyte Biol.* **2002**, *71*, 16–32. [PubMed]
2. Jimenez, C.; Leets, I.; Puche, R.; Anzola, E.; Montilla, R.; Parra, C.; Aguilera, A.; Garcia-Casal, M.N. A single dose of vitamin A improves haemoglobin concentration, retinol status and phagocytic function of neutrophils in preschool children. *Brit. J. Nutr.* **2010**, *103*, 798–802. [CrossRef] [PubMed]
3. Maggini, S.; Wenzlaff, S.; Hornig, D. Essential role of vitamin C and zinc in child immunity and health. *J. Int. Med. Res.* **2010**, *38*, 386–414. [CrossRef] [PubMed]
4. Prasad, A.S. Zinc: Role in immunity, oxidative stress and chronic inflammation. *Curr. Opin. Clin. Nutr.* **2009**, *12*, 646–652. [CrossRef] [PubMed]
5. Wintergerst, E.S.; Maggini, S.; Hornig, D.H. Immune-enhancing role of vitamin C and zinc and effect on clinical conditions. *Ann. Nutr. Metab.* **2006**, *50*, 85–94. [CrossRef] [PubMed]
6. Cherayil, B.J. Iron and immunity: Immunological consequences of iron deficiency and overload. *Arch. Immunol. Ther. Exp.* **2010**, *58*, 407–415. [CrossRef] [PubMed]
7. Ekiz, C.; Agaoglu, L.; Karakas, Z.; Gurel, N.; Yalcin, I. The effect of iron deficiency anemia on the function of the immune system. *Hematol. J.* **2005**, *5*, 579–583. [CrossRef] [PubMed]
8. Munow, M.; van der Gaag, E.J. Ailing Toddlers: Is There a Relation between Behavior and Health? Book of Abstracts 27th Annual Meeting of the European Society for Pediatric Infectious Diseases; 2009; p. 764. Available online: http://www.scirp.org/%28S%28351jmbntvnsjt1aadkposzje%29%29/reference/ReferencesPapers.aspx?ReferenceID=962833 (accessed on 18 May 2017).
9. National Institute for Public Health and the Environment (RIVM)/the Kingdom of the Netherlands. Dutch Food Composition Database 2014. Available online: http://nevo-online.rivm.nl/ (accessed on 12 May 2014).
10. German, J.B. Dietary lipids from an evolutionary perspective: Sources, structures and functions. *Matern. Child Nutr.* **2011**, *7*, 2–16. [CrossRef] [PubMed]
11. Batovska, D.; Todorova, I.; Tsvetkova, I.; Najdenski, H. Antibacterial study of the medium chain fatty acids and their 1-monoglycerides: Individual effects and synergistic relationships. *Pol. J. Microbiol.* **2009**, *58*, 43–47. [PubMed]
12. Dietary Reference Intakes: Energy, Proteins, Fats and Digestible Carbohydrates. Health Council Neth. Available online: https://www.narcis.nl/publication/RecordID/oai:cris.maastrichtuniversity.nl:publications%2Fdc7e056b-a54d-471d-a496-ec334fd5ad1e (accessed on 13 June 2013).
13. Brink, E.J.; Breedveld, B.C.; Peters, J.A.C. Aanbevelingen Voor Vitamines, Mineralen en Spoorelementen. Factsheet The Netherlands Nutrition Centre. Available online: http://www.voedingscentrum.nl/Assets/Uploads/voedingscentrum/Documents/Professionals/Pers/Factsheets/Factsheet%20Aanbevelingen%20voor%20vitamines,%20mineralen%20en%20spoorelementen.pdf (accessed on 15 December 2016).
14. Ten Velde, L.G.H.; Leegsma, J.; van der Gaag, E.J. Recurrent upper respiratory tract infections in children;the influence of green vegetables, beef, whole milk and butter. *Food Nutr. Sci.* **2013**, *4*, 71–77. [CrossRef]
15. Steenbruggen, T.G.; Hoekstra, S.J.; van der Gaag, E.J. Could a change in diet revitalize children who suffer from unresolved fatigue? *Nutrients* **2015**, *7*, 1965–1977. [CrossRef] [PubMed]
16. Shrapnel, W.S.; Calvert, G.D.; Nestle, P.J.; Truswell, A.S. Diet and coronary heart disease. *Natl. Heart Found. Aust. Med. J. Aust.* **1992**, *156*, S9–S16.
17. Gidding, S.S.; Dennison, B.A.; Birch, L.L.; Daniels, S.R.; Gillman, M.W.; Lichtenstein, A.H.; Rattay, K.T.; Steinberger, J.; Stettler, N.; van Horn, L. Dietary recommendations for children and adolescents: A guide for practitioners. *Pediatrics* **2006**, *117*, 544–559. [CrossRef] [PubMed]
18. The Netherlands Nutrition Centre. Verzadigd vet. Available online: http://www.voedingscentrum.nl/encyclopedie/verzadigd-vet.aspx (accessed on 15 May 2016).
19. Muskiet, F.A.J.; Muskiet, M.H.A.; Kuipers, R.S. Het faillissement van de verzadigd vethypothese van cardiovasculaire ziektes. *Ned. Tijdschr. Klin. Chem. Labgeneesk* **2012**, *37*, 192–211. (In Dutch).
20. Siri-Tarino, P.W.; Sun, Q.; Hu, F.B.; Krauss, R.M. Meta-analysis of prospective cohort studies evaluating the association of saturated fat with cardiovascular disease. *Am. J. Clin. Nutr.* **2010**, *91*, 535–546. [CrossRef] [PubMed]

21. Kratz, M.; Baars, T.; Guyenet, S. The relationship between high-fat dairy consumption and obesity, cardiovascular, and metabolic disease. *Eur. J. Nutr.* **2013**, *52*, 1–24. [CrossRef] [PubMed]

22. Kinosian, B.; Glick, H.; Garland, G. Cholesterol and coronary heart disease predicting risks by levels and ratios. *Ann. Intern. Med.* **1994**, *121*, 641–647. [CrossRef] [PubMed]

23. The Netherlands Nutrition Centre. Cholesterol. Available online: http://www.voedingscentrum.nl/encyclopedie/cholesterol.aspx (accessed on 16 May 2016).

24. Department of Health and Human Services. National Heart Lung and Blood Institute. Expert Panel on Integrated Guidelines for Cardiovascular Health and Risk Reduction in Children and Adolescents. Available online: https://www.nhlbi.nih.gov/files/docs/guidelines/peds_guidelines_full.pdf (accessed on 15 January 2017).

25. The Netherlands National Health Care Institute. Farmacotherapeutisch kompas. Available online: https://www.farmacotherapeutischkompas.nl/ (accessed on 5 January 2014).

26. U.S. Department of Health and Human Services. National Center for Health Statistics, Z-Score Data Files. Available online: https://www.cdc.gov/growthcharts/zscore.htm (accessed on 14 February 2014).

27. Kubo, T.; Takahashi, K.; Furujo, M.; Hyodo, Y.; Tsuchiya, H.; Hattori, M.; Fujinaga, S.; Urayama, K. Usefulness of non-fasting lipid parameters in children. *J. Pediatr. Endocr. Metab.* **2017**, *30*, 77–83. [CrossRef] [PubMed]

28. Mensink, R.P.; Zock, P.L.; Kester, A.D.; Katan, M.B. Effects of dietary fatty acids and carbohydrates on the ratio of serum total to HDL cholesterol and on serum lipids and apolipoproteins: A meta-analysis of 60 controlled trials. *Am. J. Clin. Nutr.* **2003**, *77*, 1146–1155. [PubMed]

29. Huth, P.J.; Park, K.M. Influence of dairy product and milk fat consumption on cardiovascular disease risk: A review of the evidence. *Adv. Nutr.* **2012**, *3*, 266–285. [CrossRef] [PubMed]

30. Lewington, S.; Whitlock, G.; Clarke, R.; Sherliker, P.; Emberson, J.; Halsey, J.; Qizilbash, N.; Peto, R.; Collins, R. Blood cholesterol and vascular mortality by age, sex, and blood pressure: A meta-analysis of individual data from 61 prospective studies with 55,000 vascular deaths. *Lancet* **2007**, *370*, 1829–1839. [CrossRef] [PubMed]

31. Skeaf, C.M.; Miller, J. Dietary fat and coronary heart disease: Summary of evidence from prospective cohort and randomized controlled trails. *Ann. Nutr. Metab.* **2009**, *55*, 173–201. [CrossRef] [PubMed]

32. Jakobsen, M.U.; O'Reilly, E.J.; Heitmann, B.L.; Pereira, M.A.; Bälter, K.; Fraser, G.E.; Goldbourt, U.; Hallmans, G.; Knekt, P.; Liu, S. Major types of dietary fat and risk of coronary heart disease: A pooled analysis of 11 cohort studies. *Am. J. Clin. Nutr.* **2009**, *89*, 1425–1432. [CrossRef] [PubMed]

33. Musunuru, K. Atherogenic dyslipidemia: Cardiovascular risk and dietary intervention. *Lipids* **2010**, *45*, 907–914. [CrossRef] [PubMed]

34. Yakoob, M.Y.; Shi, P.; Willet, W.C.; Rexrode, K.M.; Campos, H.; Orav, E.J.; Hu, F.B.; Mozaffarian, D. Circulating Biomarkers of dairy fat and risk of incident diabetes mellitus among men and women in the United States in two large prospective cohorts. *Circulation* **2016**, *133*, 1645–1654. [CrossRef] [PubMed]

35. Ramsden, C.E.; Hibbeln, J.R.; Majchrzak, S.F.; Davis, J.M. N-6 fatty acid-specific and mixed polyunsaturate dietary interventions have different effects on CHD risk: A meta-analysis of randomised controlled trials. *Brit. J. Nutr.* **2010**, *104*, 1586–1600. [CrossRef] [PubMed]

36. Simopoulos, A.P. The importance of the Omega-6/Omega-3 fatty-acid ratio in cardiovascular disease and other chronic diseases. *Exp. Biol. Med.* **2008**, *233*, 674–688. [CrossRef] [PubMed]

37. Ahmed, F. Health: Edible advice. *Nature* **2010**, *468*, S10–S12. [CrossRef] [PubMed]

38. Cohen, J.H.; Kristal, A.R.; Standford, J.L. Fruit and vegetable intakes and prostate cancer risk. *J. Natl. Cancer Inst.* **2000**, *92*, 61–68. [CrossRef]

39. Ambrosone, C.B.; McCann, S.E.; Freudenheim, J.L.; Marshall, J.R.; Zhang, Y.; Shields, P.G. Breast cancer risk in premenopausal women is inversely associated with consumption of broccoli, a source of isothiocyanates, but is not modified by GST genotype. *J. Nutr.* **2004**, *134*, 1134–1138. [PubMed]

40. Zhang, P.Y.; Xu, X.; Li, X.C. Cardiovascular diseases: Oxidative damage and antioxidant protection. *Eur. Rev. Med. Pharmacol. Sci.* **2014**, *18*, 3091–3096. [PubMed]

41. The Netherlands Nutrition Centre. Hoeveel en wat kan ik per dag eten? Available online: http://www.voedingscentrum.nl/nl/schijf-van-vijf/eet-niet-teveel-en-beweeg/hoe-eet-ik-niet-te-veel.aspx (accessed on 21 March 2014).

42. Haug, A.; Høstmark, A.T.; Harstad, O.M. Bovine milk in human nutrition—A review. *Lipids Health Dis.* **2007**, *6*, 25. [CrossRef] [PubMed]

43. Snijder, M.B.; van der Heijden, A.A.W.A.; van Dam, R.M.; Stehouwer, C.D.A.; Hiddink, G.J.; Nijpels, G.; Heine, R.J.; Bouter, L.M.; Dekker, J.M. Is higher dairy consumption associated with lower body weight and fewer metabolic disturbances? *Am. J. Clin. Nutr.* **2007**, *85*, 989–995. [PubMed]

44. Rautiainen, S.; Wang, L.; Lee, I.M.; Manson, J.E.; Buring, J.E.; Sesso, H.D. Dairy consumption in association with weight change and risk of becoming overweight or obese in middle-aged and older woman: A prospective cohort study. *Am. J. Clin. Nutr.* **2016**, *103*, 979–988. [CrossRef] [PubMed]

15

A Socio-Ecological Examination of Weight-Related Characteristics of the Home Environment and Lifestyles of Households with Young Children

Virginia Quick [1,*], Jennifer Martin-Biggers [1], Gayle Alleman Povis [2], Nobuko Hongu [2], John Worobey [1] and Carol Byrd-Bredbenner [1]

[1] Department of Nutritional Sciences, Rutgers University, 26 Nichol Avenue, New Brunswick, NJ 08901, USA; jmartin@aesop.rutgers.edu (J.M.-B.); worobey@rci.rutgers.edu (J.W.); bredbenner@aesop.rutgers.edu (C.B.-B.)

[2] Department of Nutritional Sciences, University of Arizona, 406 Shantz Building, 1177 E. 4th Street, Tucson, AZ 85721, USA; gpovis@email.arizona.edu (G.A.P.); hongu@email.arizona.edu (N.H.)

* Correspondence: vquick@njaes.rutgers.edu

Abstract: Home environment and family lifestyle practices have an influence on child obesity risk, thereby making it critical to systematically examine these factors. Thus, parents ($n = 489$) of preschool children completed a cross-sectional online survey which was the baseline data collection conducted, before randomization, in the HomeStyles program. The survey comprehensively assessed these factors using a socio-ecological approach, incorporating intrapersonal, interpersonal and environmental measures. Healthy intrapersonal dietary behaviors identified were parent and child intakes of recommended amounts of 100% juice and low intakes of sugar-sweetened beverages. Unhealthy behaviors included low milk intake and high parent fat intake. The home environment's food supply was found to support healthy intakes of 100% juice and sugar-sweetened beverages, but provided too little milk and ample quantities of salty/fatty snacks. Physical activity levels, sedentary activity and the home's physical activity and media environment were found to be less than ideal. Environmental supports for active play inside homes were moderate and somewhat better in the area immediately outside homes and in the neighborhood. Family interpersonal interaction measures revealed several positive behaviors, including frequent family meals. Parents had considerable self-efficacy in their ability to perform food- and physical activity-related childhood obesity protective practices. This study identified lifestyle practices and home environment characteristics that health educators could target to help parents promote optimal child development and lower their children's risk for obesity.

Keywords: socio-ecological model; home environment; parents; child; nutrition; diet; physical activity; sleep; obesity

1. Introduction

The high prevalence of obesity, especially among young children, continues to be of great public health concern given obesity's long-term negative health effects on child growth, development and lifelong health [1–3]. Research suggests the pervasiveness of obesity is at least partly due to myriad socio-ecological factors that, unlike genetic factors, may be modifiable via public health interventions [4]. The socio-ecological model considers the complex interplay between intrapersonal factors (e.g., values, self-efficacy, outcome expectations), interpersonal factors (e.g., social norms, social support), and environmental factors (e.g., physical environment related to food and physical activity availability and accessibility). Understudied socioecological factors critical to childhood obesity prevention are the weight-related aspects of the home environment and family interpersonal factors and lifestyle patterns [5,6].

The socio-ecological model is a graphic depiction of the ecological theory of a specific health behavior or outcome [4,5]. It illustrates how the health and well-being of an individual is determined by multiple influences that interact at both the macro-level and micro-level environments [7]. At the macro-level, factors such as social norms, economic policies and advertising have a more indirect influence on behaviors. Micro-level factors, such as an individual's physical and social environment (i.e., interpersonal level) and personal factors (i.e., intrapersonal level), more directly influence behaviors. In obesity research, socio-ecological theory is conceptualized as being influenced by factors across multiple levels: individual and family characteristics, and characteristics of the home, community, and region [8]. Environments that do not support healthy weight-management behaviors (e.g., access to safe parks and sidewalks for physical activity) make it difficult for individuals to engage in behaviors that prevent, limit, or reverse weight gain. To date, obesity interventions focused on prevention of weight gain in children under 5 years of age have shown limited effectiveness in reducing or limiting weight gain [9]. A systematic review of obesity prevention interventions among preschool children suggest the failure to show an intervention effect may be partly due to the lack of focus on social and environmental factors within which diet and physical activity behaviors are enacted [10].

The currently available research on the prevention and treatment of obesity among preschool-aged children and adults highlight the importance of considering the environment [11]. The micro-level of the home is the prominent shared environment of parents and their children. Parents act as 'gate keepers' of the home and role models for their children; they strongly influence food and physical activity behaviors and practices that may increase or decrease their child's obesity risk [12–21]. Additionally, physical attributes of the home environment (e.g., availability of healthy foods) and parental behaviors (e.g., parent feeding practices) have been found to be associated with preschool children's weight-related behaviors (e.g., physical activity, dietary patterns) [22]. Prior research has suggested that a number of intra- and inter-personal factors in the home environment are also associated with children's overweight status, such as parent overweight status [23], limited daily physical activity [24], frequent family meals [25], low household availability of fruits and vegetables [26], greater daily television viewing time [25], and less parental modeling of healthy behaviors [27].

Given the home environment (intra- and inter-personal factors) may greatly influence child obesity risk, it is critical to systematically examine these factors. Few studies have comprehensively assessed the home environment and lifestyles of parents of preschool-aged children using a socio-ecological approach with reliable and validated intrapersonal, interpersonal, and environmental measures [28], which are necessary for understanding the potential influencers of obesity risk on families with young children [29]. To expand our understanding, the objective of this study was to utilize a baseline dataset collected prior to randomization to describe the socio-ecological factors related to the obesogenic home environments of parents with preschool-aged children (2 to 5 years of age) in a program called HomeStyles [30–33].

2. Materials and Methods

Details of the protocol for the HomeStyles program are reported elsewhere [34] and are described in brief in this section. The Institutional Review Board at the authors' universities approved this study (ethical approval code is #11-294Mc). All participants gave informed consent.

2.1. Sample & Recruitment

Parents of preschool children (ages 2 to <6 years) who resided in the catchment areas of New Jersey and Arizona in the U.S. were recruited to participate in a program that would help them build closer family bonds and raise healthier families. Recruitment notices were distributed as flyers, posters, and/or email announcements to community centers, workplaces, schools, daycare programs, doctor's offices, and places of worship. In-person recruiting was conducted at these sites and community events. To be eligible to participate, parents had to have at least one preschool child, be able to read and write English or Spanish at about the 4th to 5th grade level, be the key decision maker with regard to family food purchases and preparation, and have consistent access to the Internet. Recruited participants began by completing a brief online eligibility screener survey. Those who were eligible were then directed to complete the online baseline survey. The online baseline survey dataset utilized in this study was collected before parents began the intervention.

2.2. Instruments

2.2.1. Survey Development & Implementation

Development of the online survey and implementation is described in detail elsewhere [34]. In brief, the survey included an array of valid, reliable measures assessing parent and household psychographic characteristics (e.g., personal organization, family conflict) as well as parent and child weight-related behaviors (i.e., diet, physical activity, sleep) and parent weight-related cognitions (e.g., values, self-efficacy) that are described further below. Measures were selected to yield an understanding of intrapersonal and interpersonal/social behaviors and cognitions and environmental conditions in and near participants' homes pertaining to diet and physical activity. All measures were self-report and underwent rigorous selection or development procedures to ensure they were valid and reliable, matched the goals of HomeStyles, and acceptable and accurately interpreted by the target audience [5,6,35,36]. Prior to data collection, the survey was pre-tested ($n = 48$) to identify refinements needed to improve clarity and verify accuracy of scale scoring algorithms. The survey was also pilot tested ($n = 550$) to confirm scale unidimensionality and internal consistency, and further reviewed by a panel of experts to confirm measures were of integrity and suitability to the study purpose [6]. After undergoing rigorous testing, recruitment and implementation of the survey was conducted online over a 15-month period [34]. Parents with more than one preschool child were instructed to report data for one "target" child, defined as the child born closest to a randomly selected date specified in the survey (i.e., noon on 1 June). The measures in the survey, including scale type, number of items, possible score range, and Cronbach's alpha (as applicable), are organized by level of the socio-ecological model as presented in Table 1.

2.2.2. Sociodemographic Characteristics

Sociodemographic characteristics of the sample (e.g., parent race/ethnicity, education level, age, sex) were collected. Family socio-economic status was assessed with both the 4-item Family Affluence Scale [37,38] and annual median household income based on U.S. Census Bureau zip code data. Parents rated their own and their child's health status (poor, fair, good, very good, or excellent) using the Centers for Disease Control and Prevention's Health-Related Quality of Life questionnaire [39,40].

2.2.3. Intrapersonal Factors

Intrapersonal measures included three scales assessing the extent of parents' personal organization [41], their need for cognition (e.g., enjoyment of thinking) [42,43], and control of stress [44]. Intrapersonal weight-related assessments included food frequency questionnaires evaluating dietary intake (e.g., fruits and vegetables, milk, sugar-sweetened beverages, fat) [45–50], physical activity level [51–53], screentime [54–56], and sleep duration [57,58] of parents and children.

2.2.4. Interpersonal/Social Factors

Interpersonal/social characteristics assessed included household chaos [41,59], family conflict [60], family support for healthy eating and physical activity, frequency of family meals [61], frequency of eating family meals in various locations (e.g., in the car) [54,62,63], and frequency with which television or other media devices were used during family meals [6,22,54]. Other interpersonal/social characteristics included appraisals of the emotional environment at family mealtime [22,62–64], meal planning behaviors [65], self-efficacy for preparing family meals [66], and parental modeling of healthy eating behaviors and self-efficacy for childhood obesity-protective practices [6,55,67–70]. Interpersonal/social characteristics associated with physical activity included frequency of parent and child actively playing together [6], parental modeling of physical activity [22,50–52,71], and parental encouragement of and self-efficacy for promoting children's physical activity [6,22,52,67,68,72,73]. The importance and value parents placed on dietary and physical activity practices and cognitions linked to obesity prevention [66,72,74] also were evaluated.

2.2.5. Environmental Factors

Food-frequency questionnaires evaluated the typical availability of fruit/vegetable juice, salty/fatty snacks, sugar-sweetened beverages, and milk in the home [46,47,50,75,76]. The availability of space and supports for physical activity inside the home, immediately outside the home (yard), and neighborhood, along with perceived neighborhood safety and frequency of outdoor active play, were appraised with the HOP-Up (Home Opportunities for Physical activity check-Up) Checklist [77]. The home media environment (i.e., media devices in the home and child bedroom [22,54–56], amount of daily screentime children were allowed [22,54–56], and total time TV was on daily [78]) served as a proxy for sedentary behavior supports.

2.3. Data Analysis

Descriptive statistics (means, standard deviations, percentages, actual score ranges) were computed to describe the sociodemographic characteristics of study participants and intrapersonal, interpersonal/social, and environmental factors. Internal consistency for continuous scales were also measured (when applicable) using Cronbach's alpha. SPSS software version 24.0 (IBM Corporation, Chicago, IL, USA) was used for all analyses.

3. Results

Of the 1221 individuals who responded to recruitment advertisements, were eligible for the study, and gave informed consent, 489 (40%) completed the baseline survey. [34]. The mean parent age was 32.34 ± 5.71 SD years and the vast majority were female (93%). More than half were white (58%), resided in New Jersey (53%), had earned a baccalaureate degree or higher (51%), and spoke English at home (87%). Slightly more than one-third of participants did not have paid employment (36%) or worked full time (38%), with the remainder working part-time.

Most households had 1 (30%) or 2 children (42%) children less than 18 years old and at least one of these children between the ages of 2 and <6 years. The target children were approximately evenly divided by sex (48% female) and had an average age of 3.85 ± 1.05 SD years. A plurality was white (49%) and most were the biological offspring of the participating parent (91%).

Most participants lived in dual parent households (82%) and had spouses/partners who had at least some post-secondary education (78%) and worked full-time (84%). A total of 17%, 58%, and 25% were low, middle, and high family affluence level [33,34], respectively. Annual median household income was based on U.S. Census Bureau zip code data for each participant's home (mean $63,654.84 ± 24,787.07 SD).

As displayed in Table 1, intrapersonal parent measure scores indicate that participants were somewhat disorganized personally, were fairly neutral about whether they had a need for cognition, and were able to handle most stresses. On average, parents reported good to very good health status. Intake of 100% fruit/vegetable juice and milk servings were low at slightly more than half a serving daily, which was lower than the nearly three-quarters of a serving of sugar-sweetened beverages daily intake. Fat intake exceeded one-third of total daily calories. Overall, physical activity level was low while sedentary screentime was high (~6 h/day).

Table 1. HomeStyles Study Measures and Baseline Scores (*n* = 489).

Measures	# of Items	Scale Type	Possible Score Range	Cronbach's Alpha	Mean ± SD	Actual Score Range
Intrapersonal Factors						
Parents						
Personal Organization [41]	4	5-point agreement rating A	1-5	0.64	2.60 ± 0.94	1-5
Need for Cognition [42,43]	1	5-point agreement rating A	1-5	*	3.39 ± 0.97	1-5
Control of Stress [44]	2	4-point frequency rating B	1-4	0.76	3.39 ± 0.76	1-4
Health Status [37,38]	1	5-point excellence rating C	1-5	*	3.45 ± 0.94	1-5
100% Fruit/Vegetable Juice (servings/day) [45,47-50]	2	9-point servings drank scale D	0-2.3	*	0.57 ± 0.57	0-2.29
Milk (servings/day) [45,47-50]	1	9-point servings drank scale D	0-8	*	0.57 ± 0.45	0-1.14
Sugar-sweetened Beverages [46,50] (servings/day)	4	9-point servings eaten scale D	0-4.6	*	0.71 ± 0.81	0-4.57
% Total Calories from Fat [45,47-49]	17	5-point servings eaten scale E	0-100	*	36.66 ± 6.00	22.10-56.90
Physical Activity Level [51-53]	3	8-point exercise scale F	0-42	*	13.8 ± 9.87	0-42
Screentime [6,56] (minutes/day)	1	minutes/day	0-1440	*	354.69 ± 279.54	0-1425
Sleep Duration (minutes/day) [57,58] ¥	1	hours/day	0-24	*	7.08 ± 1.21	4-12
Children						
Health Status [37,38]	1	5-point excellence rating C	1-5	*	4.36 ± 0.77	2-5
Fruit/Vegetable Juice (servings/day) [45-50,76]	2	9-point servings drank scale D	0-2.3	*	0.75 ± 0.56	0-2.29
Milk (servings/day) [45-50,76]	1	9-point servings drank scale D	0-8	*	0.85 ± 0.35	0-1.14
Sugar-sweetened Beverage (servings/day) [45-50,76]	2	9-point servings drank scale D	0-2.3	*	0.28 ± 0.42	0-2.29
Physical Activity Level [51-53]	3	8-point Exercise scale F	0-42	*	25.83 ± 11.53	0-42
Screentime minutes/day [6,56]	1	minutes	0-1440	*	294.57 ± 261.98	
Sleep Duration (hours/day) [57,58] †	1	hours	0-24	*	10.68 ± 1.41	8-15
Interpersonal/Social Factors						
Household Chaos [41,57]	2	5-point agreement rating A	1-5	0.86	2.51 ± 1.07	1-5
Family Conflict [60]	5	5-point agreement rating A	1-5	0.86	1.99 ± 0.76	1-5
Family Support for Healthy Eating and Physical Activity [61]	4	5-point frequency rating G	1-5	0.79	3.55 ± 1.35	1-5
Food-Related						
Family Meal frequency/week [61]	3	0-7 days for breakfast, lunch, dinner; score is sum of 3 meals	0-21	*	12.40 ± 5.02	0-21

Table 1. *Cont.*

Measures	# of Items	Scale Type	Possible Score Range	Cronbach's Alpha	Mean ± SD	Actual Score Range
Family Meal Location [54,62,63]						
In Car (days/week)	1	0–7 days	0–7	*	0.55 ± 1.4	0–7
At Fast Food Restaurant (days/week)	1	0–7 days	0–7	*	0.88 ± 1.27	0–7
At Dining Table (days/week)	1	0–7 days	0–7	*	4.64 ± 2.5	0–7
In Front of TV (days/week)	1	0–7 days	0–7	*	2.36 ± 2.52	0–7
Media Device Use at Family Meals [6,22,52] (days/week)	1	0–7 days	0–7	*	1.69 ± 2.4	0–7
TV Use at Family Meals & Snacking Occasions [6,22,52] (days/week)	1	0–7 days	0–7	*	3.50 ± 2.67	0–7
Family Mealtime Emotional Environment [22,63]	2	5-point agreement rating [A]	1–5	0.62	4.06 ± 0.85	1–5
Family Meals are Planned [65,66]	2	5-point agreement rating [A]	1–5	0.77	3.38 ± 1.02	1–5
Parent Family Meal Preparation Self-Efficacy [66]	2	5-point agreement rating [A]	1–5	0.56	3.95 ± 0.9	1–5
Parent Modeling of Healthy Eating [55,69,70]	4	5-point agreement rating [A]	1–5	0.74	3.61 ± 0.81	1–5
Parent Self-efficacy for Food-Related Childhood Obesity-Protective Practices [6,67,68]	6	5-point confidence rating [H]	1–5	0.81	3.78 ± 0.71	1–5
Physical Activity-Related						
Parent: Child Co-Physical Activity (days/week) [6]	2	8-point modeling scale [I]	0–7	0.68	3.64 ± 1.85	0–7
Parent Modeling of Physical Activity (days/week) [22,54,55,70]	2	8-point modeling scale [I]	0–7	0.59	3.20 ± 1.31	0–6.67
Parent Modeling of Sedentary Activity (days/week) [22,54,55,70]	2	8-point modeling scale [I]	0–7	0.72	3.51 ± 2.33	0–7
Parent Encouragement of Child Physical Activity [6,22,55,72,73]	5	5-point agreement rating [A]	1–5	0.85	4.02 ± 0.67	1–5
Parent Self-Efficacy for Physical-Activity Related Childhood Obesity-Protective Practices [6,67,68]	3	5-point confidence rating [H]	1–5	0.84	3.49 ± 1.01	1–5
Parent Values Related to Obesity-Protective Practices						
Healthy Eating Outcome Expectations [66,74]	6	5-point agreement rating [A]	1–5	0.92	4.55 ± 0.54	2–5
Physical Activity Outcome Expectations [66,74]	6	5-point agreement rating [A]	1–5	0.94	4.44 ± 0.61	2–5
Value Placed on Modeling Physical Activity [6,22,71–73]	2	5-point agreement rating [A]	1–5	0.73	3.86 ± 0.86	1–5
Valued Placed on Not Modeling Sedentary Behavior [6]	1	5-point agreement rating [A]	1–5	*	3.81 ± 0.97	1–5
Value Placed on Physical Activity for Children [72,73]	2	5-point agreement rating [A]	1–5	0.71	3.70 ± 0.88	1–5
Environmental Factors						
Household Food Availability [46,47,50,75,76]						

Table 1. *Cont.*

Measures	# of Items	Scale Type	Possible Score Range	Cronbach's Alpha	Mean ± SD	Actual Score Range
100% Fruit/Vegetable Juice (servings/household member/week)	2	9-point servings scale[J]	0–8	*	3.19 ± 2.06	0–8
Salty/fatty snacks (servings/household member/week)	4	9-point servings scale[J]	0–32	*	7.9 ± 7.19	0–32
Sugar-sweetened Beverages (servings/household member/week)	4	9-point servings scale[J]	0–8	*	1.62 ± 1.8	0–8
Milk (servings/household member/week)	1	9-point servings scale[J]	0–8	*	6.60 ± 2.04	0–8
Physical Activity Environment [77]						
Indoor Home Space & Supports For Physical Activity	6	Varies by item; 2 items are counts; 1 item is a 5-point agreement rating;[A] 3 items are 5-point occurrence ratings[K]	1–5	0.74	3.31 ± 0.87	1–5
Outdoor/Yard Space & Supports For Physical Activity[‡]	4	5-point agreement rating[A]	1–5	0.75	4.31 ± 0.7	1–5
Neighborhood Space & Supports For Physical Activity[§]	4	5-point agreement rating[A]	1–5	0.88	4.01 ± 0.99	0.50–5
Neighborhood Environment Safety	2	5-point agreement rating[A]	1–5	0.42	3.41 ± 0.87	1–5
Frequency of Active Play Outdoors	2	5-point occurrence ratings[K]	1–5	0.54	2.55 ± 0.97	1–5
Media Environment						
Total Number of Inactive Media Devices (including TV) in the Home [22,54,55]	6	Total devices[L]	0–66	*	10.51 ± 4.53	1–27
Total Number of Inactive Media Devices (including TV) in Children's Bedrooms	7	Total # of media device types[M]	0–7	*	1.32 ± 1.57	0–7
Time Children are Allowed to Watch TV/Movies & Use Inactive Media Devices (e.g., computers, tablets, smart phones) [6] (minutes/day)	1	minutes	0–1440	*	475.98 ± 701.11	0–1440
Total Time TV is on When No One is Watching [6,22,78] (minutes/day)	1	minutes	0–1440	*	130.18 ± 214.95	0–1410

* Not applicable. ¥ n = 477. † n = 448. ‡ n = 437. § n = 482. ^ 5-point Agreement Rating: strongly disagree, disagree, neither agree nor disagree, agree, strongly agree; scored 1 to 5 respectively with scoring reversed for negatively worded statements; scale score equals average of item scores; higher scale score indicates greater expression of the trait. B 4-point Frequency Rating: not at all, several days, more than half the days, nearly every day; scored 1 to 4; higher score indicates greater frequency. C 5-point Excellence Rating: poor, fair, good, very good, excellent; scored 1 to 5 respectively; higher score indicates better health. D 9-point Beverage Servings Rating: <1 time/week, 1 day/week, 2 days/week, 3 days/week, 4 days/week, 5 days/week, 6 days/week, 7 days/week, >1 time/day; scored 0 to 8 respectively; higher score indicates greater frequency. E 5-point Fatty Food Servings Rating: 1 time/month or less, 2 to 3 times/month, 1 to 2 times/week, 3 to 4 times/week, 5 or more times/week; scored 0 to 4 respectively; scale scoring algorithm is protected by copyright and described in detail elsewhere [79]; higher score indicates greater intake. F 8-point Exercise Days/week: 0, 1, 2, 3, 4, 5, 6, and 7; days/week weighted by exercise intensity (weights of 1, 2, 3 for walking, moderate, and vigorous activity, respectively) and summed to create scale score; higher scale score indicates greater activity level. G 5-point Frequency Rating: never, rarely, sometimes, most of the time, always; scored 1 to 5; higher score indicates greater frequency. H 5-point Confidence Rating: not at all confident, not confident, confident, quite confident, very confident; scored 1 to 5 respectively; higher scale score indicates greater confidence. I 8-point Modeling Days/week: 0 (almost never), 1, 2, 3, 4, 5, 6, and 7; days averaged to create scale score; higher score indicates more frequent modeling. J 9-point Household Servings Rating: <1 time/week, 1 day/week, 2 days/week, 3 days/week, 4 days/week, 5 days/week, 6 days/week, 7 days/week, >1 time/day; scored 0 to 8 respectively; higher score indicates greater frequency. K 5-point Occurrence Rating: almost never, 1-2 times/week; 3 to 4 times/week, 5 to 6 times/week, every day; scored 1 to 5 respectively; scale score equals average of item scores; higher scale score indicates greater occurrence of behavior. L 11-point Media Device Count: 1 = 1 to 10 = 10, 11 = more than 10; scale score equals sum of items; higher score indicates greater number of media devices. M Response for each media device in child's bedroom was 0 = no and 1 = yes; scale score equals sum of items; higher score indicates greater number of different device types.

Child intake of fruit/vegetable juice, milk, and sugar-sweetened beverages all equaled less than one serving per day. Physical activity was moderate while sedentary screentime was high (~5 h/day). Sleep averaged 7 h nightly for parents (~62% meeting sleep recommendations of 7 or more hours per night) and total sleep duration for children (daytime naps and nighttime sleep) was nearly 11 h (62% meeting sleep recommendations (11–14 h/day for 2 year olds; 10–13 h/day for 3–5 year olds).

Psychographic household measures indicated that participants' had somewhat chaotic households and tended to feel their families got along fairly well, disagreeing that they had family conflict. Family meals were eaten nearly twice per day and were eaten at a dining table more often than other locations. On average, TV was watched during family meals or while snacking on half the days in a week. Parents agreed that family meals had a positive emotional environment. They somewhat agreed that they planned family meals, had self-efficacy for preparing family meals, modeled healthy eating behaviors to children, and had self-efficacy for food-related childhood obesity-protective practices. With regard to physical activity, parents agreed that they encouraged children to be physically active, but actively played with children or modeled physical activity to children less than half of the days in a week. Parents strongly agreed that healthy eating and physical activity behaviors lead to positive outcomes, however the value placed on modeling healthy physical activity behaviors tended to be somewhat neutral.

The household food environment provided about 3 servings of 100% fruit/vegetable juice and 1.5 servings of sugar-sweetened beverages per household member per week. Approximately 7 servings of both milk and salty/fatty snacks were available weekly per person. Physical activity space and supports for children inside the home were moderate, with outdoor/yard and neighborhood space and supports for physical activity ratings being higher. Neighborhood safety ratings tended to be neutral, and participants reported the frequency of child active play outdoors occurred 2 to 3 times per week. Households were replete with 'inactive' media devices, and the time spent with these devices equaled about 8 h daily.

4. Discussion

Healthy intrapersonal behaviors identified in this study population include parent and child intakes of 100% fruit/vegetable juice that mirror recommendations of 4 to 6 ounces per day [80,81], with these intake levels corroborated by the household environment's availability of 100% fruit/vegetable juice servings/household member/week. Another positive feature is the intake and household availability of sugar-sweetened beverages (e.g., soft drinks, fruit drinks) were fairly low, contributing only about 90 and 29 calories (and 18 and 6 grams of sugar) to parent and child daily intake, respectively; values which are lower than the per capita intakes found in nationally representative studies [82]. An area in great need of improvement is milk intake and availability in the household, which were far below recommendations for both parents and children [80], thereby potentially placing parents at risk of osteoporosis [83] and children at risk for decreased bone mineralization and associated sequelae [83]. These low milk intakes during childhood are especially worrisome given that milk intake tends to drop off as children, especially females, enter adolescence [82]. Also of concern are the household availability of more than 1 serving/person daily of salty/fatty snacks and the percentage of total calories contributed by fat to parents' diets. Indeed, parents' fat intake exceeded the upper limit of the Acceptable Macronutrient Distribution Ranges (AMDRs) [84] and was somewhat higher than the mean intake of U.S. adults [85].

Physical activity levels, time spent in sedentary activity, and the physical activity and media environment were found to be less than ideal. Much like in national reports [85], adults in this study had limited physical activity, scoring less than one-third of the maximum score possible. One-third of parents reported walking at least 10 minutes continuously and/or engaging in moderate exercise at least 5 times per week, but only 10% engaged in vigorous activity 5 or more times per week. Children had more physical activity, but achieved only about 60% of the highest score possible. Unlike parents, half of the children walked at least 10 minutes continuously, two-thirds engaged in moderate exercise, and 40% received vigorous exercise at least 5 times per week. Environmental supports for active play inside homes were moderate. That is, children had restricted space inside homes to vigorously play (e.g., the amount of active play space for half of the children was insufficient for doing more than 3 continuous somersaults or cartwheels before hitting furniture), few toys that helped them be active inside (37% had less than 5 toys supporting active play inside the home), and engaged in active play inside the home few days per week (one-third actively played indoors less than 3 times weekly). Supports and space for physical activity outdoors and in the neighborhood were higher than indoors. Almost all parents agreed or strongly agreed that the yard or area immediately outside their homes had plenty of room for kids to play games, and more than 8 out of 10 agreed or strongly agreed that there were outdoor areas like parks, pools, and playgrounds nearby where their children could play. However, the frequency of playing outdoors averaged less than 3 to 4 times weekly. (Data were collected year round from both New Jersey and Arizona, hence seasonality should not be an influence on this frequency). The relatively infrequent outdoor play may reflect the young age of the children studied and their need for adult supervision as well as the fairly neutral ratings parents gave their neighborhood for being safe from crime and biting insects and animals.

Parents and children reported 5 to 6 h of daily screentime; children exceeded the 2016 recommendations from the American Academy of Pediatrics by 5 times [86]. The home media environment was clearly conducive to sedentary behavior—children were allowed to watch television or use 'inactive' media devices nearly 8 h daily and television was on for 2 h, even when no one was watching. Despite recommendations to make children's bedrooms media free [86], 56% of children had at least one media device in their bedrooms.

Adequate sleep appears protective against excess weight gain [87–92]. The nightly sleep duration recommendation for adult is 7 to 9 h per night [93]. Nearly two-thirds of parents surveyed met these recommendations, while the remainder got less than the recommendations. The mean sleep time for parents in this study, however, is higher than the 6 h and 31 min average nightly duration for U.S. adults [94]. A comparison of children's sleep with age-specific recommendations [93] indicated that 28% got less daily sleep than recommended for their age group.

Measures of interpersonal or family social interactions indicated several positive behaviors. For example, frequent family meals eaten in a positive emotional environment without distractions, such as television and angry discussions, are associated with healthier dietary intakes [87,95–101]. Parents in this study reported that their families ate together almost twice daily and mealtimes were fairly calm (e.g., low stress, infrequent arguments). Most meals were eaten at a dining or kitchen table, a location associated with fewer problems with child behaviors at mealtime [102], which likely contributed to the positive emotional atmosphere reported. However, television and media devices were used fairly often while eating, and meals were eaten in front of the television more than two days per week.

Although observational learning is an important way that children learn [103,104], parents were neutral about whether they modeled healthy eating to their children. Scores on scales assessing parent modeling of healthy physical activity behaviors, sedentary activity behaviors, and active play with their children indicated that they exhibited these behaviors fewer than three days per week. Parents tended to agree that they valued modeling physical activity and not modeling sedentary behavior to children. Opportunities for parents to learn how to put these values into action are warranted.

Outcome expectations and self-efficacy are key predictors of behavior [104–106]. Parents were firm in their beliefs that healthy eating and physical activity improved health. Their self-efficacy scores for engaging in food-related and physical activity-related childhood obesity protective practices showed that they were confident to very confident in their ability to perform these practices. Providing opportunities for parents to increase their self-efficacy to be "very confident" could help them increase implementation of these childhood obesity protective behaviors.

Although this is one of few studies that has comprehensively assessed obesity-related factors associated with home environment and lifestyle practices among parents of preschool aged children using a socio-ecological approach, findings should be interpreted in the light of study limitations. The cross-sectional study design does not allow for inference of causality in the observed associations. Additionally, the study sample only included parents of preschool-aged children in two geographical areas of the U.S., so findings may not be generalizable to families with children of different ages or living in other areas of the country including geography (rural vs. urban). There also is a potential for self-selection bias as participants were recruited for a behavioral intervention. Lastly, all information from participants was self-reported and may be subject to both reporting error and bias. Future research should examine the relationship of socioecological factors related to the home obesogenic environment with child weight status to determine factors predictive of childhood obesity.

5. Conclusions

In conclusion, this study identified socioecological factors related to the obesogenic home environment of parents with preschool-aged children that could be improved to promote optimal child development while lowering the risk of childhood obesity. However, parents had a constellation of characteristics that likely would make it a challenge for them to orchestrate changes to weight-related characteristics of their home environments and lifestyles. That is, parents indicated they tended to be disorganized (e.g., late for appointments, put off chores, not dependable) and did not enjoy dealing with situations requiring a lot of thinking. Additionally, they reported high stress levels—on at least half the days in a week they felt unable to control important things in their life and felt difficulties were piling up so high they could not overcome them. They also reported households were somewhat chaotic (i.e., a real "zoo", noisy). On a positive note, these families had low family conflict (e.g., fighting, criticizing). These findings suggest that obesity prevention interventions for parents of preschool children need to address not only obesity-protective behaviors (e.g., diet, physical activity, sleep, parent behavior modeling) and cognitions associated with behavior change (e.g., self-efficacy, values), but also should take into consideration behavioral characteristics (e.g., parent organizational skills, need for cognition, stress, household organization) that may affect their ability to realize the benefits of the intervention.

Acknowledgments: This study was funded by USDA NIFA #2011-68001-30170.

Author Contributions: C.B.-B., J.W. and N.H. conceived and designed the study. J.M.-B., C.B.-B. and G.A.P. collected data. V.Q., J.M.-B. and C.B.-B. analyzed the data. All authors were involved in manuscript preparation and revision and approved the final manuscript.

References

1. Finkelstein, E.; Trogdon, J.; Cohen, J.; Dietz, W. Annual medical spending attributalbe to obesity: Payer-and service-specific estimates. *Health Aff.* **2009**, *28*, w822–w831. [CrossRef] [PubMed]

2. Pi-Sunyer, F. The obesity epidemic: Pathophysiology and consequences of obesity. *Obes. Res.* **2002**, *10*, 97S–104S. [CrossRef] [PubMed]

3. Ogden, L.; Carroll, M.; Jit, B.; Flegal, K. Prevalence of childhood and adult obesity in the United States. *JAMA* **2014**, *311*, 806–814. [CrossRef] [PubMed]

4. Fairburn, C.; Brownell, K. *Eating Disorders and Obesity*; Guilford Press Inc.: New York, NY, USA, 2002.

5. Martin-Biggers, J.M.; Worobey, J.; Byrd-Bredbenner, C. Interpersonal Characteristics in the Home Environment Associated with Childhood Obesity. In *Recent Advances in Obesity in Children*; Avid Science Publications: Berlin, Germany, 2016; Available online: www.avidscience.com/wp-content/uploads/2016/05/OIC-15-03_May-06-2016.pdf (accessed on 10 April 2017).

6. Martin-Biggers, J. Home Environment Characteristics Associated with Obesity Risk in Preschool-Aged Children and Their Mothers. Ph.D. Thesis, Rutgers, The State University of New Jersey, New Brunswick, NJ, USA, 2016.

7.   Story, M.; Kaphingst, K.; Robinson-O'Brien, R.; Glanz, K. Creating healthy food and eating environments: Policy and environmental approaches. *Annu. Rev. Public Health* **2008**, *29*, 253–272. [CrossRef] [PubMed]

8.   Hawkins, S.; Cole, T.; Law, C. An ecological systems approach to examine risk factors for early childhood overweight: Findings from the UK millenium cohort. *J. Epidemiol. Community Health* **2009**, *63*, 147–155. [CrossRef] [PubMed]

9.   Wang, Y.; Wu, Y.; Wilson, R.; Bleich, S.; Cheskin, L.; Weston, C.; Showell, N.; Fawole, O.; Lau, B.; Segal, J. *Childhood Obesity Prevention Programs: Comparitive Effectiveness Review and Meta-Analysis*; Prepared by the John Hopkins University Evidence-based Practice Center under Contract No. 290-2007-10061-I; Agency for Healthcare Research and Quality: Rockville, MD, USA, 2013.

10.   Monasta, L.; Batty, G.; Macaluso, A.; Ronfani, L.; Lutje, V.; Bavcar, A.; van Lenthe, F.; Brug, J.; Cattaneo, A. Interventions for the prevention of overweight and obesity in preschool children: A systematic review of randomized controlled trials. *Obes. Rev.* **2011**, *12*, e107–e118. [CrossRef] [PubMed]

11.   Monasta, L.; Batty, G.; Cattaneo, A.; Lutje, V.; Ronfani, L.; Van Lenthe, F.; Brug, J. Early-life determinants of overweigth and obesity: A review of systematic reviews. *Obes. Rev.* **2010**, *11*, 695–708. [CrossRef] [PubMed]

12.   Ogata, B.; Hayes, D. Position of the Academy of Nutrition and Dietetics: Nutrition guidance for healthy children ages 2 to 11 years. *J. Acad. Nutr. Diet.* **2014**, *114*, 1257–1276. [CrossRef] [PubMed]

13.   Birch, L.; Davison, K. Family environmental factors influencing the developing behavioral controls of food intake and childhood overweight. *Pediatr. Clin. N. Am.* **2001**, *48*, 893–907. [CrossRef]

14.   Brustad, R. Attraction to physical activity in urban schoolchildren: Parental socialization and gender influences. *Res. Q. Exerc. Sport* **1996**, *67*, 316–323. [CrossRef] [PubMed]

15.   Demsey, J.; Kimiecik, J.; Horn, T. Parental influence on children's moderate to vigorous physical activity participation: An expectancy-value approach. *Pediatr. Exerc.* **1993**, *5*, 151–167. [CrossRef]

16.   Gruber, K.; Haldeman, L. Using the family to combat childhood and adult obesity. *Prev. Chronic Dis.* **2009**, *6*, A106. [PubMed]

17.   Lau, R.; Quadrell, J.; Hartman, K. Development and change of young adults' preventive health beliefs and behavior: Influence from parents and peers. *J. Health Soc. Behav.* **1990**, *31*, 240–259. [CrossRef] [PubMed]

18.   Patterson, T.; Sallis, J.; Nader, P.; Kaplan, R.; Rupp, J. Familial similarities of changes in cognitive, behavioral and physiological variables in a cardiovascular health promotion program. *J. Pediatr. Psychol.* **1989**, *14*, 277–292. [CrossRef] [PubMed]

19.   Sahay, T.; Ashbury, F.; Roberts, M.; Rootman, I. Effective components for nutrition interventions: A review and application of the literature. *Health Promot. Pract.* **2006**, *7*, 418–427. [CrossRef] [PubMed]

20.   Skouteris, H.; McCabe, M.; Winburn, B.; Newbreen, V.; Sacher, P.; Chadwick, P. Parental influence and obesity prefention in pre-schoolers: A systematic review of interventions. *Obes. Rev.* **2011**, *12*, 315–328. [CrossRef] [PubMed]

21.   Wyse, R.; Campbell, E.; Nathan, N.; Wolfenden, L. Associations between characteristics of the home food environment and fruit and vegetable intake in preschool children: A cross-sectional study. *BMC Public Health* **2011**, *11*, 938. [CrossRef] [PubMed]

22.   Spurrier, N.; Magarey, A.; Golley, R.; Curnow, F.; Sawyer, M. Relationships between the home environment and physical activity and dietary patterns of preschool children: A cross-sectional study. *Int. J. Behav. Nutr. Phys. Act.* **2008**, *5*, 31. [CrossRef] [PubMed]

23.   Whitaker, R.; Wright, J.; Pepe, M.; Seidel, K.; Dietz, W. Predicting obesity in young adulthood from childhood and parental obesity. *N. Engl. J. Med.* **1997**, *337*, 869–873. [CrossRef] [PubMed]

24.   Trost, S.; Sirard, J.; Dowda, M.; Pfeiffer, K.; Pate, R. Physical activity in overwegith and nonoverweight preschool children. *Int. J. Obes. Relat. Metab. Disord.* **2003**, *27*, 834–839. [CrossRef] [PubMed]

25.   Anderson, S.; Whitaker, R. Household routines and obesity in US preschool-aged children. *Pediatrics* **2010**, *125*, 420–428. [CrossRef] [PubMed]

26.   Rolls, B.; Ello-Martin, J.; Tohill, B. What can intervention studies tell us about the relationship between fruit and vegetable consumption and weight management. *Nutr. Rev.* **2004**, *62*, 1–17. [CrossRef] [PubMed]

27.   He, M.; Piche, L.; Harris, S. Screen-related sedentary behaviors: children's and parents' attitudes, motivations, and practices. *J. Nutr. Educ. Behav.* **2010**, *42*, 17–25. [CrossRef] [PubMed]

28.   Glanz, K. Measuring food environments: A historical perspective. *Am. J. Prev. Med.* **2009**, *36*, S93–S98. [CrossRef] [PubMed]

29. Pinard, C.; Yaroch, A.; Hart, M.; Serrano, E.; McFerre, M.; Estabrooks, P. Measures of the home environment related to childhood obesity: A systematic review. *Public Health Nutr.* **2012**, *15*, 97–109. [CrossRef] [PubMed]

30. Martin-Biggers, J.; Beluska, K.; Quick, V.M.; Byrd-Bredbenner, C. Cover Lines Using Positive, Urgent, Unique language Entice Moms to Read Health Communications. *J. Health Commun.* **2015**, *20*, 766–772. [CrossRef] [PubMed]

31. Martin-Biggers, J.; Spaccarotella, K.; Delaney, C.; Koenings, M.; Alleman, G.; Hongu, N.; Worobey, J.; Byrd-Bredbenner, C. Development of the intervention materials for the homestyles childhood obesity prevention program for parents of preschoolers. *Nutrients* **2015**, *7*, 6628–6669. [CrossRef] [PubMed]

32. Martin-Biggers, J.; Spaccarotella, K.; Hongu, N.; Worobey, J.; Byrd-Bredbenner, C. Translating it into real life: Cognitions, barriers and supports for key weight-related behaviors of parents of preschoolers. *BMC Public Health* **2015**, *15*, 189. [CrossRef] [PubMed]

33. Delaney, C.; Barrios, P.; Lozada, C.; Soto-Balbuena, K.; Martin-Biggers, J.; Byrd-Bredbenner, C. Applying common Latino magazine cover line themes to health communication. *Hisp. J. Behav. Sci.* **2016**, *38*, 546–558. [CrossRef]

34. Byrd-Bredbenner, C.; Martin-Biggers, J.; Koenings, M.; Quick, V.; Hongu, K.; Worobey, J. Homestyles, A web-based childhood obesity prevention program for families with preschool children: Protocol for a randomized controlled trial. *JMIR Res. Protoc.* **2017**, *6*, e73. [CrossRef] [PubMed]

35. Martin-Biggers, J.; Cheng, C.; Spaccarotella, K.; Byrd-Bredbenner, C. The Physical Activity Environment in Homes and Neighborhoods. In *Recent Advances in Obesity in Children*; Avid Science Publications: Berlin, Germany, 2016. Available online: www.avidscience.com/wp-content/uploads/2016/05/OIC-15-04_May-06-2016.pdf (accessed on 10 April 2017).

36. Byrd-Bredbenner, C.; Maurer Abbot, J. Food choice influencers of mothers of young children: Implications for nutrition educators. *Top. Clin. Nutr.* **2008**, *25*, 198–215. [CrossRef]

37. Hartley, J.; Levin, K.; Currie, C. A new version of the HBSC Family Affluence Scale—FAS III: Scottish qualitative findings from the international FAS developments study. *Child Indicat. Res.* **2016**, *9*, 233–245. [CrossRef] [PubMed]

38. Currie, C.; Mollcho, M.; Boyce, W.; Holstein, B.; Torsheim, T.; Richter, M. Researching health inequalities in adolescents: The development of the health behavior in school-aged children (HBSC) family affluence scale. *Soc. Sci. Med.* **2008**, *66*, 1429–1436. [CrossRef] [PubMed]

39. Centers for Disease Control and Prevention. HRQOL Concepts. Why Is Quality of Life Important? Available online: www.cdc.gov/hrqol/concept.htm (accessed on 9 May 2016).

40. Centers for Disease Control and Prevention. HRQOL-14 Healthy Days Measure. Available online: www.cdc.gov/hrqol/hrqol14_measure.htm (accessed on 9 May 2016).

41. Matheny, A.; Wachs, T.; Ludwig, J.; Phillips, K. Bringing order out of chaos: Psychometric characteristics of the confusion, hubbub, and order scale. *J. Appl. Dev. Psychol.* **1995**, *16*, 429–444. [CrossRef]

42. Cacioppo, J.; Petty, R. The need for cognition. *J. Personal. Soc. Psychol.* **1982**, *42*, 116–131. [CrossRef]

43. Cacioppo, J.; Petty, R.; Kao, C.F. The efficient assessment of need for cognition. *J. Personal. Assess.* **1984**, *48*, 306–307. [CrossRef] [PubMed]

44. Cohen, S.; Kamarck, T.; Mermelstein, R. A global measure of perceived stress. *J. Health Soc. Behav.* **1983**, *24*, 385–396. [CrossRef] [PubMed]

45. Wakimoto, P.; Block, G.; Mandel, S.; Medina, N. Development and reliability of brief dietary assessment tools for Hispanics. *Perv. Chronic Dis.* **2006**, *3*, A95.

46. Nelson, M.; Lytle, L. Development and evaluation of a brief screener to estimate fast-food and beverage consumption among adolescents. *J. Am. Diet. Assoc.* **2009**, *109*, 730–734. [CrossRef] [PubMed]

47. Block, G.; Gillespie, C.; Rosenbaum, E.H.; Jenson, C. A rapid food screener to assess fat and fruit and vegetable intake. *Am. J. Prev. Med.* **2000**, *18*, 284–288. [CrossRef]

48. Block, G.; Hartman, A.; Naughton, D. A reduced dietary questionnaire: Development and validation. *Epidemiology* **1990**, *1*, 58–64. [CrossRef] [PubMed]

49. Block, G.; Thompson, F.; Hartman, A.; Larkin, F.; Guire, K. Comparison of two dietary questionnaires validated against multiple dietary records collected during a 1-year period. *J. Am. Diet Assoc.* **1992**, *92*, 686–693. [PubMed]

50. West, D.; Bursac, Z.; Quimby, D.; Prewit, T.; Spatz, T.; Nash, C.; Mays, G.; Eddings, K. Self-reported sugar-sweetened beverage intake among college students. *Obesity* **2006**, *14*, 1825–1831. [CrossRef] [PubMed]

51. Quick, V.; Byrd-Bredbenner, C.; Shoff, S.; White, A.; Lohse, B.; Horacek, T.; Kattlemann, K.; Phillips, B.; Hoerr, S.; Greene, G. A streamlined, enhanced self-report physical activity measure for young adults. *Int. J. Health Promot. Educ.* **2016**, *54*, 245–254. [CrossRef]

52. Lee, P.; Macfarlane, D.; Lam, T.; Stewart, S. Validity of the international physical activity questionnaire short form (IPAQ-SF): A systematic review. *Int. J. Behav. Nutr. Phys. Act.* **2011**, *8*, 115. [CrossRef] [PubMed]

53. Craig, C.; Marshall, A.; Sjostrom, M.; Bauman, A.E.; Booth, M.L.; Ainsworth, B.E.; Pratt, M.; Ekelund, U.; Yngve, A.; Sallis, J.F.; et al. International Physical Activity Questionnaire: 12-country reliability and validity. *Med. Sci. Sport Exerc.* **2003**, *35*, 1381–1395. [CrossRef] [PubMed]

54. Bryant, M.; Ward, D.; Hales, D.; Vaughn, A.; Tabak, R.; Stevens, J. Reliability and validity of the Healthy Home Survey: A tool to measure factors within homes hypothesized to relate to overweight in children. *Int. J. Behav. Nutr. Phys. Act.* **2008**, *5*, 23. [CrossRef] [PubMed]

55. Gattshall, M.; Shoup, J.; Marshall, J.; Crane, L.; Estabrooks, P. Validation of a survey instrument to assess home environments for physical activity and healthy eating in overweight children. *Int. J. Behav. Nutr. Phys. Act.* **2008**, *5*, 3. [CrossRef] [PubMed]

56. Owen, N.; Sugiyama, T.; Eakin, E.; Gardiner, P.; Tremblay, M.; Sallis, J. Adults' sedentary behavior determinants and interventions. *Am. J. Prev. Med.* **2011**, *41*, 189–196. [CrossRef] [PubMed]

57. Buysse, D.; Reynolds, C.; Monk, T.; Berman, S.; Kupfer, D. The Pittsburgh Sleep Quality Index: A new instrument for psychiatric practice and research. *Psychiatry Res.* **1989**, *28*, 193–213. [CrossRef]

58. Carpenter, J.; Andrykowski, M. Psychometric evaluation of the Pittsburgh Sleep Quality Index. *J. Psychosom. Res.* **1998**, *45*, 5–13. [CrossRef]

59. Coldwell, J.; Pike, A.; Dunn, J. Household chaos—Links with parenting and child behaviour. *J. Child Psychol. Psychiatry* **2006**, *47*, 1116–1122. [CrossRef] [PubMed]

60. Moos, R.; Moos, B. *Family Environment Scale Manual: Development, Applications, Research*, 3rd ed.; Consulting Psychologists Press: Palo Alto, CA, USA, 1994.

61. Koszewski, W.; Behrends, D.; Nichols, M.; Sehi, N.; Jones, G. Patterns of family meals and food and nutrition intake in limited resource families. *Fam. Consum. Sci. Res. J.* **2011**, *39*, 431–441. [CrossRef]

62. Neumark-Sztainer, D.; Story, M.; Hannan, P.; Moe, J. Overweight status and eating patterns among adolescents: Where do youths stand in comparison to the Healthy People 2010 Objectives? *Am. J. Public Health* **2002**, *92*, 844–851. [CrossRef] [PubMed]

63. Neumark-Sztainer, D.; Wall, M.M.; Story, M.; Perry, C.L. Correlates of unhealthy weight-control behaviors among adolescents: Implications for prevention programs. *Health Psychol.* **2003**, *22*, 88–98. [CrossRef] [PubMed]

64. Neumark-Sztainer, D.; Story, M.; Hannan, P.; Perry, C.; Irving, L. Weight-Related Concerns and Behaviors Among Overweight and Nonoverweight Adolescents Implications for Preventing Weight-Related Disorders. *Arch. Pediatr. Adolesc. Med.* **2002**, *156*, 171–178. [CrossRef] [PubMed]

65. Neumark-Sztainer, D.; Larson, N.; Fulkerson, J.; Eisenberg, M.; Story, M. Family meals and adolescents: What have we learned from Project EAT (Eating Among Teens)? *Public Health Nutr.* **2010**, *13*, 1113–1121. [CrossRef] [PubMed]

66. Byrd-Bredbenner, C.; Maurer Abbot, J.; Cussler, E. Relationship of social cognitive theory concepts to mothers' dietary intake and BMI. *Matern. Child Nutr.* **2011**, *7*, 241–252. [CrossRef] [PubMed]

67. Kiernan, M.; Moore, S.; Schoffman, D.; Lee, K.; King, A.; Taylor, C.; Kiernan, N.; Perri, M. Social support for healthy behavior: Scale psychometrics and prediction of weight loss among women in a behavioral program. *Obesity* **2012**, *20*, 756–764. [CrossRef] [PubMed]

68. Ball, K.; Crawford, D. An investigation of psychological, social and environmental correlates of obesity and weight gain in young women. *Int. J. Obes.* **2006**, *30*, 1240–1249. [CrossRef] [PubMed]

69. Wardle, J.; Sanderson, S.; Guthrie, C.A.; Rapoport, L.; Plomin, R. Parental feeding style and the inter-generational transmission of obesity risk. *Obes. Res.* **2002**, *10*, 453–462. [CrossRef] [PubMed]

70. Ogden, J.; Reynolds, R.; Smith, A. Expanding the concept of parental control: A role for overt and covert control in children's snacking behaviour? *Appetite* **2006**, *47*, 100–106. [CrossRef] [PubMed]

71. Earls, F.; Brooks-Gunn, J.; Raudenbush, S.; Sampson, R. *Project on Human Development in Chicago Neighborhoods (PHDCN): Home and Life Interview, Wave 2, 1997–2000*; Instruments for ICPSR 13630; Inter-University Consortium for Political and Social Research: Ann Arbor, MI, USA, 2005.

72. Sallis, J.F.; Prochaska, J.J.; Taylor, W.C.; Hill, J.O.; Geraci, J.C. Correlates of physical activity in a national sample of girls and boys in Grades 4 through 12. *Health Psychol.* **1999**, *18*, 410–415. [CrossRef] [PubMed]

73. Trost, S.G.; Sallis, J.F.; Pate, R.R.; Freedson, P.S.; Taylor, W.C.; Dowda, M. Evaluating a model of parental influence on youth physical activity. *Am. J. Prev. Med.* **2003**, *25*, 277–282. [CrossRef]

74. AbuSabha, R.; Achterberg, C. Review of self-efficacy and locus of control for nutrition- and health-related behavior. *J. Am. Diet. Assoc.* **1997**, *97*, 1122–1132. [CrossRef]

75. Martin-Biggers, J.; Koenings, M.; Quick, V.; Abbot, J.; Byrd-Bredbenner, C. Appraising nutrient availability of household food supplies using Block dietary screeners for individuals. *Eur. Clin. Nutr.* **2015**, *69*, 1028–1034. [CrossRef] [PubMed]

76. Hunsberger, M.; O'Malley, J.; Block, T.; Norris, J. Relative validation of Block Kids Food Screener for dietary assessment in children and adolescents. *Matern. Child Nutr.* **2012**, *11*, 260–270. [CrossRef] [PubMed]

77. Cheng, C.; Martin-Biggers, J.; Quick, V.; Spaccarotella, K.; Byrd-Bredbenner, C. Validity and reliability of HOP-Up: A questionnaire to evaluate physical activity environments in homes with preschool-aged children. *Int. J. Behav. Nutr. Phys. Act.* **2016**, *13*, 91. [CrossRef] [PubMed]

78. Lapierre, M.; Piotrowski, J.; Linebarger, D. Background television in the homes of US children. *Pediatrics* **2012**, *130*, 839–846. [CrossRef] [PubMed]

79. Block, G.; Clifford, C.; Naughton, M.; Henderson, M.; McAdams, M. A brief dietary screen for high fat intake. *J. Nutr. Educ.* **1989**, *21*, 199–207. [CrossRef]

80. United States Department of Agriculture. ChooseMyPlate.gov. Available online: https://www.choosemyplate.gov/ (accessed on 9 February 2017).

81. American Academy of Pediatrics Committee on Nutrition, Policy statement: The use and misuse of fruit juices in pediatrics. *Pediatrics* **2006**, *107*, 1210–1213.

82. Lasater, G.; Piernas, C.; Popkin, B. Beverage patterns and trends among school-aged children in the US, 1989–2008. *Nutr. J.* **2011**, *10*, 103. [CrossRef] [PubMed]

83. Committee to Review Dietary Reference Intakes for Vitamin D and Calcium; Food and Nutrition Board; Institute of Medicine; National Academy of Sciences. *Dietary Reference Intakes for Calcium and Vitamin D*; National Academies Press: Washington, DC, USA, 2011.

84. Food and Nutrition Board; Institute of Medicine; National Academy of Sciences. *Dietary Reference Intakes for Energy, Carbohydrate. Fiber, Fat, Fatty Acids, Cholesterol, Protein, and Amino Acids*; National Academies Press: Washington, DC, USA, 2005.

85. U.S. Department of Health and Human Services; Centers for Disease Control and Prevention; National Center for Health Statistics. *Health, United States, 2015 with Special Feature on Racial and Ethnic Health Disparities*; U.S. Government Printing Office: Hyattsville, MD, USA, 2015.

86. Council on Communications and Media; American Academy of Pediatrics. Media and young minds. *Pediatrics* **2016**, *138*, e20162591.

87. Golem, D.; Martin-Biggers, J.; Koenings, M.; Finn Davis, K.; Byrd-Bredbenner, C. An integrative review of sleep for nutrition professionals. *Adv. Nutr.* **2014**, *5*, 742–759. [CrossRef] [PubMed]

88. Hiscock, H.; Scalzo, K.; Canterford, L.; Wake, M. Sleep duration and body mass index in 0–7-year old. *Arch. Dis. Child.* **2011**, *96*, 735–739. [CrossRef] [PubMed]

89. Bell, J.F.; Zimmerman, F.J. Shortened nighttime sleep duration in early life and subsequent childhood obesity. *Arch. Pediatr. Adolesc. Med.* **2010**, *164*, 840–845. [CrossRef] [PubMed]

90. Taveras, E.; Rifas-Shiman, S.; Oken, E.; Gunderson, E.; Gillman, M. Short Sleep Duration in Infancy and Risk of Childhood Overweight. *Arch. Pediatr. Adolesc. Med.* **2008**, *165*, 305–311. [CrossRef] [PubMed]

91. Cappuccio, F.P.; Taggart, F.M.; Ngianga-Bakwin, K.; Currie, A.; Peile, E.; Stranges, S.; Miller, M.A. Meta-analysis of short sleep duration and obesity in children and adults. *Sleep* **2008**, *31*, 619–626. [CrossRef] [PubMed]

92. Chaput, J.-P.; Brunet, M.; Tremblay, A. Relationship between short sleeping hours and childhood overweight/obesity: Results from the 'Québec en Forme' Project. *Int. J. Obes.* **2006**, *30*, 1080–1085. [CrossRef] [PubMed]

93. Hirshkowitz, M.; Whiton, K.; Albert, S.; Alessi, C.; Bruni, O.; DonCarlos, L.; Hazen, N.; Herman, J.; Hillard, P.; Katz, E.; et al. National Sleep Foundation updated sleep duration recommendations: Final report. *Sleep Health* **2015**, *1*, 233–243. [CrossRef]

94. National Sleep Foundation. *International Bedroom Poll: Summary of Findings*; National Sleep Foundation: Arlington, VA, USA, 2013.

95. Burnier, D.; Dubois, L.; Girard, M. Arguments at mealtime and child energy intake. *J. Nutr. Educ. Behav.* **2011**, *43*, 473–481. [CrossRef] [PubMed]

96. Neumark-Sztainer, D.; Hannan, P.J.; Story, M.; Croll, J.; Perry, C. Family meal patterns: Associations with sociodemographic characteristics and improved dietary intake among adolescents. *J. Am. Diet Assoc.* **2003**, *103*, 317–322. [CrossRef] [PubMed]

97. Ayala, G.; Baquero, B.; Arrendondo, E.; Campbell, N.; Larios, M.; Elder, J. Association between family variables and Mexican American children's dietary behaviors. *J. Nutr. Educ. Behav.* **2007**, *39*, 62–69. [CrossRef] [PubMed]

98. Gillman, M.; Rifas-Shiman, S.; Frazier, L.; Rockett, H.; Camargo, C.; Field, A.; Berkey, C.; Colditz, G. Family dinner and diet quality among older children and adolescents. *Arch. Fam. Med.* **2000**, *9*, 235–240. [CrossRef] [PubMed]

99. Guthrie, J.; Lin, B.; Frazao, E. Role of food prepared away from home in the American diet, 1977–78 versus 1994–96: Changes and consequences. *J. Nutr. Educ. Behav.* **2002**, *34*, 140–150. [CrossRef]

100. Boutelle, K.; Fulkerson, J.; Neumark-Sztainer, D.; Story, M.; French, S. Fast food for family meals: Relationships with parent and adolescent food intake, home food availability, and weight status. *Public Health Nutr.* **2007**, *10*, 16–23. [CrossRef] [PubMed]

101. McIntosh, W.; Kubena, K.; Tolle, G.; Dean, W.; Jan, J.; Anding, J. Mothers and meals. The effects of mothers. meal planning and shopping motivations on children's participation in family meals. *Appetite* **2010**, *55*, 623–628. [CrossRef] [PubMed]

102. Anderson, S.; Must, A.; Curtin, C.; Bandini, L. Meals in our household: Reliability and initial validation of a questionnaire to assess child mealtime behaviors and family mealtime environments. *J. Acad. Nutr. Diet* **2012**, *112*, 276–284. [CrossRef] [PubMed]

103. Bandura, A. *Social Learning Theory*; Prentice-Hall: Englewood Cliffs, NJ, USA, 1977.

104. Kelder, S.; Hoelscher, D.; Perry, C. How individuals, environments, and health behavior interact; Social Cognitive Theory. In *Health Behavior and Health Education. Theory, Research, and Practice*, 4th ed.; Glanz, K., Rimer, B., Viswanath, K., Eds.; Jossey-Bass: San Francisco, CA, USA, 2015.

105. Montano, D.; Kasprzyk, D. Theory of reasoned action, theory of planned behavior, and the integrated behavioral model. In *Health Behavior and Health Education. Theory, Research, and Practice*, 4th ed.; Glanz, K., Rimer, B., Viswanath, K., Eds.; Jossey-Bass: San Francisco, CA, USA, 2015.

106. Bandura, A. *Self-Efficacy: The Exercise of Control*; W.H. Freeman: New York, NY, USA, 1997.

16

Snacking Quality is Associated with Secondary School Academic Achievement and the Intention to Enroll in Higher Education

Paulina Correa-Burrows [1],*, Yanina Rodríguez [1], Estela Blanco [2], Sheila Gahagan [2] and Raquel Burrows [1]

[1] Institute of Nutrition and Food Technology, University of Chile, Santiago 7830490, Chile; yanirod77@hotmail.com (Y.R.); rburrows@inta.uchile.cl (R.B.)

[2] Division of Child Development and Community Health, University of California, San Diego, CA 92093, USA; esblanco@ucsd.edu (E.B.); sgahagan@ucsd.edu (S.G.)

* Correspondence: paulina.correa@inta.uchile.cl

Abstract: Although numerous studies have approached the effects of exposure to a Western diet (WD) on academic outcomes, very few have focused on foods consumed during snack times. We explored whether there is a link between nutritious snacking habits and academic achievement in high school (HS) students from Santiago, Chile. We conducted a cross-sectional study with 678 adolescents. The nutritional quality of snacks consumed by 16-year-old was assessed using a validated food frequency questionnaire. The academic outcomes measured were HS grade point average (GPA), the likelihood of HS completion, and the likelihood of taking college entrance exams. A multivariate analysis was performed to determine the independent associations of nutritious snacking with having completed HS and having taken college entrance exams. An analysis of covariance (ANCOVA) estimated the differences in GPA by the quality of snacks. Compared to students with healthy in-home snacking behaviors, adolescents having unhealthy in-home snacks had significantly lower GPAs (M difference: -40.1 points, 95% confidence interval (CI): -59.2, -16.9, $d = 0.41$), significantly lower odds of HS completion (adjusted odds ratio (aOR): 0.47; 95% CI: 0.25–0.88), and significantly lower odds of taking college entrance exams (aOR: 0.53; 95% CI: 0.31–0.88). Unhealthy at-school snacking showed similar associations with the outcome variables. Poor nutritional quality snacking at school and at home was associated with poor secondary school academic achievement and the intention to enroll in higher education.

Keywords: adolescents; unhealthy eating; snacks; academic performance; diet quality

1. Introduction

In spite of efforts by public agencies to monitor the types of food sold in school settings or regulate food advertising aimed at young people, their exposure to energy-dense foods (those with a high caloric concentration per bite) at and away from school remains high [1]. A recent study on the consumption of fast food in 36 developed and developing countries showed that more than 50% of adolescents consume fast food frequently or very frequently [2]. In Latin America, the Global School-based Health Survey (GSHS) showed that two-thirds of adolescents (13–17 years old) in Argentina, Chile and Uruguay reported daily intake of sugar-sweetened beverages [3]. In the early 2010s, among European 15-year-old, daily soft drink consumption was more than 40% in England, the Netherlands, Belgium, Slovakia and Slovenia [4].

Evidence is available on the role of Western-type diets (WD) in limiting cognitive abilities in critical brain maturation periods (i.e., infancy and childhood) [5,6]. Animal models show that exposure to a high-fat, high-sugar (HFS) diet in adolescence is related to impairment in hippocampal learning and memory processes, regardless of weight status [7,8]. One important mechanism that is proposed to underlie HFS-induced impaired hippocampal function is the reduced synthesis, secretion, and action of the brain-derived neurotrophic factor (BDNF). BDNF facilitates synaptic efficacy by converting changes in electrical activity to long-lasting changes in synaptic function, which is a suggested key process for memory formation [9]. Reduced levels of BDNF in association with impaired memory function has been well documented in the literature [10,11].

Impairment of memory consolidation and memory performance is a risk factor for learning difficulties and poor academic progress [12]. Thus, a diet of poor nutritional value may compromise students' ability to perform well in school. Longitudinal and cross-sectional studies, mostly conducted in developed countries, have examined the relationship between diet and school grades [13–15], as well as the relationship between diet and performance on standardized academic tests [16–18]. Results collectively suggest that better educational outcomes are associated with regular consumption of nutritious breakfasts, lower intake of energy-dense, nutrient-poor foods, and maintaining a healthy diet [19].

The effect of WDs on academic results can be used to strengthen health promotion strategies. While the connection between unhealthy diet and poor academic performance (as measured by school grades and standardized test scores) in elementary and middle schoolers has been well described, less is known about the relationship between dietary habits and postsecondary educational aspirations—that is, the intention to pursue higher education after secondary school. The increasing number of HS graduates seeking entrance to higher education institutions, including in non-industrialized nations, has made this a particularly important topic for students, families and policymakers.

Since the question of how WD foods may compromise students' intention to pursue higher education is also of interest to non-academic audiences, we used a translational-research approach to provide evidence that can be translated from research and applied to practice and policy. Thus, we examined the relationship of nutritional quality of snacks with academic outcomes using functional cognition measures like grade point average (GPA), high school (HS) completion, and college entrance examination participation rates. Our decision to concentrate on snacks rather than overall diet or meals such as breakfast, lunch or supper was based on wanting to focus on food choices made by adolescents rather than consumption of foods over which they may have little volition. We hypothesized that students habitually eating unhealthy snacks would have lower grades and be less likely to complete HS and take college admission exams.

2. Materials and Methods

2.1. Study Design and Population

We studied 16–17-year-old adolescents living in Santiago, Chile, from low-to-middle socioeconomic status (SES), who were part of an infancy cohort. Participants were recruited at 4 months from public healthcare facilities in the southeast area of Santiago ($n = 1791$). They were born at term of uncomplicated vaginal births, weighed >3.0 kg, and were free of acute or chronic health problems. At 6 months, infants free of iron deficiency anemia ($n = 1657$) were randomly assigned to receive iron supplementation or no added iron (ages 6–12 months). They were assessed for developmental outcomes in infancy, and at 5, 10 and 15 years [20]. At 16–17 years, those with complete data in each wave ($n = 678$) were also assessed for obesity risk and the presence of cardiovascular risk factors in a half-day evaluation that included assessment of dietary habits and nutritional content of food intake. Ethical approval was obtained by the institutional review boards of the University of Michigan, Institute of Nutrition and Food Technology (INTA), University of Chile, and the University of California, San Diego. Participants and their primary caregiver provided informed and written consent, according to the norms for Human Experimentation, Code of Ethics of the World Medical Association (Declaration of Helsinki, 1995).

2.2. Nutritional Quality of Snacking at Age 16

Nutritional quality of in-school and at-home snacking was measured considering the amount of saturated fat, fiber, sugar and salt in the food. Assessment was performed with a food frequency questionnaire, validated using three 24 h recalls to include weekends [21,22]. A section of this questionnaire was specially designed to assess the usual diet during the snack time at school and at home, by asking about the frequency of food consumption within the past three months. A list of 50 foods and beverages was used. The frequency of food consumption was assessed by a multiple response grid; respondents were asked to estimate how often a particular food or beverage was consumed. Categories ranged from "never" to "five or more times a week". The electronic version of the Chilean Food Composition Tables/Database was used to assess the quality of snacks composition [23]. Food items were classified as unhealthy (poor nutritional value items, high in fat, sugar, salt and calories), unhealthy-to-fair (highly processed items although low in fat) and healthy (nutrient rich foods). We assigned adjustment weights to each food item conditioned to its nutritional quality. A score ranging from 0–10 was computed by adjusting the frequency of food consumption to the nutritional quality of foods consumed during the snack time. For each snacking type (in-school or at-home), participants had a continuous score, with higher scores representing healthier snacking habits. We applied quartile cutoffs for the Chilean adolescent population (comprising students of high-, middle- and low-SES) to classify the nutritional quality of in-home and at-school snacking of participants into three groups: unhealthy ($\leq$4.3 or $\leq$25th percentile), unhealthy-to-fair (from 4.4 to 5.9 or >25th percentile and <75th percentile) and healthy ($\geq$6.0 or $\geq$75th percentile) [21].

2.3. Academic Outcomes

The academic outcomes measured were HS GPA, the likelihood of HS completion, and the likelihood of taking college entrance exams. Data on GPA and high school completion were obtained from publicly available records at the Academic Assessment Unit of the Ministry of Education of Chile. Following the Ministry of Education criteria, GPA (on a scale of 1–7) was transformed into standardized scores (ranging from 210–825), and adjusted by type of secondary education (academic, vocational or adult school). Data on college examination rates were derived from publicly available information from the Assessment and Measurement Department of the University of Chile, which administers the tests for college entrance on behalf of the Ministry of Education. Although the exams for college admission are non-mandatory for HS graduates (only for those aiming at enrolling in higher education), more than 85% of Chilean HS graduates take the tests and, thus, have plans for future schooling [24].

2.4. Weight Status at Age 16

A research physician used standardized procedures to measure the adolescent's height (cm) and weight (kg) in duplicate. Body mass index (BMI = kg/m^2) at age 16 was evaluated and z-scores were estimated according to the World Health Organization (WHO) 2007 references [25]. Weight status was defined as follows: underweight (BMI-z < -1 SD), normal weight (BMI-z from -1 SD to 1 SD), overweight (BMI-z from 1 SD to <2 SD) and obesity (BMI-z $\geq$ 2 SD).

2.5. Physical Activity at Age 16

Physical activity has been found to be associated with academic achievement in studies conducted in Chile [26,27]; therefore, it could be a relevant confounder for the association between diet and academic results. We approached physical activity habits with scheduled, repetitive and planned exercise, accounting for the number of weekly hours devoted to Physical Education (PE), and extracurricular sports. To measure this, we used a questionnaire that was validated in a previous study using accelerometry-based activity monitors in both elementary and high school children [28]. The questionnaire was administered by a researcher to all students at the time they attended the anthropometric examination. Participants were asked: (1) On average, over the past week, how often did you engage in PE? (2) On average, over the past week, how often did you engage in extracurricular sports, either school- or non-school-organized? (3) On those days, on average, how long did you engage in such activities? With this information, we estimated the average hours per week of scheduled physical activity. Participants having $\leq$90 min of weekly scheduled physical activity, which is the mandatory time for school-based PE, were considered to be physically inactive.

2.6. Other Covariates Collected in Previous Waves

Parental educational attainment is an important measure of human capital level among populations and, also, is an important predictor of children's educational outcomes [29]. In infancy, participant's mother and father were asked to report the highest schooling level they have been enrolled in, as well as the highest grade they completed at that level. In our analysis, five standard hierarchic levels were defined according to the 2011 International Standard Classification of Education: (1) no education completed; (2) first level (primary school or 1st–8th); (3) secondary level (first phase or 9th–10th); (4) secondary level (second phase or 11th–12th); and (5) post-secondary non-tertiary educations or short-cycle tertiary education [30]. Then, we merged these categories into two: incomplete secondary education (1 + 2 + 3), and complete secondary education or higher (4 + 5). In health research, parental education has been often used as proxy for socioeconomic background [31]. Also, because the literature describes correlations between children's educational outcomes and family structure [32], we include a variable denoting whether the participant was raised in a fatherless family. This information was reported by the participant's parents or guardian. Finally, to control potential design biases, we used a categorical variable denoting whether the participant had received iron supplementation or no added iron at 6–12 months.

2.7. Statistical Analysis

Data were processed using Stata SE for Windows 12.0 (Lakeway Drive College Station, TX, USA). All categorical data were expressed as absolute and relative frequencies, while continuous data were expressed as means and standard deviations. Statistical analysis included χ^2 for categorical variables, and analysis of variance (ANOVA) with Bonferroni correction for comparison of means. We tested for effect measure modification (interaction) by weight status and physical activity, in the association between quality of snacking and academic outcomes using two-way ANOVA. The interaction of quality of snacking with weight status and physical activity was non-significant at $p < 0.05$ and, therefore, we did not stratify the analysis. Unadjusted logistic models were used to explore cross-sectional patterns of variation in academic behavior across snack categories (unhealthy and unhealthy-to-fair vs. healthy). Next, the models were adjusted for sex, weight status, physical activity, familial background and a variable to control potential design biases. Odds ratios are presented in the tables with 95% CI to evaluate the strength and precision of the associations. Analysis of covariance (ANCOVA) was used to determine whether high school GPA differed by nutritional quality of snacking, accounting for the same potential confounders. Because GPA scores do not have an intrinsic meaning, the effect size for difference was estimated using Cohen's *d* coefficients. A $p < 0.05$ denoted statistical significance.

3. Results

As shown in Table 1, our sample was composed of 16.8-year-old (0.3 SD) adolescents (47% males). Eighty-four percent completed HS (*n* = 571) and were allowed to take the exams for college admission. Of them, 68% (*n* = 388) took the college entrance exam. High school GPA ranged from 269–795 points, and mean value was 481.1 (92.3 SD) points. Mean value of BMI-z was 0.65 (1.2 SD). Of the participants, 25% and 14% were overweight and obese, respectively. In the sample, 60% were physically inactive.

Table 1. Descriptive statistics of the sample: adolescent students from Santiago, Chile ($n = 678$).

Variables	Mean or n	SD or Percentage
Chronological age		
Age (years)	16.8	0.3
In-home snacking		
Healthy	180	26.55
Unhealthy-to-fair	337	49.71
Unhealthy	161	23.74
At-school snacking		
Healthy	183	26.99
Unhealthy-to-fair	302	44.54
Unhealthy	193	28.47
Academic outcomes		
Graduated high school	571	84.09
Took college admission exams * ($n = 571$)	387	67.76
High school GPA (score) ($n = 571$)	481.1	92.3
Sex		
Male	357	52.58
Anthropometrics		
BMI (z-score)	0.65	1.2
Weight status		
Normal	417	61.42
Overweight	167	24.59
Obesity	95	14.99
Physical activity		
Weekly scheduled PA $\leq$ 90 min	403	59.35
Parental education		
Maternal education: incomplete secondary	240	35.40
Paternal education: incomplete secondary	192	28.32
Family structure		
Fatherless family	274	40.4
Iron supplementation in infancy		
No added Fe (6–12 months)	286	42.18

* Only those students graduating from high school ($n = 571$) are allowed to take the exams for college admission. BMI: Body-Mass Index. Normal weight: BMI-z from -1 SD to $+1$ SD. Overweight: BMI-z from >1 SD to 2 SD. Obesity: BMI-z $\geq$ 2 SD. GPA: grade point average; SD: standard deviation; PA: physical activity.

The share of students completing the secondary education significantly increased with better nutritional quality of at-school ($\chi^2 = 6.73$, $p < 0.05$) and in-home ($\chi^2 = 7.19$, $p < 0.05$) snacking (Figure 1). Likewise, the proportion of students taking the exams for higher education was significantly higher among participants having healthy in-home ($\chi^2 = 12.40$, $p < 0.01$) and at-school ($\chi^2 = 11.66$, $p < 0.01$) snacking (Figure 2).

Table 2 shows the estimated cross-sectional association between graduating HS and the nutritional quality of in-home and at-school snacking. After adjusting for sex, weight status, physical activity, parental education, family structure and iron supplementation in infancy, unhealthy snacking significantly reduced the odds of completing the secondary education. For instance, students having unhealthy in-home snacks were 53% (odds ratio (OR): 0.47, 95% CI: 0.25–0.88) less likely to complete HS than students having healthy in-home snacks. Odds were lower but non-significant among students eating foods of unhealthy-to-fair nutritional quality at home compared to those eating healthy snacks at home. When school snacking was the exposure, we also found a positive significant association of nutritional quality of snacks with the likelihood of getting the HS diploma (aOR: 0.49, 95% CI: 0.27–0.89). In all these models, sex and physical activity were also related to the chances of HS graduation.

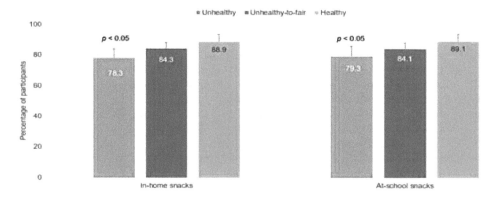

Figure 1. Proportion of students getting their high school diploma (outcome) by nutritional quality of in-home and at-school snacking (exposure) ($n = 678$). Error bars are 95% CI (upper limit). CI: confidence interval.

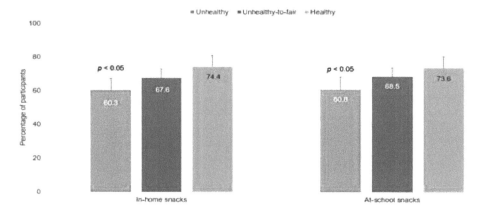

Figure 2. Proportion of participants taking the exams for college admission (outcome) by nutritional quality of in-home and at-school snacking (exposure) ($n = 571$). Only those students graduating from high school ($n = 571$) are allowed to take the exams for college admission. Error bars are 95% CI (upper limit).

Table 2. Estimated cross-sectional association between achieving the high school diploma (outcomes) and nutritional quality of in-home and at-school snacking (exposure) in students from Santiago, Chile, after adjusting other influences ($n = 678$).

	In-Home Snacking				At-School Snacking			
	OR	95% CI	aOR	95% CI	OR	95% CI	aOR	95% CI
Unhealthy	0.44 **	0.25–0.82	0.47 *	0.25–0.88	0.47 *	0.26–0.83	0.49 *	0.27–0.89
Unhealthy-to-fair	0.67	0.39–1.16	0.70	0.39–1.24	0.65	0.37–1.13	0.67	0.37–1.20
Male	(…)	–	0.42 ***	0.27–0.67	(…)	–	0.43 ***	0.27–0.68
Overweight	(…)	–	0.88	0.52–1.46	(…)	–	0.89	0.53–1.48
Obesity	(…)	–	0.81	0.44–1.49	(…)	–	0.81	0.44–1.49
Physically inactive	(…)	–	0.37 ***	0.22–0.61	(…)	–	0.37 ***	0.22–0.63
Maternal education	(…)	–	0.66	0.42–1.02	(…)	–	0.66	0.42–1.02
Paternal education	(…)	–	0.91	0.55–1.47	(…)	–	0.91	0.56–1.48
Fatherless family	(…)	–	0.77	0.51–1.20	(…)	–	0.77	0.50–1.19
No added Fe	(…)	–	0.89	0.57–1.37	(…)	–	0.89	0.58–1.38

OR: Odds ratio. aOR: adjusted OR. (…) Non-observed variables. Overweight: BMI-z from >1 SD to <2 SD. Obesity: BMI-z $\geq$ 2 SD. Physically inactive: $\leq$90 min/week of scheduled exercise. Maternal and paternal education: incomplete high school. * $p < 0.05$; ** $p < 0.01$; *** $p < 0.001$.

Similarly, among students who completed HS, the odds of taking the college entrance exam were significantly lower for those having unhealthy in-home snacks compared to those having healthy in-home snacks (Table 3). After controlling other influences, students who reported consumption of unhealthy in-home snacks were 47% less likely (aOR: 0.53; 95% CI: 0.31–0.88) to take the college entrance exam, compared to students eating healthy snack items. In addition, students eating in-home snacks of unhealthy-to-fair nutritional quality had lower odds of taking the college entrance exam, compared to those with healthier habits, though the association was non-significant. When school snacking was the exposure, the odds of taking the examination for college were also lower in students eating unhealthy snacks (aOR: 0.57; 95% CI: 0.35–0.90) compared to those eating healthy at-school snacks. In all these models, the odds of taking the college entrance exam were significantly associated with sex, maternal education and family structure.

The nutritional quality of snacking was also significantly related with students' final GPA as shown in Figure 3. After accounting for the effect of sex, weight status, physical activity, parental education, family structure and iron supplementation in infancy (Table 4), the group snacking on unhealthy foods at home had a final GPA of 490.0 points, on average, whereas participants having healthy snacks at home had a final GPA of 530.1 points (GPA mean difference = −40.1 points; 95% CI: −59.2; −16.9, d = 0.43). When comparing those having unhealthy-to-fair snacks vs. those having healthy snacks at home the GPA mean difference was −27.9 points (95% CI: −43.5; −8.2, d = 0.30). It is worth noting that Cohen's d coefficients around 0.20 are considered of interest in educational research when they are based on measures of academic achievement [33]. Lastly, the same pattern was observed when the main exposure was the nutritional quality of at-school snacking.

Table 3. Estimated cross-sectional association between taking the exams for higher education (outcome) and nutritional quality of in-home and at-school snacking (exposure) in students from Santiago, Chile, after adjusting other influences (n = 571).

	In-Home Snacking				At-School Snacking			
	OR	95% CI	aOR	95% CI	OR	95% CI	aOR	95% CI
Unhealthy	0.46 **	0.29–0.71	0.53 *	0.31–0.88	0.49 ***	0.32–0.74	0.57 *	0.35–0.90
Unhealthy-to-fair	0.68 *	0.47–0.98	0.75	0.48–1.15	0.71	0.49–1.04	0.81	0.51–1.27
Male	(...)	–	0.66 *	0.45–0.96	(...)	–	0.66 *	0.45–0.97
Overweight	(...)	–	0.99	0.64–1.52	(...)	–	0.99	0.65–1.55
Obesity	(...)	–	0.97	0.56–1.66	(...)	–	0.97	0.57–1.67
Physically inactive	(...)	–	0.85	0.57–1.25	(...)	–	0.84	0.57–1.24
Maternal education	(...)	–	0.63 *	0.42–0.92	(...)	–	0.63 *	0.42–0.92
Paternal education	(...)	–	0.75	0.49–1.13	(...)	–	0.76	0.50–1.15
Fatherless family	(...)	–	0.68 *	0.48–0.99	(...)	–	0.68 *	0.47–0.98
No added Fe	(...)	–	0.84	0.59–1.21	(...)	–	0.84	0.58–1.21

OR: Odds ratio. aOR: adjusted OR. (...) Non-observed variables. Overweight: BMI-z from >1 SD to <2 SD. Obesity: BMI-z ≥ 2 SD. Physically inactive: ≤90 min/week of scheduled exercise. Maternal and paternal education: incomplete high school. * $p < 0.05$; ** $p < 0.01$; *** $p < 0.001$.

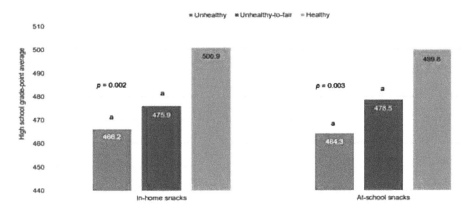

Figure 3. Mean high school grade point average (GPA) by nutritional quality of in-home and at-school snacking (n = 571). GPA expressed as standardized score, according to the Chilean Ministry of Education. a, significantly different from the group having healthy snacks at home or at school. p value estimated with Analysis of Variance (ANOVA) with Bonferroni adjustment.

Table 4. Cross-sectional association between academic attainment in high school (outcome) and nutritional quality of in-home snacking and at-school (exposure) in students from Santiago, Chile, after adjusting other influences ($n = 571$).

	In-Home Snacking			At-School Snacking		
Mean GPA	Mean	Mean		Mean	SD	
Unhealthy (1)	490.0	473.2		473.2	90.2	
Unhealthy-to-fair (2)	502.2	486.8		486.8	89.3	
Healthy (3)	530.1	512.4		512.4	93.6	
Comparison of mean GPA [§]	Mean diff.	95% CI	d [†]	Mean diff.	95% CI	d [†]
(1) vs. (2)	−12.2	−32.7; 4.6	0.09	−13.6	−33.2; 2.4	0.15
(1) vs. (3)	−40.1 ***	−59.2; −16.9	0.41	−39.2 ***	−57.0; −17.1	0.44
(2) vs. (3)	−27.9 ***	−43.5; −8.2	0.30	−25.6 *	−40.6; −4.9	0.31

GPA: Grade point average (expressed in score according to the Ministry of Education). [§] ANCOVA: * $p < 0.05$; *** $p < 0.001$. Models were adjusted for sex, weight status, familial background and iron supplementation in infancy. [†] Cohen's d coefficients account for the effect of different sample sizes. ESs around 0.20 are of policy interest when they are based on measures of academic achievement [33]. ANCOVA: analysis of covariance.

4. Discussion

4.1. Main Findings

This study explored whether the nutritional quality of in-home and at-school snacking among high school students in Santiago, Chile, was cross-sectionally associated with secondary school academic achievement and the intention to enroll in higher education. Although numerous studies have approached the effects of short-term exposure to a WD on academic outcomes [19], very few have focused on foods consumed during snack times. We found that unhealthy snacking was correlated with lower high school GPA and rate of graduation, as well as a reduced likelihood of taking college admission exams. When controls for sex and other potentially confounding variables (e.g., weight status, physical activity, familial background, etc.) were entered into the models, unhealthy snacking continued to be associated with worse academic results.

Our findings are consistent with previous research that found evidence of a relationship between a healthy diet and academic achievement. The results of a population-based study of 4th and 8th grade Chilean school children—students from subsidized, partially subsidized, and private schools—showed a positive cross-sectional association between performance in language and mathematics as measured by Chile's standardized System for the Assessment of Educational Quality test and the nutritional quality of school snacking, regardless of sex, SES, and other educational influences [17]. Similarly, in a subset ($n = 395$) of the current sample, Correa et al. [18] observed that, among students taking college entrance exams, unhealthy dietary habits of 16-year-old were associated with lower performance on college examination tests when compared to the performance of students with healthy dietary habits.

Cross-sectional studies conducted in adolescents from other countries also found that participants having healthy dietary habits performed better at school compared to those having unhealthy dietary habits. For instance, the native and foreign language attainment among 14- and 15-year-old Icelandic students, as well as their mathematics achievement, were negatively influenced by poor dietary habits [13,15]. Norwegian 9th and 10th graders with a high intake of sugar-sweetened soft drinks, candies, chocolate, chips, pizza, hot dogs, and hamburgers were up to 6 times more likely to manifest learning difficulties in mathematics. Conversely, a diet of fresh fruits at least once daily reduced the chances of difficulties in these areas [14]. Also in 15- to 17-year-old Norwegian adolescents, high academic achievement was associated with a high intake of fruits and berries, and a low intake of sugar-sweetened beverages [34]. Unfavorable academic performance, as measured by a standardized test, was positively associated with unhealthy dietary patterns in 6- to 13-year-old Taiwanese students. The likelihood of underperforming on the test was 1.63 times higher for students with greater consumption of low-quality foods (e.g., sweets and fried foods) than it was for students with low intake of such items. Fu et al. also showed that students with poor academic performance were less likely to regularly eat foods that are rich in protein, vitamins and minerals [35].

Diet is also an important influence on other determinants of academic success. Among adolescent students from Iceland, having an optimal diet was cross-sectionally associated with decreased odds of behavioral problems in the classroom [36]. Likewise, in 15- and 16-year-old male students from Oslo (Norway), intake of >4 glasses/day of sugar-sweetened soft drinks more than doubled the probability of having behavioral problems at school, compared to students drinking <1 glass of sugary drinks per day [37]. Among female students in Oslo with excessive intake of sugar-sweetened soft drinks, the chances of conduct problems at school were 4.1 times higher compared to the reference group. In males, soft drink consumption was also related to hyperactivity and higher levels of mental distress, both of which are associated with academic difficulties [38].

It is likely that the effect on academic results of excessive consumption of foods high in saturated fats and simple sugars is mediated by the effect of these macronutrients on brain health and cognitive function. In developmental stages such as adolescence, the brain is particularly vulnerable to the effects of excessive intake of saturated fats and simple carbohydrates [5,6]. Diet-induced impairment in learning and hippocampus-dependent memory processes have been widely documented [7,8,39,40]. In addition to reducing production of neurotrophins such as BDNF, other WD-induced effects have been reported on this brain structure, including overexpression of proinflammatory cytokines, mitochondrial damage due to oxidative stress, and altered blood–brain barrier permeability [7,8,10,39]. Also, insulin resistance and hyperleptinemia have been linked to impaired hippocampal synaptic plasticity and poor cognitive functioning [41–43]. Furthermore, evidence suggests that juvenile exposure to a WD may be more harmful than such exposure in adulthood. A 3-week juvenile WD regimen induced similar weight gain and metabolic alterations as did a 12-week adult WD regimen. Juvenile exposure, however, also affected memory consolidation and flexible memory expression while promoting exaggerated pro-inflammatory cytokine expression in the hippocampus after an immune challenge, and it diminished hippocampal neurogenesis [8,39].

While the cross-sectional design of our study prevents definitive conclusions about causality and the direction of the associations depicted here, it is worth noting that research conducted in both animals and humans described short-term effects of Western-type dietary habits on hippocampal-dependent learning and memory. In animals, it is well established that a WD causes rapid impairments of hippocampal-based tasks, with diet-related cognitive effects observed after only 72 h [44,45]. Studies in humans are limited but they confirm that a WD impacts hippocampal memory tasks following a relatively short exposure. Healthy 20-year-old college students from Australia consuming a HFS breakfast (30% saturated fats plus 18% refined sugars), over four consecutive days, showed significantly poorer memory recall compared to control students consuming a healthier breakfast of similar palatability and food types, but significantly lower in saturated fats and refined sugars (5% saturated fats plus 10% sugars). Since these changes in memory performance were linked to shifts in blood glucose across breakfast, authors suggest that this could be one potential mechanism by which a WD affects hippocampal function [46]. In a similar manner, in sedentary men aged 25–45 years, Edwards et al. found decreased power of attention and increased simple reaction time after seven days of consuming a diet comprising 74% kcal. from fat [47]. It is less clear for how long the cognitive effects of a WD will remain and, thus, further investigations should address that question. Although experimental studies in humans show that improvements in memory can occur following reductions in energy intake and fat [48], or shift to a diet low in saturated fats and refined sugars [49], observational longitudinal studies conducted in Anglo-Saxon countries suggest that unhealthy dietary practices in developmental periods have a lasting association with cognitive and educational outcomes that seem to persist over time, regardless of later changes in diet [16,50–52].

Our results also showed that a significant share (73%) of participants in the sample ate snacks of intermediate or poor nutritional value. This is consistent with population surveys conducted nationally and internationally. In Chile, adolescents (aged 14 years to 18 years) ranked first in the consumption of refined sugar (121 g/day) and second in the consumption of saturated fats (12.7 mL-g/day) compared to other age groups. In this age group, the consumption of sugar-sweetened soft drinks was 254 mL/day, according to the latest National Food Consumption Survey [53]. This survey also reported that 97% of children and adolescents aged 6 years to 18 years need to improve the quality of their diets. The World Health Organization's Health Behaviour in School-aged Children (HBSC) survey found that in Scotland, 35% of adolescents eat sweets or chocolate every day, and 18% eat chips every day. In addition, 20% of Scottish female adolescents and 27% of their male counterparts consume sugary soft drinks daily [54]. Among US high schoolers, 22% of males and 17% of females report consumption of sugar-sweetened soft drinks ≥ 2 times per day [55].

4.2. Implications for Practice

Our results are of interest for a number of reasons. Translating research knowledge to practice and policy is much needed in the field of health promotion [56,57]. The idea of testing the connection between diet and cognition using functional cognitive measures such as GPA, graduation rates, and rates of taking college entrance exams was aimed at bridging the gap between research and policymaking. Although evidence on the consequences of unhealthy diets on learning and cognition is growing, the failure to implement effective interventions persists. A more informed approach to this connection can influence healthcare practitioners, educators and parents.

In addition, lower academic results have been associated with several health-risk behaviors in youths. In US adolescent populations, over the past three decades, cross-sectional and longitudinal studies demonstrate links connecting poor academic performance with sedentary lifestyle, alcohol/tobacco abuse, sexually risky behaviors, and violence [58]. All of these risk behaviors have been regarded as important contributors to poor health status in adulthood and multiple social problems. Since the influence of academic performance on future health is known [59], the relationship of diet and academic results may be an important public health tool. It is also important to identify the nutrients and dietary patterns that most influence cognitive health and academic performance.

The fact that adolescents struggle to make healthy dietary choices is not new information. Youthful anomalous health decision-making has been attributed to an aversion to forced choices; the inclination to rely on taste, brands, and convenience as primary drivers of food decisions; and the tendency to discount the value of delayed rewards or penalties [60]. Also, sufficient nutrition knowledge does not necessarily correspond to responsible dietary behavior [61]. Thus, associating healthy dietary choices with school performance can perhaps enhance the value of healthy eating and boost motivation. After all, academic achievement, academic behavior, and academic performance are closely linked to expectations of better postsecondary opportunities and subsequent job status [62,63].

Our results that show an association between a healthy diet and improved cognitive and educational outcomes should be a matter of interest to support nutrition interventions designed for adolescents. To date, the majority of interventions that emphasize the relationship between diet type and cognition and academics have been designed for infants and young children [6,19,52], who are less independent in their food choices. For health promotion purposes, unhealthy dietary habits during adolescence are usually said to be related to early onset of cardiometabolic disorders, including high blood pressure, type-2 diabetes and coronary heart disease, while arguments based on the potential cognitive impact of diet are still lacking. We have seen that adolescents are also exposed to the detrimental cognitive effects of a diet high in saturated fats and refined sugars. Moreover, adolescence is a transitional period with subcortical regions associated with reward-seeking and emotion developing earlier than prefrontal control regions [64]. Greater emotional reactivity and sensitivity may in part explain unhealthy dietary habits among teenagers. Sociocultural changes, the need to fit in, food availability and the quest for independent decision-making also contribute to unhealthy food choices that are common during adolescence [65], making this period one of tremendous importance in terms of cognitive development.

A further implication of these findings is that they can potentially play a major role in health promotion by educational agencies and schools. Dietary habits that comport with food guidelines might help pave the way for students on the path to higher education. Chilean high school students perform far below the Organization for Economic Co-operation and Development (OECD) average in mathematics, reading and science, with less than 2% of 15-year-old scoring in the group of top performers [63]. Evidence shows that students who fail to reach baseline levels of performance in these areas have difficulties with academic readiness, persistence and higher education completion [66]. Nonetheless, 80% of Chilean parents expect their children to obtain a college degree [63].

4.3. Limitations and Strengths

This research provides results that support a connection between nutritious dietary intake and higher academic achievement. Given that most studies have been conducted in the developed world, one strength of this study is that it provides evidence that may be useful for countries undergoing nutritional and epidemiological transitions. Second, the use of a translational research approach to explore the diet–learning–cognition connection and provide applicable results is a positive contribution. Further, to our best knowledge, this is the first study to investigate the association of nutrition and academic achievement on HS students' postsecondary education intentions.

Despite these strengths, several limitations persist that should be considered when interpreting these results. Our sample is not representative of the Chilean adolescent population, as it consisted of adolescents from low and middle SES families. However, data from these socioeconomic groups may be especially important: population-based surveys conducted in Chile show that the prevalence of unhealthy dietary habits, physical inactivity, and excess weight is higher in adolescents from low and middle SES families compared to adolescents from high SES families [53,67]. This means that students from low and middle SES families are more exposed to risk factors for difficulties related to progressing from high school to higher education. Encouraging healthy dietary habits and, in particular, intake of healthy snacks, might smooth the pathway to college. Second, although we accounted for the effect of important confounders (including parental education and family structure), we were not able to consider other key influences, such as family support-related variables, general motivational factors (e.g., achievement motivation), and students' interests in specific subject areas, which may also impact their academic functioning. A third limitation is the cross-sectional nature of the study. Since data on snack quality for each participant was recorded only once, it would be difficult to infer the temporal association between this exposure and the academic outcomes. Thus, only association, and not causation, can be inferred from our study. While our results may be useful to inform new hypotheses, a more complex investigation, such as a longitudinal study or crossover intervention trial, should be conducted to test the temporality of these associations, i.e., that the exposure to Western-type food items precede academic difficulties. Finally, future studies should replicate and extend this analysis in other young populations.

5. Conclusions

Poor nutritional quality snacking at school and at home was associated with poor secondary school academic achievement and lower intention to enroll in higher education. Both types of snacking showed similar associations with these educational outcomes. These results may have important implications for the promotion of healthy lifestyles by educational agencies and schools. Also, associating healthy snacking with educational outcomes can perhaps enhance the value of having responsible health behaviors and boost motivation for a healthy way of life.

Acknowledgments: The authors wish to acknowledge the ongoing commitment of participants and their families. We also thank all the people who contributed to the development of this project, especially, Professors Betsy Lozoff and Marcela Castillo. This study was funded by the National Heart, Blood, and Lung Institute, National Institutes of Health (USA) under grant R01HL088530-2980925, and the National Council for Scientific Research and Technology (CONICYT) (Chile) under grants PAI 79140003 and FONDECYT 1160240. They had no role in the design of the study; in the collection, analyses, or interpretation of data; in the writing of the manuscript, and in the decision to publish the results.

Author Contributions: P.C.-B., R.B. and S.G. conceived and designed the study. R.B., P.C.-B. and Y.R. performed the field study. P.C.-B. and R.B. analyzed the data and wrote the paper. Y.R., E.B. and S.G. performed critical analysis of manuscript draft. E.B. and S.G. edited language. All authors read and approved the final manuscript.

References

1. Fraser, B. Latin American countries crack down on junk food. *Lancet* **2013**, *382*, 385–386. [CrossRef]
2. Braithwaite, I.; Stewart, A.; Hancox, R.; Beasley, R.; Murphy, R.; Mitchell, E.A. Fast-food consumption and body mass index in children and adolescents: An international cross-sectional study. *BMJ Open* **2014**, *4*, e005813. [CrossRef] [PubMed]
3. Ministerio de Salud. Global School-Based Health Survey (Chile). Available online: http://www.who.int/chp/gshs/2013_Chile_GSHS_fact_sheet.pdf (accessed on 10 October 2016).
4. Currie, C.; Zanotti, C.; Morgan, A.; Barnekow, V. Social Determinants of Health and Well-Being among Young People. Health Behaviour in School-Aged Children (HBSC) Study: International Report from the 2009/2010 Survey. WHO Regional Office for Europe: Copenhagen. Available online: http://www.euro.who.int/__data/assets/pdf_file/0003/163857/Social-determinants-of-health-and-well-being-among-young-people.pdf (accessed on 2 November 2016).
5. Benton, D. The influence of children's diet on their cognition and behavior. *Eur. J. Nutr.* **2008**, *47*, 25–37. [CrossRef] [PubMed]
6. Nyaradi, A.; Li, J.; Hickling, S.; Foster, J.; Oddy, W. The role of nutrition in children's neurocognitive development, from pregnancy through infancy. *Front. Hum. Neurosci.* **2013**, *7*, 97. [CrossRef] [PubMed]
7. Boitard, C.; Cavaroc, A.; Sauvant, J.; Aubert, A.; Castanon, N.; Layé, S.; Ferreira, G. Impairment of hippocampal-dependent memory induced by juvenile high-fat diet intake is associated with enhanced hippocampal inflammation in rats. *Brain Behav. Immun.* **2014**, *40*, 9–17. [CrossRef] [PubMed]
8. Valladolid-Acebes, I.; Fole, A.; Martín, M.; Morales, L.; Cano, M.; Ruiz-Gayo, M.; Del Olmo, N. Spatial memory impairment and changes in hippocampal morphology are triggered by high-fat diets in adolescent mice. Is there a role of leptin? *Neurobiol. Learn. Mem.* **2013**, *106*, 18–25. [CrossRef] [PubMed]
9. Lynch, M. Long-term potentiation and memory. *Physiol. Rev.* **2004**, *84*, 87–136. [CrossRef] [PubMed]
10. Kanoski, S.; Davidson, T. Western diet consumption and cognitive impairment: Links to hippocampal dysfunction and obesity. *Physiol. Behav.* **2011**, *103*, 59–68. [CrossRef] [PubMed]
11. Beilharz, J.; Maniam, J.; Morris, M. Diet-induced cognitive deficits: The role of fat and sugar, potential mechanisms and nutritional interventions. *Nutrients* **2015**, *7*, 6719–6738. [CrossRef] [PubMed]
12. Blankenship, T.; O'Neill, M.; Ross, A.; Bell, M. Working memory and recollection contribute to academic achievement. *Learn. Individ. Differ.* **2015**, *43*, 164–169. [CrossRef] [PubMed]
13. Sigfúsdóttir, I.; Krisjánsson, A.; Allegrante, J. Health behaviours and academic achievement in Icelandic school children. *Health Educ. Res.* **2007**, *22*, 70–80. [CrossRef] [PubMed]
14. Kristjánsson, A.; Sigfúsdóttir, I.; Allegrante, J. Health behavior and academic achievement among adolescents: The relative contribution of dietary habits, physical activity, body mass index, and self-esteem. *Health Educ. Behav.* **2010**, *37*, 51–64. [CrossRef] [PubMed]
15. Øverby, N.; Lüdemann, E.; Høigaard, R. Self-reported learning difficulties and dietary intake in Norwegian adolescents. *Scand. J. Public Health* **2013**, *41*, 754–760. [CrossRef] [PubMed]
16. Feinstein, L.; Sabates, R.; Sorhaindo, A.; Emmett, P. Dietary patterns related to attainment in school: The importance of early eating patterns. *J. Epidemiol. Commun. Health* **2008**, *62*, 734–739. [CrossRef] [PubMed]
17. Correa-Burrows, P.; Burrows, R.; Orellana, Y.; Ivanovic, D. The relationship between unhealthy snacking at school and academic outcomes: A population study in Chilean schoolchildren. *Public Health Nutr.* **2015**, *18*, 2022–2030. [CrossRef] [PubMed]
18. Correa-Burrows, P.; Burrows, R.; Blanco, E.; Reyes, M.; Gahagan, S. Nutritional quality of diet and academic performance in Chilean students. *Bull. World Health Org.* **2016**, *94*, 185–192. [CrossRef] [PubMed]
19. Burrows, T.; Goldman, S.; Pursey, K.; Lim, R. Is there an association between dietary intake and academic achievement? A systematic review. *J. Hum. Nutr. Diet.* **2016**, *30*, 117–140. [CrossRef] [PubMed]

20. Lozoff, B.; Castillo, M.; Clark, K.; Smith, J.; Sturza, J. Iron supplementation in infancy contributes to more adaptive behavior at 10 years of age. *J. Nutr.* **2014**, *144*, 838–845. [CrossRef] [PubMed]

21. Burrows, R.; Díaz, E.; Schiaraffia, V.; Gattas, V.; Montoya, A.; Lera, L. Dietary intake and physical activity in school age children. *Rev. Med. Chile* **2008**, *136*, 53–63.

22. Gattas, V.; Burrows, R.; Burgueño, M. Validity Assessment of A Food Frequency Questionnaire in Chilean School-Age Children. In Proceedings of the XVI Congress of the Latin-American Society of Pediatric Research and the XXII Pan-American Meeting of Pediatrics, Santiago, Chile, 25–30 April 2007.

23. Ministerio de Salud. *Tablas Chilenas de Composición Química de los Alimentos*; Ministerio de Salud: Santiago, Chile, 2010.

24. Departamento de Evaluación, Medición y Registro Educacional (DEMRE). Prueba de Selección Universitaria. Informe Técnico. Volumen IV. Proceso de Admisión 2016. Unidad de Desarrollo y Análisis. Universidad de Chile. Available online: http://psu.demre.cl/estadisticas/documentos/informes/2016-vol-4-informe-tecnico-admision-2016.pdf (accessed on 19 September 2016).

25. De Onis, M.; Onyango, A.; Borghi, E.; Siyam, A.; Nishida, C.; Siekmann, J. Development of a WHO growth reference for school-aged children and adolescents. *Bull. World Health Org.* **2007**, *85*, 660–667. [CrossRef] [PubMed]

26. Correa-Burrows, P.; Burrows, R.; Orellana, Y.; Ivanovic, D. Achievement in mathematics and language is linked to regular physical activity: A population study in Chilean youth. *J. Sports Sci.* **2014**, *32*, 1631–1638. [CrossRef] [PubMed]

27. Burrows, R.; Correa-Burrows, P.; Orellana, Y.; Almagiá, A.; Lizana, P.; Ivanovic, D. Scheduled physical activity is associated with better academic performance in Chilean school-age children. *J. Phys. Act. Health* **2014**, *11*, 1600–1606. [CrossRef] [PubMed]

28. Godard, C.; Rodríguez, M.; Díaz, N.; Lera, L.; Salazar, G.; Burrows, R. Value of a clinical test for assessing physical activity in children. *Rev. Med. Chile* **2008**, *136*, 1155–1162.

29. Dobow, E.; Boxer, P.; Huesmann, L. Long-term effects of parents' education on children's educational and occupational success: Mediation by family interactions, child aggression, and teenage aspirations. *Merrill Palmer Q.* **2009**, *55*, 224–249. [CrossRef] [PubMed]

30. United Nations Educational, Scientific and Cultural Organization (UNESCO). International Standard Classification of Education. ISCED 2011. Available online: http://www.uis.unesco.org/Education/Documents/isced-2011-en.pdf (accessed on 19 September 2016).

31. Braveman, P.; Cubbin, C.; Egerter, S.; Chideya, S.; Marchi, K.S.; Metzler, M.; Posner, S. Socioeconomic status in health research: One size does not fit all. *JAMA* **2005**, *294*, 2879–2888. [CrossRef] [PubMed]

32. Ginther, D.; Pollak, R. Family structure and children's educational outcomes: Blended families, stylized facts, and descriptive regressions. *Demography* **2004**, *41*, 671–696. [CrossRef] [PubMed]

33. Hedges, L.; Hedberg, E. Intraclass correlation values for planning group-randomized trials in education. *Educ. Eval. Policy Anal.* **2007**, *29*, 60–87. [CrossRef]

34. Stea, T.; Tortsveit, M. Association of lifestyle habits and academic achievement in Norwegian adolescents: A cross-sectional study. *BMC Public Health* **2014**, *14*, 829. [CrossRef] [PubMed]

35. Fu, M.; Cheng, L.; Tu, S.; Pan, W. Association between unhealthful eating patterns and unfavorable overall school performance in children. *J. Am. Diet Assoc.* **2007**, *107*, 1935–1943. [CrossRef] [PubMed]

36. Øverby, N.; Høigaard, R. Diet and behavioral problems at school in Norwegian adolescents. *Food Nutr. Res.* **2012**, *56*. [CrossRef] [PubMed]

37. Lien, L.; Lien, N.; Heyerdahl, S.; Thoresen, M.; Bjertness, E. Consumption of soft drinks and hyperactivity, mental distress, and conduct problems among adolescents in Oslo, Norway. *Am. J. Public Health* **2006**, *96*, 1815–1820. [CrossRef] [PubMed]

38. Polderman, T.; Boomsma, D.; Bartels, M.; Verhulst, F.; Huizink, A. A systematic review of prospective studies on attention problems and academic achievement. *Acta Psychiatr. Scand.* **2010**, *122*, 271–284. [CrossRef] [PubMed]

39. Boitard, C.; Etchamendy, N.; Sauvant, J.; Ferreira, G. Juvenile but not adult exposure to high fat diet impairs relational memory and hippocampal neurogenesis in mice. *Hippocampus* **2012**, *22*, 2095–2100. [CrossRef] [PubMed]

40. Mellendijk, L.; Wiesmann, M.; Kiliaan, A. Impact of nutrition on cerebral circulation and cognition in the metabolic syndrome. *Nutrients* **2015**, *7*, 9416–9439. [CrossRef] [PubMed]

41. Stranahan, A.; Norman, E.; Lee, K.; Mattson, M. Diet-induced insulin resistance impairs hippocampal synaptic plasticity and cognition in middle-aged rats. *Hippocampus* **2008**, *18*, 1085–1088. [CrossRef] [PubMed]

42. Irving, A.; Harvey, J. Leptin regulation of hippocampal synaptic function in health and disease. *Philos. Trans. R. Soc. B Biol. Sci.* **2013**, *369*. [CrossRef] [PubMed]

43. Lee, S.; Zabolotny, J.; Huang, H.; Lee, H.; Kim, Y. Insulin in the nervous system and the mind: Functions in metabolism, memory, and mood. *Mol. Metab.* **2016**, *5*, 589–601. [CrossRef] [PubMed]

44. Murray, A.; Knight, N.; Cochlin, L.; McAleese, S.; Deacon, R.; Rawlins, J.; Clarke, K. Deterioration of physical performance and cognitive function in rats with short-term high-fat feeding. *FASEB J.* **2009**, *23*, 4353–4360. [CrossRef] [PubMed]

45. Beilharz, J.E.; Maniam, J.; Morris, M.J. Short exposure to a diet rich in both fat and sugar or sugar alone impairs place, but not object recognition memory in rats. *Brain Behav. Immun.* **2014**, *37*, 134–141. [CrossRef] [PubMed]

46. Edwards, L.; Murray, A.; Holloway, C.; Clarke, K. Short-term consumption of a high-fat diet impairs whole-body efficiency and cognitive function in sedentary men. *FASEB J.* **2011**, *25*, 1088–1096. [CrossRef] [PubMed]

47. Attuquayefio, T.; Stevenson, R.; Oaten, M.; Francis, H. A four-day Western-style dietary intervention causes reductions in hippocampal-dependent learning and memory and interoceptive sensitivity. *PLoS ONE* **2017**, *12*, e0172645. [CrossRef] [PubMed]

48. Attuquayefio, T.; Stevenson, R. A systematic review of longer-term dietary interventions on human cognitive function: Emerging patterns and future directions. *Appetite* **2015**, *95*, 554–570. [CrossRef] [PubMed]

49. Nilsson, A.; Tovar, J.; Johansson, M.; Radeborg, K.; Björck, I. A diet based on multiple functional concepts improves cognitive performance in healthy subjects. *Nutr. Metab.* **2013**, *10*, 49. [CrossRef] [PubMed]

50. Smithers, L.; Golley, R.; Mittinty, M.; Lynch, J. Do dietary trajectories between infancy and toddlerhood influence IQ in childhood and adolescence? Results from a prospective birth cohort study. *PLoS ONE* **2013**, *8*, e58904. [CrossRef] [PubMed]

51. Theodore, R.; Thompson, J.; Waldie, K.; Mitchell, E. Dietary patterns and intelligence in early and middle childhood. *Intelligence* **2009**, *37*, 506–513. [CrossRef]

52. Nyaradi, A.; Li, J.; Hickling, S.; Whitehouse, A.; Foster, J.; Oddy, W. Diet in the early years of life influences cognitive outcomes at 10 years: A prospective cohort study. *Acta Paediatr.* **2013**, *102*, 1165–1173. [CrossRef] [PubMed]

53. Ministerio de Salud. Encuesta Nacional de Consumo Alimentario. Informe Final de Resultados. Subsecretaría de Salud Pública; Ministerio de Salud: Santiago de Chile. Available online: web.minsal. cl/sites/default/files/ENCA-INFORME_FINAL.pdf (accessed on 27 January 2017).

54. Currie, C.; Van der Sluijs, W.; Whitehead, R.; Currie, D.; Rhodes, G.; Neville, F.; Inchley, J. HBSC 2014 Survey in Scotland National Report. Child and Adolescent Health Research Unit (CAHRU). University of St Andrews: Fife. Available online: www.hbsc.org/news/index.aspx?ni=3272 (accessed on 27 January 2017).

55. Kann, L.; Kinchen, S.; Shankil, S.; Zaza, S. Youth risk behavior surveillance. United Sates 2013. *MMWR CDC Surveill. Summ.* **2014**, *63*, 29–35.

56. Spoth, R.; Rohrbach, L.; Greenberg, M.; Hawkins, J. Addressing core challenges for the next generation of type 2 translation research and systems: The translation science to population impact (TSci impact) framework. *Prev. Sci.* **2013**, *14*, 319–351. [CrossRef] [PubMed]

57. Biglan, A. The ultimate goal of prevention and the larger context for translation. *Prev. Sci.* **2016**. [CrossRef] [PubMed]

58. Bradley, B.; Greene, A. Do health and education agencies in the United States share responsibility for academic achievement and health? A review of 25 years of evidence about the relationship of adolescents' academic achievement and health behaviors. *J. Adolesc. Health* **2013**, *52*, 523–532. [PubMed]

59. Baker, D.; Leon, J.; Smith-Greenaway, E.; Collins, J.; Movit, M. The education effect on population health: A reassessment. *Popul. Dev. Rev.* **2011**, *37*, 307–332. [CrossRef] [PubMed]

60. Just, D.; Mancino, L.; Wansink, B. *Could Behavioral Economics Help Improve Diet Quality for Nutrition Assistance Program Participants?* US Department of Agriculture: Washington, DC, USA.

61. Kersting, M.; Sichert-Hellert, W.; Vereecken, C.; Sette, S. Food and nutrient intake, nutritional knowledge and diet-related attitudes in European adolescents. *Int. J. Obes.* **2008**, *32*, 35–41. [CrossRef] [PubMed]

62. Centers for Disease Control and Prevention, National Center for Chronic Disease Prevention and Health Promotion. Health and Academic Achievement. Available online: http://www.cdc.gov/healthyschools/health_and_academics/pdf/health-academic-achievement.pdf (accessed on 2 November 2016).

63. Organization for Economic Cooperation and Development, Program for International Students Assessment. Programme for International Students Assessment 2012 Results in Focus. What 15-Year-Old Know and What They Can Do with What They Know. Available online: http://www.oecd.org/pisa/keyfindings/pisa-2012-results.htm (accessed on 7 December 2016).

64. Casey, B.; Jones, R.; Hare, T. The adolescent brain. *Ann. N. Y. Acad. Sci.* **2008**, *1124*, 111–126. [CrossRef] [PubMed]

65. Pedersen, S.; Grønhøj, A.; Thøgersen, J. Following family or friends. Social norms in adolescent healthy eating. *Appetite* **2015**, *86*, 54–60. [CrossRef] [PubMed]

66. Hakkarainen, A.; Holopainen, L.; Savolainen, H. Mathematical and reading difficulties as predictors of school achievement and transition to secondary education. *Scand. J. Educ. Res.* **2013**, *57*, 488–506. [CrossRef]

67. Ministerio de Educación. Informe de resultados Estudio Nacional Educación Física 2013. Agencia de Calidad de la Educación. Available online: http://archivos.agenciaeducacion.cl/biblioteca_digital_historica/resultados/2013/result8b_edfisica_2013.pdf (accessed on 2 November 2016).

Permissions

All chapters in this book were first published by MDPI; hereby published with permission under the Creative Commons Attribution License or equivalent. Every chapter published in this book has been scrutinized by our experts. Their significance has been extensively debated. The topics covered herein carry significant findings which will fuel the growth of the discipline. They may even be implemented as practical applications or may be referred to as a beginning point for another development.

The contributors of this book come from diverse backgrounds, making this book a truly international effort. This book will bring forth new frontiers with its revolutionizing research information and detailed analysis of the nascent developments around the world.

We would like to thank all the contributing authors for lending their expertise to make the book truly unique. They have played a crucial role in the development of this book. Without their invaluable contributions this book wouldn't have been possible. They have made vital efforts to compile up to date information on the varied aspects of this subject to make this book a valuable addition to the collection of many professionals and students.

This book was conceptualized with the vision of imparting up-to-date information and advanced data in this field. To ensure the same, a matchless editorial board was set up. Every individual on the board went through rigorous rounds of assessment to prove their worth. After which they invested a large part of their time researching and compiling the most relevant data for our readers.

The editorial board has been involved in producing this book since its inception. They have spent rigorous hours researching and exploring the diverse topics which have resulted in the successful publishing of this book. They have passed on their knowledge of decades through this book. To expedite this challenging task, the publisher supported the team at every step. A small team of assistant editors was also appointed to further simplify the editing procedure and attain best results for the readers.

Apart from the editorial board, the designing team has also invested a significant amount of their time in understanding the subject and creating the most relevant covers. They scrutinized every image to scout for the most suitable representation of the subject and create an appropriate cover for the book.

The publishing team has been an ardent support to the editorial, designing and production team. Their endless efforts to recruit the best for this project, has resulted in the accomplishment of this book. They are a veteran in the field of academics and their pool of knowledge is as vast as their experience in printing. Their expertise and guidance has proved useful at every step. Their uncompromising quality standards have made this book an exceptional effort. Their encouragement from time to time has been an inspiration for everyone.

The publisher and the editorial board hope that this book will prove to be a valuable piece of knowledge for researchers, students, practitioners and scholars across the globe.

List of Contributors

Miriam Latorre-Millán
GENUD Research group, Instituto de Investigación Sanitaria de Aragón (IIS Aragón), Universidad de Zaragoza, 50013 Zaragoza, Spain
Unidad de Endocrinología Pediátrica, Hospital Clínico Universitario Lozano Blesa, 50009 Zaragoza, Spain

Azahara I. Rupérez
GENUD Research group, Instituto de Investigación Sanitaria de Aragón (IIS Aragón), Universidad de Zaragoza, 50013 Zaragoza, Spain
Instituto Agroalimentario de Aragón (IA2), 50013 Zaragoza, Spain

Gloria Bueno
GENUD Research group, Instituto de Investigación Sanitaria de Aragón (IIS Aragón), Universidad de Zaragoza, 50013 Zaragoza, Spain
Unidad de Endocrinología Pediátrica, Hospital Clínico Universitario Lozano Blesa, 50009 Zaragoza, Spain
Instituto Agroalimentario de Aragón (IA2), 50013 Zaragoza, Spain
Centro de Investigación Biomédica en Red de Fisiopatología de la Obesidad y Nutrición (CIBEROBN), Instituto de Salud Carlos III, 28029 Madrid, Spain

Alba Santaliestra-Pasías and Luis A. Moreno
GENUD Research group, Instituto de Investigación Sanitaria de Aragón (IIS Aragón), Universidad de Zaragoza, 50013 Zaragoza, Spain
Instituto Agroalimentario de Aragón (IA2), 50013 Zaragoza, Spain
Centro de Investigación Biomédica en Red de Fisiopatología de la Obesidad y Nutrición (CIBEROBN), Instituto de Salud Carlos III, 28029 Madrid, Spain

Esther M. González-Gil
GENUD Research group, Instituto de Investigación Sanitaria de Aragón (IIS Aragón), Universidad de Zaragoza, 50013 Zaragoza, Spain
Centro de Investigación Biomédica en Red de Fisiopatología de la Obesidad y Nutrición (CIBEROBN), Instituto de Salud Carlos III, 28029 Madrid, Spain
Departamento de Bioquímica y Biología Molecular II, Instituto de Nutrición y Tecnología de los Alimentos, Centro de Investigación Biomédica, Universidad de Granada, 18016 Granada, Spain

Rocío Vázquez-Cobela
Unidad de Gastroenterología, Hepatología y Nutrición Pediátrica, Grupo de Investigación Nutrición Pediátrica, Instituto de Investigación Sanitaria de Santiago de Compostela (IDIS), Complejo Hospitalario Universitario de Santiago, 15706 Santiago de Compostela, Spain

Mercedes Gil-Campos
Centro de Investigación Biomédica en Red de Fisiopatología de la Obesidad y Nutrición (CIBEROBN), Instituto de Salud Carlos III, 28029 Madrid, Spain
Unidad de Metabolismo e Investigación Pediátrica, Hospital Universitario Reina Sofía, Instituto Maimónides de Investigación Biomédica de Córdoba (IMIBIC), 14071 Córdoba, Spain

Concepción M. Aguilera and Ángel Gil
Centro de Investigación Biomédica en Red de Fisiopatología de la Obesidad y Nutrición (CIBEROBN), Instituto de Salud Carlos III, 28029 Madrid, Spain
Departamento de Bioquímica y Biología Molecular II, Instituto de Nutrición y Tecnología de los Alimentos, Centro de Investigación Biomédica, Universidad de Granada, 18016 Granada, Spain
Instituto de Investigación Biosanitaria IBS.GRANADA, Complejo Hospitalario Universitario de Granada, 18014 Granada, Spain

Rosaura Leis
Centro de Investigación Biomédica en Red de Fisiopatología de la Obesidad y Nutrición (CIBEROBN), Instituto de Salud Carlos III, 28029 Madrid, Spain
Unidad de Gastroenterología, Hepatología y Nutrición Pediátrica, Grupo de Investigación Nutrición Pediátrica, Instituto de Investigación Sanitaria de Santiago de Compostela (IDIS), Complejo Hospitalario Universitario de Santiago, 15706 Santiago de Compostela, Spain
Unidad de Investigación en Nutrición, Crecimiento y Desarrollo Humano de Galicia (GALINUT), Universidad de Santiago de Compostela, 15706 Santiago de Compostela, Spain

Barbara Groele and Dominika Głąbska
Department of Dietetics, Faculty of Human Nutrition and Consumer Sciences, Warsaw University of Life Sciences (SGGW-WULS), 159C Nowoursynowska Street, 02-787 Warsaw, Poland

Krystyna Gutkowska and Dominika Guzek
Department of Organization and Consumption Economics, Faculty of Human Nutrition and Consumer Sciences, Warsaw University of Life Sciences (SGGW-WULS), 159C Nowoursynowska Street, 02-787 Warsaw, Poland

Megan A. McCrory
Department of Health Sciences, Programs in Nutrition, Sargent College of Health and Rehabilitation Sciences, Boston University, Boston, MA 02215, USA

Charles L. Jaret, Jung Ha Kim and Donald C. Reitzes
Department of Sociology, College of Arts and Sciences, Georgia State University, Atlanta, GA 30302, USA

Xiaoqin Wang, Zhaozhao Hui, Yue Zhang, Mei Ma, Mingxu Wang, Wei Gu, Shuangyan Lei, Ling Li, Mingyue Ma and Bin Zhang
Department of Public Health, Xi'an Jiaotong University Health Science Center, Xi'an 710061, China

Xiaoling Dai
Department of Nursing, Shaanxi Provincial Tumor Hospital, Xi'an 710061, China

Paul D. Terry
Department of Medicine, University of Tennessee Medical Center, Knoxville, TN 37996, USA

Fu Deng
Xi'an Tie Yi High School, Xi'an 710000, China

Kayla Vosburgh, Samantha Oldman, Tania Huedo-Medina and Valerie B. Duffy
Department of Allied Health Sciences, University of Connecticut, Storrs, CT 06269, USA

Sharon R. Smith
CT Children's Medical Center, University of Connecticut School of Medicine, Hartford, CT 06106 2, USA

Angie Saliba and Christelle Akl
Department of Nutrition and Food Science, Faculty of Agricultural and Food Sciences, American University of Beirut, Riad El Solh, Beirut, Lebanon

Lara Nasreddine, Nahla Hwalla and Farah Naja
Department of Nutrition and Food Science, Faculty of Agricultural and Food Sciences, American University of Beirut, Riad El Solh, Beirut, Lebanon
Nutrition, Obesity and Related Diseases (NORD), Office of Strategic Health Initiatives, American University of Beirut, Riad El Solh, Beirut, Lebanon

Hanna Perlitz, Gert B.M. Mensink, Clarissa Lage Barbosa, Almut Richter, Anna-Kristin Brettschneider, Franziska Lehmann, Eleni Patelakis, Melanie Frank, Karoline Heide and Marjolein Haftenberger
Department of Epidemiology and Health Monitoring, Robert Koch Institute, 12101 Berlin, Germany

Elli Jalo, Henna Vepsalainen and Mikael Fogelholm
Department of Food and Nutrition, University of Helsinki, 00014 Helsinki, Finla

Hanna Konttinen
Department of Food and Nutrition, University of Helsinki, 00014 Helsinki, Finland
Sociology, University of Helsinki, 00014 Helsinki, Finland

Jean-Philippe Chaput
Children's Hospital of Eastern Ontario Research Institute, Ottawa, ON K1H 8L1, Canada

Gang Hu and Peter T. Katzmarzyk
Pennington Biomedical Research Center, Baton Rouge, LA 70808, USA

Carol Maher
Alliance for Research In Exercise Nutrition and Activity (ARENA), School of Health Sciences, University of South Australia, Adelaide, SA 5001, Australia

José Maia
CIFI2D, Faculdade de Desporto, University of Porto, 4200-450 Porto, Portugal

Olga L. Sarmiento
School of Medicine, Universidad de los Andes, Bogotá 11001000, Colombia

Martyn Standage
Department for Health, University of Bath, Bath BA2 7AY, UK

Catrine Tudor-Locke
Department of Kinesiology, School of Public Health and Health Sciences, University of Massachusetts Amherst, MA 01003, USA

Hye Ah Lee and Hyesook Park
Department of Preventive Medicine, School of Medicine, Ewha Womans University, Seoul 07985, Korea

Hyo Jeong Hwang
Biomaterials Research Institute, Sahmyook University, Seoul 01795, Korea

Se Young Oh
Department of Food & Nutrition, Research Center for Human Ecology, College of Human Ecology, Kyung Hee University, Seoul 02447, Korea

Eun Ae Park, Su Jin Cho and Hae Soon Kim
Department of Pediatrics, School of Medicine, Ewha Womans University, Seoul 07985, Korea

Alicia Beltran, Teresia M. O'Connor, Sheryl O. Hughes, Debbe Thompson, Janice Baranowski, Theresa A. Nicklas and Tom Baranowski
USDA/ARS Children's Nutrition Research Center, Department of Pediatrics, Baylor College of Medicine, Houston, TX 77030, USA

Amy L. Lovell and Clare R. Wall
Discipline of Nutrition and Dietetics, Faculty of Medical and Health Sciences, University of Auckland, Auckland 1142, New Zealand

Tania Milne
Faculty of Medical and Health Sciences, University of Auckland, Auckland 1142, New Zealand

Yannan Jiang and Rachel X. Chen
Department of Statistics, Faculty of Science, University of Auckland, Auckland 1142, New Zealand

Cameron C. Grant
Department of Paediatrics, Child and Youth Health, University of Auckland, Grafton 1023, New Zealand
Centre for Longitudinal Research He Ara ki Mua, University of Auckland, Auckland 1743, New Zealand
General Paediatrics, Starship Children's Hospital, Auckland District Health Board, Auckland, Auckland 1142, New Zealand

Ewa Sicińska, Barbara Pietruszka, Olga Januszko and Joanna Kałuża
Department of Human Nutrition, Faculty of Human Nutrition and Consumer Sciences, Warsaw University of Life Sciences (WULS—SGGW), 159c Nowoursynowska str., 02-776 Warsaw, Poland

Kyung Min Kwon
Department of Food and Nutrition, College of Human Ecology, Seoul National University, 1 Gwanak-ro, Gwanak-gu, Seoul 08826, Korea

Jae Eun Shim
Department of Food and Nutrition, Daejeon University, 62 Daehak-ro, Dong-gu, Daejeon 34520, Korea

Daejeon Dong-gu Center for Children's Food Service Management, Daejeon University, 62 Daehak-ro, Dong-gu, Daejeon 34520, Korea

Minji Kang
Research Institute of Human Ecology, College of Human Ecology, Seoul National University, 1 Gwanak ro, Gwanak-gu, Seoul 08826, Korea

Hee-Young Paik
Department of Food and Nutrition, College of Human Ecology, Seoul National University, 1 Gwanak-ro, Gwanak-gu, Seoul 08826, Korea
Research Institute of Human Ecology, College of Human Ecology, Seoul National University, 1 Gwanak ro, Gwanak-gu, Seoul 08826, Korea

Ellen José van der Gaag and Judith van der Kraats
Ziekenhuisgroep Twente, Hengelo, Geerdinksweg 141, Hengelo 7555 DL, The Netherlands

Romy Wieffer
Isala Zwolle, Dokter van Heesweg 2, Zwolle 8025 AB, The Netherlands

Virginia Quick, Jennifer Martin-Biggers, Gayle, John Worobey and Carol Byrd-Bredbenner
Department of Nutritional Sciences, Rutgers University, 26 Nichol Avenue, New Brunswick, NJ 08901, USA

Alleman Povis and Nobuko Hongu
Department of Nutritional Sciences, University of Arizona, 406 Shantz Building, 1177 E. 4th Street, Tucson, AZ 85721, USA

Paulina Correa-Burrows, Yanina Rodríguez and Raquel Burrows
Institute of Nutrition and Food Technology, University of Chile, Santiago 7830490, Chile

Estela Blanco and Sheila Gahagan
Division of Child Development and Community Health, University of California, San Diego, CA 92093, USA

Index